Oxford Case Histories
in General Surgery

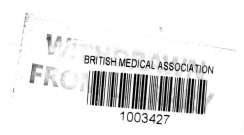

Oxford Case Histories

Series Editors:

Sarah Pendlebury and Peter Rothwell

Published:

Neurological Case Histories (Sarah T Pendlebury, Philip Anslow, and Peter M Rothwell)

Oxford Case Histories in Anaesthesia (Jon McCormack and Keith Kelly)

Oxford Case Histories in Cardiology (Rajkumar Rajendram, Javed Ehtisham, and Colin Forfar)

Oxford Case Histories in Gastroenterology and Hepatology (Alissa J. Walsh, Otto C. Buchel, Jane Collier, and Simon P.L. Travis)

Oxford Case Histories in General Surgery (Judith Ritchie and K. Raj Prasad)

Oxford Case Histories in Geriatric Medicine (Sanja Thompson, Nicola Lovett, John Grimley Evans, and Sarah Pendlebury)

Oxford Case Histories in Respiratory Medicine (John Stradling, Andrew Stanton, Najib M. Rahman, Annabel H. Nickol, and Helen E. Davies)

Oxford Case Histories in Rheumatology (Joel David, Anne Miller, Anushka Soni, and Lyn Williamson)

Oxford Case Histories in TIA and Stroke (Sarah T. Pendlebury, Ursula G. Schulz, Aneil Malhotra, and Peter M. Rothwell)

Oxford Case Histories in Neurosurgery (Harutomo Hasegawa, Matthew Crocker, and Pawan Singh Minhas)

Oxford Case Histories in Oncology (Harutomo Hasegawa, Matthew Crocker, and Pawan Singh Minhas)

Oxford Case Histories in General Surgery

Edited by

Judith E. Ritchie
General surgical registrar,
Yorkshire and the Humber Deanery, UK

K. Raj Prasad
Consultant hepatobiliary surgeon, Leeds Teaching Hospitals
NHS Trust, UK

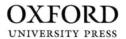
OXFORD
UNIVERSITY PRESS

OXFORD
UNIVERSITY PRESS

Great Clarendon Street, Oxford, OX2 6DP,
United Kingdom

Oxford University Press is a department of the University of Oxford.
It furthers the University's objective of excellence in research, scholarship,
and education by publishing worldwide. Oxford is a registered trade mark of
Oxford University Press in the UK and in certain other countries

First Edition published in 2018
Impression: 1

Published in the United States of America by Oxford University Press
198 Madison Avenue, New York, NY 10016, United States of America

British Library Cataloguing in Publication Data
Data available

Library of Congress Control Number: 2017952351

ISBN 978-0-19-874981-3

Printed and bound by
CPI Group (UK) Ltd, Croydon, CR0 4YY

A note from the series editors

Case histories have always had an important role in medical education, but most published material has been directed at undergraduates or residents. The *Oxford Case Histories* series aims to provide more complex case-based learning for clinicians in specialist training and consultants, and is now well-established in aiding preparation for entry and exit-level specialty examinations and revalidation. Each case book follows the same format with approximately 50 cases, each comprising a brief clinical history and investigations, followed by questions on differential diagnosis and management, and detailed answers with discussion. At the end of each book, cases are listed by mode of presentation, aetiology, and diagnosis.

We are grateful to our colleagues in the various medical specialties for their enthusiasm and hard work in making the series possible.

Sarah Pendlebury and Peter Rothwell

From reviews of other books in the series:

Oxford Case Histories in Neurosurgery
'This book provides a great method for learning and preparing for neurosurgery examinations. The cases cover all relevant topics in neurosurgery, and the questions following the cases go to the core of the subject, highlighting the important points for students. The discussion section in particular is very informative, going over the differential diagnosis and citing the scientific basis for the answers. The strengths of the book are the simple and concise explanations and the discussions of related topics. This is useful not only for examinees, but also for practicing neurosurgeons.'

Ramsis Farid Ghaly, MD, Doody's Notes

Oxford Case Histories in Cardiology

'Clearly the three authors have put a huge amount of time and effort into this book to make sure it is relevant, accurate and up to date. Overall, this book will be an excellent aid to those preparing for post-graduate exams in general medicine and cardiology, but will also be of relevance to senior medical students with more than a passing interest in cardiology.'

Cardiology News

Oxford Case Histories in Respiratory Medicine

'It is like having your favourite clinical teacher share his/her accumulated clinical nouse in a way that makes the apparently ordinary case stimulating and full of subtlety . . . I thoroughly enjoyed this book and recommend it to specialist registrars and consultants in respiratory medicine—go out and get a copy for your department.'

British Journal of Hospital Medicine

Foreword

It is a pleasure to write the Foreword to the *Oxford Case Histories in General Surgery*. The book provides a case-based format around real-life cases covering the subspecialties of general surgery (upper gastro-intestinal, hepatobiliary, pancreatic, endocrine, breast, and colorectal surgery) in both elective and emergency situations. Each section presents a clinical vignette followed by a series of questions based on the vignettes relating to aetiology, diagnosis, investigations, and modalities of treatment, including references for further reading. The questions are presented in logical order and the answers are extremely comprehensive, including tables, algorithms, flow diagrams, and excellent-quality images, which are clear and well labelled. The book is written by both surgical trainees and established consultants, the authorship of each chapter being overseen by a consultant in the relevant speciality. The editors and authors are to be congratulated on a clearly written, up to date, and well-presented text. This book will appeal to clinical students starting out on the wards, as well as foundation doctors and core surgical trainees studying for the MRCS. It will also provide good revision reading for the Intercollegiate Examination in General Surgery. Not only will it guide the candidate through the hurdle of examinations, but it will be invaluable in everyday clinical practice. There is a need for a book like this on the market. I can thoroughly recommend it. I wish it the success that it deserves.

Andrew T Raftery
Consultant Surgeon (retired)
Medical Author
Sheffield 2017

Preface

Oxford Case Histories in General Surgery aims to bring the different subspecialties of general surgery to life for its readers by adopting a case-based discussion format around real-life cases. It is most relevant to those who are just starting out in general surgery, including medical students, surgical care practitioners, foundation doctors, and those entering core surgical training. Each case presents a clinical vignette comprising focussed and relevant clinical and diagnostic information followed by a case-based discussion that covers relevant clinical material pertinent to the core surgical element of the Intercollegiate Surgical Curriculum. The case-based discussion format is an important learning tool, as it allows focussed application of textbook knowledge to clinical practice and incorporates that with current evidence-based approaches to clinical and surgical management.

The book presents interesting and clinically relevant case scenarios from the subspecialties of upper gastrointestinal, hepatobiliary, pancreatic, endocrine, breast, and colorectal surgery. Furthermore, the cases in these chapters are grouped by the elective and emergency nature in which they most commonly present clinically. In addition to these subspecialty chapters, there is also an emergency surgery chapter that presents additional case presentations that are commonly encountered on the acute surgical take. This chapter also includes trauma surgery and kidney transplantation, which doctors will be exposed to on the acute surgical take if they work at major trauma or transplant centres during their training. The authorship of each chapter has been overseen by a consultant who works in that subspecialty to ensure the material is factually accurate and up to date.

We hope that you find this book interesting, engaging, and useful for your own learning and clinical practice.

Acknowledgements

We would like to thank everyone who has been involved in the preparation and production of this book. We start by thanking each and every author for their commitment, motivation, and hard work. We also thank those who have proofread and given valuable academic input, in particular Mr Matthew Lee, Mr Jonathan Wild, Dr Suneil Raju, Dr Qaiser Jalal, Professor Richard Nelson, and Mr Simon Boyes. We would also like to thank Mr Manoj Valluru for his technical support in formatting the images. We are grateful for the support we have had in obtaining appropriate radiological images for the cases, for which we would like to thank Dr Anthony Blakeborough and Dr Mathew Kaduthodil.

We would particularly like to thank the team at Oxford University Press for their constant support, expert guidance, and unwavering patience during the preparation of the book. And last but not least we thank the friends and family members whose faith and support underlie every step of this journey.

Contents

Abbreviations *xvii*

Contributors *xxi*

Blood test reference ranges *xxiii*

1 UGI surgery *1*

Corinne Owers and Roger Ackroyd

  1.1 Elective: gastro-oesophageal reflux disease *1*

  1.2 Elective: metabolic (bariatric) surgery *9*

  1.3 Elective: gastro-oesophageal cancer *19*

  1.4 Emergency: upper gastrointestinal bleeding *29*

  1.5 Emergency: perforated duodenal ulcer *37*

  1.6 Emergency: complications of UGI resectional surgery *43*

  1.7 Emergency: complications of metabolic surgery *51*

2 Hepatobiliary surgery *57*

K. Raj Prasad and Imeshi Wijetunga

  2.1 Elective: colorectal liver metastasis *57*

  2.2 Elective: hepatocellular carcinoma *69*

  2.3 Elective: cholangiocarcinoma *79*

  2.4 Emergency: symptomatic gallstones *87*

  2.5 Emergency: acute ascending cholangitis *99*

  2.6 Emergency: complications following laparoscopic cholecystectomy *109*

3 Pancreatic surgery *117*

Judith Ritchie and Ahmed Al-Mukhtar

  3.1 Elective: pancreatic cystic mass *117*

  3.2 Elective: pancreatic cancer *129*

  3.3 Elective: chronic pancreatitis *143*

  3.4 Emergency: acute pancreatitis *155*

  3.5 Emergency: pancreatic trauma *167*

4. Colorectal surgery *177*
Peter Webster, Judith Ritchie, and Veerabhadram Garimella

4.1 Elective: constipation *177*

4.2 Elective: anal fistula *185*

4.3 Elective: colorectal cancer *191*

4.4 Elective: faecal incontinence *201*

4.5 Elective: fissure in ano *207*

4.6 Elective: haemorrhoids *211*

4.7 Elective: hernias *215*

4.8 Elective: inflammatory bowel disease *223*

4.9 Emergency: pilonidal abscesses *229*

4.10 Emergency: anorectal sepsis *235*

4.11 Emergency: acute diverticulitis *243*

4.12 Emergency: ischaemic bowel (acute mesenteric ischaemia) *253*

4.13 Emergency: large bowel obstruction *265*

4.14 Emergency: rectal bleeding *275*

4.15 Emergency: rectal prolapse *283*

5 Breast surgery *291*
Jenna Morgan and Lynda Wyld

5.1 Elective: breast lump *291*

5.2 Elective: nipple discharge *299*

5.3 Elective: breast cancer *307*

5.4 Emergency: breast abscess *317*

6 Endocrine surgery *323*
Jenna Morgan and Saba Balasubramanian

6.1 Elective: goitre and thyroid cancer *323*

6.2 Elective: parathyroid disease *337*

6.3 Elective: adrenal lesion *347*

6.4 Emergency: peri-operative management of the thyroid patient *353*

7 Emergency surgery *363*
*Jonathan Wild, Emma Nofal, Imeshi Wijetunga,
and Antonia Durham-Hall*

7.1 Emergency: acute abdominal pain *363*

7.2 Emergency: acute appendicitis *381*

7.3 Emergency: sigmoid volvulus *393*

7.4 Emergency: small bowel obstruction *403*

7.5   Emergency: obstructed groin hernia *415*

7.6   Emergency: blunt abdominal trauma *423*

7.7   Emergency: necrotizing soft-tissue infection *437*

7.8   Emergency: kidney transplant *445*

7.9   Emergency: cutaneous abscesses *455*

Index *461*

Abbreviations

AAST	American Association for the Surgery of Trauma scoring systems
ACE	Angiotensin converting enzyme
AFP	Alpha-fetoprotein
AJCC	American Joint Committee on Cancer
ALP	Alkaline phosphatase
APC	Argon plasma coagulation
APD	Automated peritoneal dialysis
ASA	American Society of Anaesthesiologists
AV	Arteriovenous
AXR	Abdominal X-ray/radiograph
BP	Blood pressure
BSD	Brainstem death
BSP	Breast Screening Programme
CAPD	Continuous ambulatory peritoneal dialysis
CBD	Common bile duct
CCK	Cholecystokinin
CCrISP	Care of the Critically Ill Surgical Patient
CEA	Carcinoembryonic antigen
CEPOD	Confidential Enquiry into Peri-Operative Deaths
CKD	Chronic kidney disease
CLO	Campylobacter-like organism
COPD	Chronic obstructive pulmonary disease
CPEX	Cardiopulmonary exercise testing
CRLM	Colorectal liver metastases
CRP	C reactive protein
CT	Computed tomography
CVP	Central venous pressure
CVVH	Continuous veno-venous haemofiltration
CVVHD	Continuous veno-venous haemodialysis
CXR	Chest X-ray/radiograph
DCIS	Ductal carcinoma *in situ*
DBD	Donation after brainstem death
DCD	Donation after circulatory death
DEXA	Dual X-ray absorptiometry
DIEP	Deep inferior epigastric perforator
DRE	Digital rectal examination
EAS	External anal sphincter
ECG	Electrocardiogram
EMR	Endoscopic mucosal resection
ER	Oestrogen receptor
ERCP	Endoscopic retrograde cholangiopancreaticogram
EUA	Examination under anaesthesia
EUS	Endoscopic ultrasound
FAP	Familial adenomatous polyposis
FHH	Familial hypocalciuric hypercalcaemia
FNA	Fine-needle aspiration
FOBT	Faecal occult blood test
GCS	Glasgow come scale
GOJ	Gastro-oesophageal junction
GORD	Gastro-oesophageal reflux disease

Hb	Haemoglobin	**MRCP**	Magnetic resonance cholangiopancreatography
HCC	Hepatocellular carcinoma	**MRI**	Magnetic resonance imaging
HD	Haemodialysis		
HER2	Human epidermal growth factor	**NAFLD**	Non-alcoholic fatty liver disease
HLA	Human leukocyte antigen	**NASH**	Non-alcoholic steatohepatitis
HNPCC	Hereditary non-polyposis colorectal cancer	**NELA**	National Emergency Laparotomy Audit
HPB	Hepatopancreaticobiliary	**NICE**	National Institute of Health and Clinical Excellence
HPL	Human placental lactogen		
HPT	Hyperparathyroidism	**NJ**	Nasojejunal
I131	Radioactive iodine	**NSAID**	Non-steroidal anti-inflammatory drugs
IAS	Internal anal sphincter		
IBD	Inflammatory bowel disease	**OGD**	Oesophagogastroduodeno-scopy
I-GAP	Inferior gluteal artery perforator	**OSNA**	One step nucleic acid amplification
IL-2	Interleukin 2	**PaCO2**	Partial pressure of carbon dioxide (CO_2)
ILOG	Ivor–Lewis oesophagogastrectomy		
IM	Intramuscular	**pANCA**	Perinuclear ANCA
INR	International normalised ratio	**PaO2**	Partial pressure of oxygen (O_2)
IPMN	Intrapapillary mucinous neoplasm	**PD**	Peritoneal dialysis
		PDS	Polydioxanone
IV	Intravenous	**PEC**	Percutaneous endoscopic colostomy
LCIS	Lobular carcinoma *in situ*		
LD	Latissimus Dorsi	**PEG**	Percutaneous entero-gastrostomy
LFTs	Liver function tests		
LIFT	Ligation of intersphincteric tract	**PEJ**	Percutaneous entero-jejunostomy
LRTI	Lower respiratory tract infection	**PET**	Positron emission tomography
MAP	Mean arterial pressure	**PFD**	Pelvic floor dysfunction
MCN	Mucinous cystic neoplasm	**PHPT**	Primary hyperparathyroidism
MCV	Mean corpuscular volume		
MDT	Multi-disciplinary team	**PPI**	Proton pump inhibitors
MELD	Modified end-stage liver disease	**P-POSSUM**	Portsmouth Physiological and Operative Severity Score for the enumeration of Mortality and Mortality
MEN	Multiple endocrine neoplasia		
		PR	Progesterone receptor
MIBG	Meta-iodobenzylguanide	**PSC**	Primary sclerosing cholangitis
MPH	Miles per hour		

PTC	Percutaneous trans-hepatic cholangiogram	**TDAP**	Thoracodorsal perforator flap
PTH	Parathyroid hormone	**TNM**	Tumour node metastases
PTLD	Post-transplant lymphoproliferative disorder	**TPN**	Total parenteral nutrition
		TRAM	Transverse rectus abdominis myocutaneous
RFA	Radiofrequency ablation	**TSH**	Thyroid stimulating hormone
RRT	Renal replacement therapy		
SBO	Small bowel obstruction	**TUG**	Transverse upper gracillis
S-GAP	Superior gluteal artery perforator	**UC**	Ulcerative colitis
		UKELD	UK model for end-stage liver disease
SIRS	Systemic inflammatory response syndrome	**UW solution**	University of Wisconsin solution
SMA	Superior mesenteric artery		
SNLB	Sentinel lymph node biopsy	**USS**	Ultrasound
		VIP	Vasoactive intestinal polypeptide
SNOD	Specialist nurse for organ donation		
		WBC	White blood cell
SNS	Sacral nerve stimulator	**WSCA**	Water-soluble contrast agent
STC	Slow transit constipation		
T4	Thyroxine	**VMA**	Vanillylmandelic acid
T3	Triiodothyronine	**WLE**	Wide local excision
TACE	Trans-arterial chemoembolization		

Contributors

Roger Ackroyd
Consultant upper GI and
bariatric surgeon, Sheffield
Teaching Hospitals Foundation
Trust, UK

Ahmed Al-Mukhtar
Consultant
hepatopancreaticobiliary surgeon,
Sheffield Teaching Hospitals NHS
Foundation Trust, UK

Saba Balasubramanian
Consultant endocrine and thyroid
surgeon, Sheffield Teaching
Hospitals NHS Foundation
Trust, UK

Antonia Durham-Hall
Consultant colorectal surgeon,
Doncaster and Bassetlaw NHS
Foundation Trust, UK

Veerabhadram Garimella
Consultant colorectal surgeon,
University Hospitals of North
Midlands NHS Trust, UK

Jenna Morgan
General surgical registrar,
Yorkshire and the Humber
Deanery, UK

Emma Nofal
General surgical registrar,
Yorkshire and the Humber
Deanery, UK

Corinne Owers
General surgical registrar,
Yorkshire and the Humber
Deanery, UK

K. Raj Prasad
Consultant hepatobiliary surgeon,
Leeds Teaching Hospitals NHS
Trust, UK

Judith Ritchie
General surgical registrar,
Yorkshire and the Humber
Deanery, UK

Peter Webster
Clinical research fellow, Leeds
Teaching Hospitals NHS
Trust, UK

Imeshi Wijetunga
HPB and transplant clinical
research fellow, Leeds Teaching
Hospital NHS Trust, UK

Jonathan Wild
General surgical registrar,
Yorkshire and the Humber
Deanery, UK

Lynda Wyld
Honorary consultant breast
surgeon, Doncaster and Bassetlaw
Hospitals NHS Foundation
Trust, UK
Reader in surgical oncology,
University of Sheffield, UK

Blood test reference ranges

Haematology

Hb:	120–180g/l
WCC:	$2–7.5 \times 10^9$/l
MCV:	81.8–96.3fl
Platelets:	$150–400 \times 10^9$/l

Coagulation

PT:	9.5–11.3 s

Electrolytes

Sodium:	135–145 mmol/l
Potassium:	3.5–5.0 mmol/l
Urea:	4.0–8.2 mmol/l
Creatinine:	50–110 μmol/l

Liver Function

Alkaline phosphatase:	20–140 IU/l
Bilirubin:	<20 μmol/l
ALT:	<40 IU/l
Albumin:	35–50 g/l
Amylase:	<100 IU/l
Adjusted calcium:	2.20–2.60 mmol/l
Phosphate:	0.8–1.4 mmol/l
CRP:	<10 mg/l

Thyroid function

TSH:	0.3–3.04 mu/l
Free T4:	10–23 pmol/l
Free T3:	3.5–6.5 pmol/l

Arterial blood gases

pH:	7.35–7.45
PaO_2:	10.5–14 kPa
$PaCO_2$	4.7–6 kPa
Bicarbonate:	22–28 mmol/l
Lactate:	<2 mmol/l

Tumour markers

AFP:	<7.5 U/mL
CA19.9:	<33k U/l
CEA:	<4 µg/l

Chapter 1

UGI surgery

Corinne Owers and Roger Ackroyd

Case history 1.1: Elective: gastro-oesophageal reflux disease

A 33-year-old male with a BMI of 36.2 attends the UGI outpatient clinic with a long-standing history of dyspepsia that has become progressively worse over the last 3 months. It is worse at night, and he finds himself occasionally waking from sleep with a hoarse voice and a cough. He has very occasional dysphagia to solids after a heavy meal but no haematemesis, malaena, or weight loss, and no other abdominal symptoms. He has tried over-the-counter remedies, including Gaviscon and Rennies, but finds these have only a temporary effect. Aside from a past medical history of borderline hypertension, he is fit and well with no previous surgical history. He is a smoker and drinks approximately 20 units per week, mainly at the weekends. He has a moderate caffeine intake and a relatively healthy diet, although admits to at least two takeaways per week, often curries. Physical examination and blood investigations are all unremarkable.

Questions

1. What are the main contributing factors to gastro-oesophageal reflux disease (GORD)?

2. What are the main symptoms suggestive of GORD?

3. What are the main investigations for GORD?

4. What lifestyle and medical recommendations should be made in this case?

5. What are the main selection criteria for surgery?

6. What are the advantages and disadvantages of anti-reflux surgery?

Answers

1. What are the main contributing factors to gastro-oesophageal reflux disease (GORD)?

Gastro-oesophageal reflux disease (GORD) is one of the most common diseases of the Western world, affecting up to 40% of people in the UK at some point during their lifetime. It is generally more common in males, although it can be experienced by both males and females at any age. A number of anatomical and physiological mechanisms exist to try to prevent reflux:

+ *Upper oesophageal sphincter (UOS).* This is formed by the lower part of the inferior constrictor of the pharynx, the cricopharyngeus, and the upper part of the oesophagus, which consists of circular muscle. At rest, the sphincter is usually closed, with a resting pressure of around 100 mmHg, which helps to prevent reflux of gastric contents into the upper airway.

+ *Lower oesophageal sphincter (LOS).* The LOS, although not demonstrable anatomically, is an area in the distal oesophagus that has a distinctly higher pressure than the rest of the oesophagus. This high-pressure zone relaxes during swallowing, belching, and vomiting, but is a crucial mechanism for preventing severe reflux, even in patients with a hiatus hernia.

+ *The Angle of His.* The angle formed between the oesophagus and the cardia of the stomach at the gastro-oesophageal junction (GOJ). This is created by the circular muscles around the GOJ and the crus at the hiatus, which form a valve, thereby preventing reflux. The main cause for failure of this preventative mechanism is a hiatus hernia: the hiatus becomes larger than normal, allowing part of the stomach to prolapse into the thorax due to the lower pressure of the thorax when compared to the abdomen. Hiatus hernia can be either sliding, where the GOJ moves up into the chest, or paraoesophageal, where the GOJ remains within the abdominal cavity but part of the fundus or cardia prolapses into the thorax. A sliding hiatus hernia can be managed conservatively depending on symptoms; a paraoesophageal is at a high risk of incarceration and is, therefore, usually treated with surgical repair.

Failure of one or more of these mechanisms can lead to symptoms. Other physiological or mechanical factors that can lead to the development of GORD may relate to either an abnormality of oesophageal contraction or delayed gastric emptying. The normal oesophagus functions by peristaltic waves, which push contents down into the stomach. Where failure of peristalsis or a degree of dysmotility occurs, e.g. in achalasia, contents remain within the oesophagus for longer periods of time. This prevents the LOS or Angle of His from acting as a defence mechanism, therefore reflux is a common result. Gastric banding surgery can lead to the same effect, creating an inability for the food to pass easily into the stomach, leading to oesophageal dilatation and reflux. Finally, any cause of delayed gastric emptying from intrinsic or extrinsic compression within the abdominal cavity means that food remains within the stomach for longer and there is a higher chance of reflux occurring. Diabetes is also a known cause of delayed gastric emptying, therefore optimal glucose control is imperative.

2. What are the main symptoms suggestive of GORD?

There are a number of symptoms that can be associated with GORD, but by far the most common presenting complaint is dyspepsia. The term dyspepsia is broad and encompasses symptoms of epigastric pain or discomfort, acid reflux, and burning. This can occur at any time of day or night, although many patients experience an increase in symptoms nocturnally. This may be due to a heavy meal in the evening, or that people are more sedentary than during the day. Whilst lying, the effect of gravity is negated, meaning that when reflux does occur, it can more easily reach the upper oesophagus and affect the laryngopharynx.

For patients with this condition, upper respiratory symptoms are also common. Reflux into the upper airway can lead to a nocturnal cough, which may cause them to wake at night, occasionally associated with shortness of breath, which is relieved by sitting up. Hoarseness is due to the effect of the acid on the vocal cords, and if this persists with no evidence of upper respiratory tract infection, it is often due to GORD, although this should be appropriately investigated. Occasionally, in severe cases, patients may present with recurrent chest infections.

Where reflux is severe or longstanding, sequelae such as strictures or oesophagitis may develop. Although usually benign, the development of a Schatzki ring, a band of fibrous tissue at the proximal end of the GOJ, may lead to symptoms of dysphagia, especially with solid foods. Furthermore, oesophagitis as a result of chemical change can cause severe symptoms, and features are endoscopically often indistinguishable from a malignancy.

Any patients with symptoms that persist for more than a couple of weeks should be referred for ongoing investigation.

3. What are the main investigations for GORD?

When initially investigating patients for GORD, a detailed history is paramount, as this can often provide you with significant information. Clinical investigation is often to corroborate the suspicion of GORD, and to ensure that no sequelae have developed that need ongoing management.

Appropriate investigations include:

◆ *An oesophagogastroduodenoscopy (OGD).* This is the most common first-line investigation to order. This can be carried out on an outpatient basis using local anaesthetic throat spray or intravenous sedation, and examines the oesophagus, stomach, and duodenum down to the second part of the duodenum (D2). This is often the most useful investigation, as hiatus hernia, oesophagitis, and gastroduodenitis can be diagnosed, as well as Barrett's oesophagus. This patient was found to have a hiatus hernia at OGD, which is depicted in Figure 1.1.1. At the time of examination, biopsies can be taken from any areas of concern, such as oesophagitis, and for patients with Barrett's oesophagus, surveillance of the mucosa to identify dysplastic change can lead to the early identification of oesophageal cancers. Testing for *Helicobacter pylori* should be considered at OGD, as the presence of this bacteria can mimic symptoms of GORD.

◆ A barium swallow can be a useful investigation for patients who either cannot tolerate OGD or in whom a diagnosis of reflux is

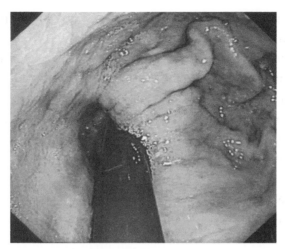

Figure 1.1.1 A photograph taken at OGD showing hiatus hernia. The tip of the endoscope is retroflexed to look back at the gastro-oesophageal junction and gastric fundus. The gastro-oesophageal junction has migrated upwards in a sliding hernia, the most common type of hiatus hernia.
Reproduced courtesy of Corinne Owers.

suspected in the absence of any other pathology on OGD. Free reflux can be demonstrated in the majority of patients, although occasionally patients require contrast to be ingested in the form of a solid (barium meal) in order to see a significant result.

- pH studies are a widely available and useful investigation. A probe is passed via the nasopharynx and remains in the lower oesophagus, approximately 6 cm from the GOJ, for 24 hours. This records the pH within the oesophagus, and allows for symptom correlation as the patient records when they have symptomatic episodes. In normal individuals, a pH of less than 4 should be present within the oesophagus for less than 4% of a 24-hour period. Any increase in these recordings would suggest a diagnosis of significant reflux.

- Oesophageal manometry is often performed alongside the pH studies. A catheter is passed into the stomach, which contains a number of pressure sensors. During both normal oesophageal contraction and swallowing, pressure measurements are taken. A diagnosis of oesophageal dysmotility is important to establish, especially when considering surgical intervention of dysphagia or dyspepsia.

4. What lifestyle and medical recommendations should be made in this case?

Before considering surgical intervention, a number of lifestyle and medical interventions should be implemented and trialled:

- *Weight loss.* Patients who are overweight are much more prone to GORD. This is likely to be due to an increase in intra-abdominal pressure leading to increased reflux. Any patient with an increased BMI should be strongly encouraged to lose weight, especially if considering anti-reflux surgery. Surgical intervention may become unnecessary if reflux improves significantly.

- Smoking, an increased caffeine intake, and alcohol are all considered to be factors that can predispose to GORD. Spicy foods, in particular, can lead to severe symptoms, especially if ingested late at night. Patients should be encouraged to adapt their diet or lifestyles, as avoidance can often lead to symptom improvement.

- Many patients find that propping themselves up at night, either with the aid of pillows or raising the head end of the bed, can help with nocturnal symptoms.

- All patients presenting with reflux should have a trial of proton pump inhibitor (PPI) or H2 receptor antagonists, such as ranitidine. These will often have been instigated by the GP. In cases of oesophagitis and Barrett's oesophagus, treatment with PPI is paramount and may need to be life-long. Occasionally the two drugs can be given in conjunction for resistant cases. In the majority of cases of simple GORD, management with medical therapies such as these, as well as simple over-the-counter anti-reflux medications, can lead to a resolution of symptoms, negating the need for surgical intervention.

- If delayed gastric emptying is suspected without the presence of compression, prokinetics such as metaclopramide or erythromycin could be considered. These help to speed peristalsis of the GI tract and move contents more swiftly from the stomach, helping to prevent GORD.

5. **What are the main selection criteria for surgery?**

Surgical intervention is usually considered for:

- Patients with complex reflux disease.
- Those where medical and lifestyle interventions have failed to adequately manage their symptoms.
- If a partial improvement is seen but there is a diagnosis that can theoretically be solved by surgery, operative intervention can occasionally be considered.

Complex reflux disease is defined by GORD alongside evidence of sequele of reflux. This may be a stricture, hiatus hernia, respiratory complications such as infection, or Barrett's oesophagus (although with Barrett's, endoscopic therapies such as argon plasma coagulation or photodynamic therapy would often be considered first).

The decision for surgery is made based on symptom correlation with UGI investigations. For patients who remain symptomatic but investigations have failed to show any pathological reflux, surgery would be of limited benefit, and may even lead to a deterioration of symptoms.

6. **What are the advantages and disadvantages of anti-reflux surgery?**

The mainstay of surgery is to increase the resting pressure in the LOS, exaggerate the Angle of His, and reduce the volume of the gastric fundus, leading to an increase in the speed of gastric emptying. This is most commonly achieved by performing a Nissen fundoplication, where the gastric fundus is wrapped around the distal oesophagus and secured, thereby reinforcing the distal oesophageal sphincter. This is commonly performed laparoscopically.

Anti-reflux surgery can be very successful at improving, if not resolving, symptoms in patients proven to have pathological reflux (i.e. a positive investigation demonstrating reflux). Patients often report a significant improvement in their quality of life, requiring fewer medications and being able to more easily manage their dietary intake. The decrease in gastric reflux can lead to a resolution of upper respiratory problems such as laryngitis, asthma, and chest infections. GORD can predispose to the development of symptomatic oesophageal strictures, as well as Barrett's oesophagus, which is a condition predisposing to adenocarcinoma of the oesophagus, therefore anti-reflux surgery can help to prevent the development of these conditions, theoretically improving longevity of patients who may otherwise have gone on to develop the disease.

Although anti-reflux surgery is very commonly performed, it is not without risk. As well as the normal complications of any operation, such as infection, bleeding, and cardiorespiratory problems, inappropriate selection of operative approach can lead to dysphagia, in particular in patients with oesophageal dysmotility. Oesophageal manometry is, therefore, essential before considering surgery, as those with a degree of dysmotility may benefit from a looser fundoplication than those with normal oesophageal function in order to prevent long-term dysphagia. Anti-reflux surgery can fail, leading to repeated operations for symptom recurrence. If the wrap is performed too tightly at the time of surgery, it may necessitate a return to theatre for loosening.

Due to surgery, the pressure at the distal GOJ is significantly increased, and this can prevent the ability to belch or vomit. Patients should, therefore, be advised to avoid carbonated drinks or beers, as ingestion of these fluids can lead to uncomfortable bloating and an increased chance of surgical failure. Increased flatulence and audible borborygmi (bowel sounds) are often the result. For patients who become obstructed in the more distal GI tract at a future date, this inability to vomit may lead to a delay in diagnosis or increased risk of perforation.

Further reading

Kahrilas PJ (2008) Gastro-oesophageal reflux disease. *New England J Med* 359: 1700–7.

Minjarez RC, Jobe BA (2006) Surgical therapy for gastro-oesophageal reflux disease. *GI Motility Online*. doi:10.1038/gimo56

Case history 1.2: Elective: metabolic (bariatric) surgery

A 54-year-old Caucasian woman is referred to the outpatient clinic from her GP for consideration of weight-management surgery. She has been significantly overweight for approximately 20 years since the birth of her first child, although she notes that she was always overweight as a child. She has a past medical history of type 2 diabetes that is controlled with oral medication and hypertension that is controlled by an angiotensin converting enzyme (ACE)-inhibitor. She suffers with depression, which she believes is secondary to her obesity as this prevents her from being able to join in with her family and causes her difficulty in her job as a nurse. She admits to being a volume eater and does have a sweet tooth. She has done a lot of research about weight-loss surgery, and has attended a community weight-management programme, although she was only able to lose 5 kg in weight. Following counselling she elected to have a laparoscopic Roux-en-Y gastric bypass procedure. The procedure went well, she proceeded to lose weight and her BMI fell from 36 to 26 within the next 12 months.

Questions

1. How do you classify morbid obesity?
2. What are the common comorbidities associated with morbid obesity?
3. What considerations should be made before offering a patient bariatric surgery?
4. What are the common operations performed during bariatric/ metabolic surgery
5. What are the main operative considerations for bariatric surgery patients?
6. What are the common metabolic side-effects associated with bariatric surgery?

Answers

1. How do you classify morbid obesity?

There are a number of classification systems for morbid obesity; the NICE classification is detailed in Table 1.2.1. Class 1, 2, and 3 obesity are associated with increasing risks of developing weight-related comorbidities (discussed in Question 2). Risk and recommendations for management can also be determined by correlating the BMI with weight circumference and comorbidities.

Table 1.2.1 NICE classification of obesity

BMI	Classification
Less than 18.5	Underweight
18.5–24.9	Normal weight
25.0–29.9	Overweight
30.0–34.9	Class 1 obesity
35.0–39.9	Class 2 obesity
Over 40	Class 3 obesity

Source: Data from 'Obesity: identification, assessment and management', *Clinical Guideline [CG189]*, NICE, Published November 2014, Copyright © 2017 National Institute for Health and Care Excellence. Available from: www.nice.org.uk/guidance/cg189/chapter/1-recommendations Reproduced courtesy of Corinne Owers

2. What are the common comorbidities associated with morbid obesity?

Obesity is a complex disease that is associated with a range of physical and psychological health problems. In the vast majority of people undergoing weight-loss surgery, the aim is to effect an improvement in their obesity-related comorbidities and psychological health, as well as increase life-expectancy, rather than to improve their physical appearance.

NICE recommends consideration of weight-loss drug therapy for patients with class 1 obesity in the presence of comorbidity, or class

2 or 3 obesity. NICE also recommends consideration for surgery in patients with class 2 obesity in the presence of comorbidity or class 3 obesity. Patients may be offered surgery on the NHS with a slightly lower BMI than recommended, as exact criteria vary around the UK in different centres.

The most common weight-related comorbidities include:

* *Type 2 diabetes.* In existence with obesity, this condition has been coined 'diabesity'. Rapid and significant improvements in glycaemic control can occur following bariatric surgery, in some cases leading to a resolution of type 2 diabetes. A recurrence of diabetes may occur if patients regain weight.

* *Hypertension*: ranging from mild to moderate, most significantly overweight patients have hypertension, often requiring significant medical treatment. Associated with hypertension are the risks of cerebrovascular accident (CVA) and myocardial infarction (MI), as well as peripheral vascular disease.

* *Obstructive sleep apnoea (OSA).* Patients experience recurrent upper airway obstruction, and obesity is thought to result in OSA through a number of neuromuscular and mechanical effects. Patients with OSA often require a non-invasive ventilation machine called a CPAP (continuous positive airway pressure) machine to provide positive airway pressure at night. Sleep can be disturbed by breathing difficulty without a CPAP mask and lead to daytime somnalescence.

* *Dyslipidaemia.*

* *Arthritis.* Hip, knee, and back arthritis are all very common and can lead to severe pain, as well as difficulty with mobilization. Orthopaedic surgeons are often reluctant to offer joint replacement to the severely obese.

* *Depression.* Up to 84% of people with obesity suffer with depression at some point in their lifetime. The psychosocial difficulties associated with obesity can lead to severe emotional and behavioural problems.

- *Infertility.* Obesity is a common cause of infertility in both males and females, which can often be reversed by significant weight loss.

- *Increased cancer risk.* Obesity has a known association with numerous types of cancer, including liver, oesophageal, stomach, breast, bowel, and kidney.

3. What considerations should be made before offering a patient bariatric surgery?

The pre-operative optimization of patients for bariatric surgery needs careful consideration by the whole of the multidisciplinary team (MDT).

First, the choice of operation must be made in conjunction with the patient. For diabetics or sweet eaters, there is some evidence that a Roux-en-Y gastric bypass may be more suitable, whereas volume eaters may be best served by a sleeve gastrectomy or gastric band (discussed in Question 4). The band is reversible unlike the other operations, but requires more follow-up. Patient preference is important, although previous abdominal surgery, abdominal hernias, and surgical preference may have some bearing on the operation performed.

Patients undergoing bariatric surgery must be committed to making significant lifestyle changes, otherwise they are likely to regain weight following surgery. Dietary advice is provided, but they must be willing to adhere to this in order to avoid problems. Smokers are strongly encouraged to quit before surgery, and in some centres, operations may be cancelled if the patients cannot demonstrate compliance. In the first year after surgery, alcohol is prohibited due to the metabolic and absorptive changes, as well as its calorific content. Given the possibility of addiction transference from food to alcohol, commitment to this is imperative.

Patients require significant support in terms of their diet, as well as their social and mental health. Patients who either have no social support, or where this is inadequate, may find themselves with more difficulty adjusting to their new lifestyle. Psychology assessment can be made and support provided, although resources are limited and this is often left to the remit of the GP in the community. Patients should be encouraged to educate themselves, wherever possible, about the expected lifestyle changes and to attend support groups.

A full pre-operative assessment must be made, including nutritional screening, as well as cardiovascular and respiratory investigations. Patients may need to undergo sleep studies and be provided with CPAP for a few months before being anaesthetized in order to minimize peri-operative anaesthetic risks. Any nutritional abnormalities should be corrected before surgery in order to prevent them from becoming worse post-operatively.

4. What are the common operations performed during bariatric/ metabolic surgery?

In the UK, the three most commonly performed procedures are:

- Laparoscopic adjustable gastric band.
- Sleeve gastrectomy.
- Roux-en-Y gastric bypass.

In the vast majority of cases, these are performed laparoscopically unless there is a specific contraindication.

Laparoscopic adjustable gastric band (LAGB) A silastic band is placed around the upper part of the stomach to form a small egg-cup sized pouch above it. This is attached to a long piece of tubing and a port, which is placed subcutaneously on the anterior abdominal wall. Using a non-coring (Huber) needle, the band can be inflated or emptied by injecting saline into the port. The higher the volume within the band, the tighter the constriction, meaning that food cannot pass through in a solid state. The band works by restriction, preventing large amounts of food from being consumed. It affects the vagus nerve inducing early satiety, and is thought to alter the hormones within the gut. Figure 1.2.1 shows a photo of a gastric band being sited laparoscopically.

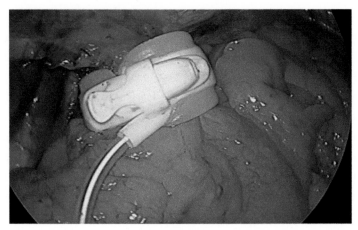

Figure 1.2.1 An intra-operative image showing an adjustable gastric band that has just been positioned around the stomach at laparoscopic surgery.

Reproduced courtesy of Corinne Owers.

Sleeve gastrectomy (SG) A bougie is passed into the stomach and down to the pylorus along the lesser curve of the stomach. Using a stapling device, the stomach is divided along the length of the bougie, creating a long, thin tube. The remainder of the stomach is removed. The sleeve also works by restriction, and is believed to alter the release of gut hormones, both of which can prevent over-eating. This procedure is illustrated in Figure 1.2.2.

Roux-en-Y gastric bypass (RYGB) With a stapling device, the stomach is divided to form a small pouch below the oesophagus. Approximately a metre down from the duodeno-jejunal (DJ) flexure, the small bowel is divided and the distal limb brought up to anastomose with the stomach pouch (alimentary limb). The proximal end of the small bowel, which is still attached to the DJ flexure and stomach (biliary limb), is then re-connected a variable distance downstream from the gastrojejunal anastomosis. Again, the RYGB has restrictive and hormonal effects, although there is also an element of malabsorption, as digestion and absorption only occur distal from the jejuno-jejunal anastomosis. This procedure is illustrated in Figure 1.2.3.

Other less commonly performed operations include the intragastric balloon, duodenal switch, biliopancreatic diversion, and Endobarrier (not approved by NICE).

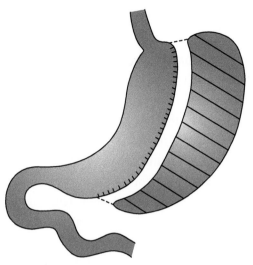

Figure 1.2.2 Illustration of the sleeve gastrectomy procedure.

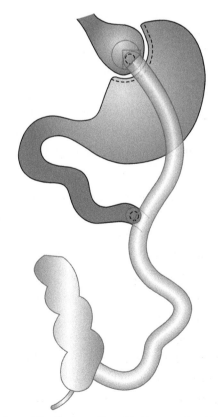

Figure 1.2.3 Illustration of the Roux-en-Y gastric bypass procedure.

5. WHAT ARE THE MAIN OPERATIVE CONSIDERATIONS FOR BARIATRIC SURGERY PATIENTS?

Bariatric surgery should only be performed in centres that are equipped to provide the high level of care required by bariatric patients, and have the necessary facilities. Bariatric chairs, beds, operating tables, CT scanners, blood pressure cuffs, gowns, transport, and wheelchairs may all become necessary as patients can often not use the standard equipment. Nursing and medical staff should be adequately trained to support patients and the psychological issues associated with obesity to prevent patients from feeling discriminated against, stigmatized, and subject to prejudice.

In the majority of cases, patients following SG and RYGB will be managed on the first night post-operatively on the high-dependency/post-operative care unit. Anaesthesia in the obese patient is associated with a number of risks, so this will necessitate careful post-operative monitoring. Risk can be attributed to the comorbidities that many patients have. Thromboembolism is more common in the obese, and one of the more common causes of death following bariatric surgery. Patients must be given adequate thromboprophylaxis, which requires higher than normal dosing of low molecular weight heparin (calculated based on their weight), as well as surgical stockings. Large stockings must be available, as standard sizes are not adequate. The bariatric population is often sedentary and hence the need for thromboprophylaxis in the hospital, as well as on discharge, is essential.

Patients require significant dietary input. Patients have to follow a pre-operative liver-shrinking diet for approximately 2 weeks before surgery, and then a staged diet after their operation. Their changing nutritional requirements, as well as the inability to eat normal textured foods, means that a specially qualified dietitian is necessary in order to support patients appropriately. Patients will present with many questions about what they can and cannot eat, both before and after surgery.

In many cases, the medications that patients were on pre-operatively may need to be changed. This could be due to an improvement in their obesity-related comorbidities, such as diabetes, but also due to an inability to swallow sometimes large volumes or, indeed, larger sized tablets. An assessment by the GP or pharmacist, who can change medications to more suitable preparations, as well as monitor their changing medication requirements, is advisable pre-operatively and needs regular reconsideration post-surgery.

6. What are the common metabolic side-effects associated with bariatric surgery?

Metabolic complications following bariatric surgery are uncommon. Side-effects, however, are experienced by a significant number of patients, but can often be managed in the community without the need for hospital admission. The majority of side-effects can be related to nutritional requirements, which can change significantly after surgery. Any nutritional deficiency can quickly lead to problems such as hair loss, poor-quality nails and teeth, skin problems, including infections, halitosis, and an increase in flatulence or burping. All patients must take a multivitamin tablet daily lifelong, as well as 3-monthly vitamin B12 injections due to surgical alteration in the anatomy of the stomach.

Dumping syndrome is associated with the RYGB and, to a lesser extent, the SG. A rapid entry of food into the duodenum causes fluid shifts, leading to hypotension, abdominal pain, diarrhoea, nausea, and vomiting. The release of insulin secondary to the 'dumping' of food can also lead to symptoms of hypoglycaemia. Although more common following sugar or carbohydrate ingestion, dumping syndrome can occur following any type of food, and can be unpleasant for the patient. This is managed by a tailored approach, simply avoiding the foods that cause dumping in that individual is often effective.

Given the amount of weight loss that is afforded to many patients following bariatric surgery, loose skin is very common and experienced to some degree in most patients. Although this may not be of concern to some, especially those who have undergone bariatric surgery in order to improve their comorbidities, for others this may lead to significant body image and psychological issues. Skin-removal surgery is not routinely offered on the NHS and, therefore, those considering this would have to seek surgery in the private sector.

Although not everyone experiences these side-effects, it is important to express to the patient that these are, in fact, normal after surgery and, with time, many of them will improve, provided they maintain a healthy balanced diet with adequate nutrition.

Further reading

Ackroyd R, Rajeswaran C, Owers C, Walker N (2014) *The Ultimate Guide to Weight Loss Surgery: All You Need To Know Regarding Weight Loss Surgery*, First edition. CreateSpace Independent Publishing.

Owers C, Ackroyd R (2014) Bariatric surgery. *Surgery (Oxford)* 32 (11): 614–8.

Schwartz AR, Patil SP, Laffan AM, Polotsky V, Schneider H, Smith PL (2008) Obesity and obstructive sleep apnea: pathogenic mechanisms and therapeutic approaches. *Proceedings of the American Thoracic Society Journal* 5 (2): 185–92.

Case history 1.3: Elective: gastro-oesophageal cancer

A 68-year-old Caucasian man attends the 2-week wait clinic with symptoms of dysphagia. He has a longstanding history of dyspepsia and was diagnosed with Barrett's oesophagus approximately 10 years earlier, but failed to attend his latest screening appointment. On questioning it appears that he has dysphagia to solids and occasional liquids, and has lost approximately 2 stone (12.75 kg) in weight over the last 6 weeks. He has a minimal appetite, although he has been trying to eat but only manages about one meal a day. He has had no change in his bowel habit, no nausea but occasionally deliberately tries to vomit food when he feels it gets stuck. His GP prescribed him some omeprazole but he does not feel this has helped his symptoms. He has a past medical history of gallstones, hypercholesterolaemia, and COPD for which he takes regular inhalers. He takes a regular statin but no other medications. On examination he looks well. His BMI is 24.5 kg/ m². Endoscopy demonstrates a non-obstructing tumour at the distal oesophagus (Figure 1.3.1). A histological diagnosis of adenocarcinoma is made from the biopsy. CT of the chest abdomen and pelvis shows no metastatic spread and the cancer was determined to be resectable.

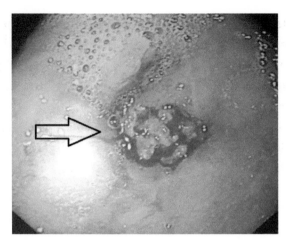

Figure 1.3.1 Image taken at diagnostic UGI endoscopy demonstrating the tumour at the distal oesophagus (see arrow).

Reproduced courtesy of Corinne Owers.

Questions

1. What are the different types of gastro-oesophageal cancers?
2. How do gastro-oesophageal tumours present and how should they be investigated?
3. What are the main operative management strategies in gastro-oesophageal cancer?
4. What are the main non-operative strategies?
5. What is the appropriate management in this case?

Answers

1. What are the different types of gastro-oesophageal cancers?

The incidence of UGI cancers varies across the world, with countries such as Japan and China having a significantly higher incidence of gastric cancer than the UK. In the Western world, oesophageal cancers appear to be migrating distally, and more cancers are arising at the gastro-oesophageal junction (GOJ) than the proximal stomach. Adenocarcinoma of the oesophagus is on the increase. The reasons for these changes are not well understood and may be partly genetic, although the significant lifestyle changes that have occurred over the last half-century, particularly in the Western world, probably have a part to play.

Oesophageal cancer This is the eighth most common malignancy worldwide, with an increasing incidence in the Western world. The commonest types are squamous and adenocarcinoma.

- *Squamous cell carcinoma (SCC).* This is common in countries with low socioeconomic status. It is not usually associated with GORD, but oesophagitis associated with dysplasia and atrophy is thought to be a precursor. Hot drinks, coarse or pickled foods, and smoking are also thought to play a part in the development of oesophageal SCC. Patients who experience corrosive or caustic injury to the oesophagus due to the ingestion of chemicals have a 1,000-fold increase in the incidence of this cancer, although there is a time delay of 20–40 years between injury and cancer presentation. Given that many of these injuries occur in childhood, there can be a number of young patients developing SCC of the oesophagus. Achalasia has also been seen to have an increased incidence of oesophageal SCC 140 times relative to the normal population. This is potentially due to the carcinogens created in fermenting food, which lies static within the oesophagus. Finally, there are a number of genetic syndromes or familial risk factors such as Plummer–Vinson syndrome and tylosis, which may have an increased disposition to oesophageal cancer, although environmental factors may also factor in the development of this disease.

♦ *Adenocarcinoma and junctional tumours.* This accounts for 72% of oesophageal tumours in the UK. In recent decades there has been a dramatic rise in the incidence of junctional adenocarcinoma, with the main aetiological factor being Barrett's oesophagus as a result of GORD. Barrett's is more prevalent in males, with the peak incidence at around 40 years of age. The peak incidence of adenocarcinoma is approximately 60 years of age. It is likely that underlying Barrett's will have been present for approximately 20 years before undergoing metaplastic change. Factors predisposing to malignant change in Barrett's include male sex, Caucasians, smoking, alcohol, obesity, the length of the Barrett's segment, and alkaline reflux.

The Siewert and Stein classification of oesophagogastric tumours is divided into three subtypes:[*]

1. Type I: adenocarcinoma of the distal oesophagus, usually arising from an area of Barrett's metaplasia, which may infiltrate the GOJ.

2. Type II: adenocarcinoma of the cardia arising from GOJ. This is also known as 'junctional carcinoma'

3. Type III: subcardial gastric adenocarcinoma, which infiltrates the GOJ and oesophagus from below.

[*]Source: Data from Griffin SM, Raimes SA, and Shenfine J, (2013) *Oesophagogastric Surgery: A Companion to Specialist Surgical Practice*, fifth edition. Saunders Ltd, Elsevier.

Gastric cancer Environmental factors are thought to be associated with the development of gastric cancer, which is supported by the apparent geographical variations in disease incidence worldwide. A poor quality or malnourished diet predispose to the development of gastric cancer, particularly in diets high in carbohydrate, low in protein, high in preservatives and salt, and low in vegetables.

In the UK, adenocarcinoma accounts for 96% of all stomach cancers. *Helicobacter pylori* has a known association with the development of squamous cell carcinoma of the stomach by causing an inflammatory reaction that can lead to chronic gastritis, mucosal atrophy, and intestinal metaplasia. Any detection of *H. pylori*, either by endoscopic, serum, or urease breath test investigations, warrants eradication therapy with antibiotics and a protein pump inhibitor (discussed in Case 1.5).

Other cancers There are a number of miscellaneous tumours of the oesophagus and stomach, which are less common but may be found histologically. These include:

+ Granular cell tumours.

+ Basaloid carcinoma.

+ Small cell carcinoma.

+ Mucoepidermoid carcinoma of the oesophagus.

+ Epithelial, mesenchymal, and neuroendocrine tumours of the stomach, including MALToma, GIST, and gastric carcinoids.

2. How do gastro-oesophageal tumours present and how should they be investigated?

Malignancies of the UGI tract can present in a number of ways. The disease does not become symptomatic until the disease process is established. Up to a quarter of cases present as an emergency to hospital. The 'red flag' symptoms that are suspicious of upper gastro-intestinal malignancy constitute the criteria for 2-week wait referral for urgent OGD or surgical assessment. These include:

+ New onset dyspepsia (in over 55-year-olds).

+ Dysphagia.

+ Chronic gastrointestinal bleeding.

+ Progressive and unintentional weight loss.

+ Persistent vomiting.

+ Iron-deficiency anaemia.

+ Epigastric mass.

Other concerning symptoms include postprandial fullness. All patients should be assessed with a thorough history and examination. First-line investigations include endoscopy, which can provide a macroscopic diagnosis, as well as providing an opportunity for obtaining tissue for histological corroboration. The likelihood of identifying areas of dysplasia, metaplasia, or early neoplasms depends on the skill and experience of the endoscopist, as well as site, size, and type of the lesion. For patients who are unable to tolerate endoscopy, barium swallow can demonstrate both severe reflux and advanced malignancies, although this may well miss early cancers.

For all cases either where tumour is strongly suspected or an endoscopic/radiological diagnosis has been made, staging imaging should be performed with a CT of the chest, abdomen, and pelvis to assess for mediastinal invasion, lymphadenopathy, and metastatic disease. PET scanning can also be of use in order to detect any signs of metastases and improve staging.

Endoscopic ultrasound (EUS) can be used to assess the depth of tumour invasion, particularly in patients who may be suitable for endoscopic mucosal resection (EMR), as opposed to a full gastro-oesophageal resection. In some patients, diagnostic laparoscopy is an appropriate investigation and allows pre-operative workup to assess for signs of peritoneal disease, which can be less reliably determined on cross-sectional imaging.

Given the magnitude of a gastro-oesophageal resection, and the advancing age and comorbidities of patients presenting with UGI malignancy, physical fitness for surgery should be determined using formal investigation such as a shuttle walk or cardiopulmonary exercise (CPEX) testing. This is often advisable before a general anaesthetic, especially in oesophageal cancers where deflation of the lung is required in order to perform the operation.

Once investigations have been performed, all patients should be referred to an UGI cancer MDT meeting so that appropriate management plans can be created. Oesophagogastric cancer resectional surgery has been centralized to regional tertiary centres in the UK in recent years, so patients will need to be referred from outlying district general hospitals for discussion.

3. What are the main operative management strategies in gastro-oesophageal cancer?

In all patients diagnosed with oesophagogastric malignancy, decision regarding operative strategy must be made in conjunction with the MDT.

- *Oesophageal.* The nature of oesophageal resection depends on the site of the tumour and the extent of the disease. Resection can be performed either laparoscopically or at open operation, although this depends on multiple factors, including surgical skill, size, site, and type of tumour, and the patient's best interests. For high tumours that are deemed resectable, either the stomach can be brought up to anastomose with the proximal end of the oesophagus or a colonic interposition graft used. Lower tumours are usually managed with an oesophagogastrectomy where the affected oesophagus and part of the upper stomach is removed. In some cases this can all be performed abdominally from below, especially where only the abdominal oesophagus is affected, or with access through both the neck and the abdomen (trans-hiatal oesophagectomy), although very often both the chest and abdominal cavities need to be opened in a two-stage operation (trans-thoracic oesophagectomy); one such approach is the Ivor–Lewis oesophagogastrectomy (ILOG). Where both the stomach and oesophagus need excision, Roux-en-Y reconstruction is often performed. In addition, two-field lymphadenectomy may be carried out to improve staging and local disease control.

- *Gastric.* The extension of any gastric resection depends on the site of the tumour and the number of involved lymph nodes. Cancers in the body and fundus require a total gastrectomy, and in these cases a Roux-en-Y reconstruction is standard to replumb both the alimentary and biliary limbs to the distal small bowel. Cancers of the distal third (antrum) and pylorus may be managed by a partial or subtotal gastrectomy. Gastric resection is performed through the abdominal cavity, and lymphadenectomy removing first- and possibly second-tier perigastric lymph nodes should be considered to improve staging and local disease control.

- *Palliative.* Where cancer is not resectable and a tumour is causing obstruction, a palliative bypass or stenting may be carried out. This allows the patients to maintain some quality of life in situations where the alternative would be to survive either on PEG/PEJ feeding or TPN. Any part of the small bowel, duodenum, stomach, or even distal oesophagus can be bypassed, although severe reflux would likely occur post-operatively. Stenting is relatively less invasive, which avoids surgical-related morbidity.

4. What are the main non-operative strategies?

Non-operative strategies are usually considered either when the tumour is very early, localized, and non-invasive, or where operative resection is not deemed appropriate.

Early, non-invasive cancers can be treated by endoscopic mucosal resection (EMR). This is a relatively new treatment, where tumours that are localized to the mucosa or submucosa can be excised using an endoscopically performed technique. This type of procedure eliminates the need for large gastro-oesophageal resectional surgery with its associated morbidity and mortality. This can be followed by treatment with photodynamic therapy or radiofrequency ablation to treat any remnant cancerous cells.

Chemoradiotherapy can have a role in both downsizing disease and palliation. More than half of patients with gastric cancer in the Western world present with inoperable disease, and only 10–20% of oesophageal cancers are deemed resectable. Neo-adjuvant chemoradiotherapy has been shown to downsize the tumour and to improve outcomes by limiting the extent of lymphatic spread. This may mean tumours either become resectable where they would otherwise be managed palliatively or it may mean a more limited resection is possible. Adjuvant chemoradiotherapy is often offered based on the histological stage of the disease following resection. Where resection is either incomplete (R1 resection) or there is lymph node involvement, this may prolong survival. Palliative chemoradiotherapy is given mainly for symptom control in cases where operative management is not an option. It has been reported to prolong survival in locally advanced oesophagogastric cancer by 3–6 months compared to best supportive care.

Palliative measures include:

◆ *Argon plasma coagulation (APC).* Another endoscopically performed procedure, APC involves directing a stream of ionized argon gas (plasma) on to the tumour and can be used to 'de-bulk' tumours in patients where resection is not feasible. This can be used either prior to, or alongside, stenting.

◆ *Stenting.* Oesophageal carcinomas (and occasionally pyloric) that are unresectable and cause obstruction can often be amenable to stenting either endoscopically or radiologically. Self-expanding stents open the lumen allowing food to pass through. A palliative option, this enables patients to maintain some quality of life by allowing them to eat and drink. Patients are counselled to risks of bleeding and perforation, as well as tumour overgrowth or dis-lodging of the stent, which may require repeat stenting.

5. What is the appropriate management in this case?

For this case, further investigations need to be performed before an appropriate management plan can be made. Although the tumour is not yet metastatic, it may be locally advanced and further assess-ment with EUS would be advisable. Given his diagnosis of COPD, he would need to undergo CPEX testing and have a pre-operative review by the anaesthetist to see if he would be suitable for extensive abdominal and thoracic surgery. Staging laparoscopy would also be suitable as, if there is any evidence of peritoneal spread, he may be left with palliative options only.

If EUS and CPEX suggest the tumour is respectable and the patient is fit for surgery, the preferred option in this case would most probably be Ivor–Lewis oesophagogastrectomy to remove the lower oesophagus and upper stomach. Depending on the histological sta-ging, he may require adjuvent chemoradiotherapy.

Following surgery he would require regular outpatient follow-up, usually 6-monthly for the first 2 years and then annually up to 5 years. Survival rates for oesophageal and gastric cancers have increased in the last decade but remain low.

Further reading

Dikken JL, van de Velde CJH, Coit DG, Shah MA, Verheij M, Cats A (2012) Treatment of resectable gastric cancer. *Therapeutic Advances in Gastroenterology* 5 (1): 48–69.

Reed CE (2009) Technique of the open Ivor Lewis esophagogastrectomy. *Operative Techniques in Thoracic and Cardiovascular Surgery* 14 (3): 160–75.

Case history 1.4: Emergency: upper gastrointestinal bleeding

A 36-year-old Caucasian female with a known history of alcohol excess and substance misuse is admitted from the emergency department with two episodes of haematemesis and marked upper abdominal pain. Due to intoxication, only a limited history could be obtained but her partner says she is under investigations by the hepatologist for abnormal liver function. She has no other medical history and takes no prescribed medications except over-the-counter medications for GORD. She is a smoker and drinks approximately 1 ltr of cider per day, with more at the weekends. Her mother died of an upper gastrointestinal cancer at 60 years of age. On examination she has a BP of 132/70 and a heart rate of 108. Respiratory rate is 10. Abdominal examination shows marked tenderness in the epigastrium but no peritonism or masses, digital rectal examination is normal with soft brown stool in the rectum. Serum haemoglobin is 104 with normal white cell count. There is a hepatitic picture on her liver function tests. Emergency OGD is performed due to the suspicion of a possible variceal bleed, given her history. One column of varices is seen but these are not bleeding. In the first part of the duodenum a bleeding ulcer is seen, which is injected with adrenaline and cauterized. She returns to the ward for alcohol detoxification and intravenous proton pump inhibitor therapy, and is discharged following this with a repeat endoscopy booked to monitor healing in 6–8 weeks.

Questions

1. What are the common causes of UGI bleeding?

2. What is the pathophysiology of variceal bleeding?

3. When dealing with UGI bleeding, how do you stratify risk?

4. What is the initial resuscitative management of a patient with an UGI bleed?

5. What is the initial endoscopic management of this patient after resuscitation?

6. What is the management after a failed endoscopy?

Answers

1. What are the common causes of UGI bleeding?

UGI bleeding is bleeding from any source proximal to the ligament of Treitz, which demarcates the duodeno-jejunal junction. It can come from a number of sources:

- *Peptic ulcer.* This is one of the most common causes, and can present either with an acute UGI haemorrhage with haematemesis or rectal bleeding (either with malaena or fresh red blood), or more insidious bleeding with iron-deficiency anaemia. Many ulcer bleeds will stop without treatment, although investigation should be considered, even in those not requiring emergency management. Peptic ulcers are mainly caused by *H. pylori* and use of non-steroidal anti-inflammatory drugs. As ulceration penetrates into the gastroduodenal mucosa, it can involve underlying blood vessels, resulting in necrosis of the arterial wall and subsequent bleeding. Ulcers in the stomach are more likely to be malignant than those in the duodenum, therefore biopsies should be taken for histological assessment, either on initial endoscopy or on repeat OGD once an initial acute bleed has settled.

- *Variceal bleed.* Varices are abnormal, distended veins that arise as a consequence of hypertension of the portal venous system and collateralization to the systemic circulation. These arise at the junction between the portal and systemic blood systems at the gastro-oesophageal junction within the stomach wall. These receive inflow from the left gastric or coronary vein and the short gastric veins. Bleeding from oesophageal varices accounts for between 5 and 11% of all cases of UGI bleeding in the UK, and is primarily managed by gastroenterologists.

- *UGI cancers.* These can either present with bleeding from the tumour or a patient with a known cancer may subsequently present with haematemesis. In many cases the bleeding can be managed endoscopically either with injection of adrenaline or APC. If the bleeding does not settle, radiological embolization can be considered, although there is an associated risk of ischaemia and infarction to surrounding tissue, as well as re-bleeding with associated morbidity. Resection of operable disease will definitively treat the bleeding, as well as the malignancy.

- *Erosive gastritis/oesophagitis.* Occasionally, erosive gastritis or oesophagitis can cause bleeding, although this is usually self-limiting. It is managed with proton pump inhibitors. *Helicobacter pylori* eradication should be considered if the patient's CLO (microbiological biopsy) is positive.

- *Mallory–Weiss tear.* Where vomiting or coughing from any cause is profuse, occasional tears in the oesophagus can result, and these can cause haematemesis, which may be massive. They are more common in alcoholics and in hyperemesis gravidarum. The tear involves the mucosa and submucosa but there is no muscular involvement (in contrast to the oesophageal perforation of Boerhaave's).

- *Dialefoy lesion.* A tortuous large-calibre vessel that protrudes into the stomach wall. Very rare cause of bleeding.

- Other rare causes include aortoenteric fistula after aortic aneurysm repair, angiectasia, and Osler–Webber–Rendu syndrome.

2. What is the pathophysiology of variceal bleeding?

Varices arise in patients with portal hypertension. The high portal pressure results in diverting the venous blood flow into a number of porto-systemic collaterals, which subsequently dilate. This most commonly results in gastro-oesophageal varices and splenomegaly. However, despite the collateral bypass, the portal hypertension persists, which is thought to be due to insufficient decompression of the portal flow and also due to splanchnic arteriolar vasodilatation. Oesophageal varices can be classified by morphology and the degree of extension into the lumen. The risk of bleeding increases in the presence of greatly elevated portal pressure.

The causes of the varices can be classified according to the site of resistance causing the portal hypertension, and these can arise at pre-hepatic, intra-hepatic, and post-hepatic levels (Table 1.4.1).

Table 1.4.1 Causes of portal hypertension

Site	Cause
Prehepatic	Portal vein thrombosis
	Extrinsic venous compression
Intra-hepatic	Primary biliary cirrhosis
	Liver cirrhosis
	Metastatic infiltration of the liver
	Sclerosing cholangitis
	Wilson disease
	A1-antitrypsin deficiency
Post-hepatic	Right-sided heart failure
	Budd–Chiari syndrome

Reproduced Courtesy of Corinne Owers.

This patient's history of liver dysfunction could be attributed to her excessive alcohol intake and intra-hepatic generation of portal hypertension from liver cirrhosis could be surmised in this circumstance, although a thorough workup would be performed to determine this once the patient is treated and stabilized.

3. When dealing with UGI bleeding, how do you stratify risk?

There are a number of scoring systems in place, which aim to stratify risk and predict adverse outcomes following UGI haemorrhage, including the risk of re-bleeding. A commonly used scoring system is the Rockall score (Table 1.4.2). A number of variables are taken into account to generate a numerical score.

The total for each variable are totalled and a risk score calculated. The risk of re-bleeding and mortality following calculation of the Rockall score can then be determined from Table 1.4.3.

Patients with a higher risk score of re-bleeding will need more intensive observation.

Table 1.4.2 Reference table for calculating the Rockall score

Variable	Score 0	Score 1	Score 2	Score 3
Age	<60	60–79	>80	
Shock	No shock	Pulse >100 BP >100 systolic	BP <100 systolic	
Comorbidity	Nil major		Cardiorespiratory disease, other major	Renal, liver or advanced malignant disease
Diagnosis	Mallory–Weiss, no lesion or no stigmata of recent bleed	All other diagnoses	UGI malignancy	
Evidence of bleeding at endoscopy	None or dark spot		Luminal blood, adherent clot, active bleeding, visible vessel	

Reproduced Courtesy of Corinne Owers.

Table 1.4.3 Reference table for determining risk of rebleeding and mortality from UGI bleeding

Risk score	Re-bleed (%)	Mortality (%)
0	5	0
3	11	3
5	24	11
6	33	17
8+	42	41

Reproduced Courtesy of Corinne Owers.

4. What is the initial resuscitative management of a patient with an UGI bleed?

In any patient presenting with an UGI bleed, an assessment of their haemodynamic stability must be made and appropriate resuscitation commenced. This will usually involve the insertion of two wide-bore cannulae and initiating immediate intravenous infusion with crystalloids. Blood investigations should be sent immediately, including full blood count, electrolytes, clotting, and crossmatch. Transfusion may be necessary. All patients who are actively bleeding should have at least six units crossmatched. O-negative blood is often required for urgent cases who need transfusing before the results of the crossmatch are available. Any clotting abnormality should be corrected and an anti-fibrinolytic drug such as tranexamic acid could also be considered. A urinary catheter should be inserted in order to better manage fluid balance and monitor end-organ perfusion.

In non-variceal bleeding, an intravenous proton pump inhibitor may be beneficial, especially if there is a suspicion of peptic ulcer bleed. Erect chest X-ray can help to rule out perforation and then, once stabilized, the patient should undergo emergency endoscopy. Therapeutic OGD is generally performed for bleeding up to two times before operative management is considered.

Variceal bleeds are often more profuse and although this is also managed endoscopically, the patient often requires more resuscitation and even temporizing measures. Protection of the airway is critical and they may require intubation to protect the airway, as aspiration is likely, which will require admission to the critical care unit. Vasoconstrictors such as octreotide, vasopressin, or one of its analogues can be given to reduce portal blood flow and therefore portal pressure, helping to slow the haemorrhage so that it can be managed endoscopically. There is evidence to suggest that administration of intravenous antibiotics can be beneficial in variceal bleeds, although not in other causes.

5. What is the initial endoscopic management of this patient after resuscitation?

As soon as the patient is adequately resuscitated and stabilized haemodynamically, emergency endoscopy should be performed. At endoscopy, two or three treatment modalities should be used in order to decrease the chances of a re-bleed. These modalities include:

- Adrenaline.
- Clips.
- Haemospray.
- Ablation (Goldprobe, APC).
- Banding.

Endoscopic approaches differ slightly in variceal and non-variceal bleeding:

Non-variceal bleeding The majority of non-variceal bleeds are the result of bleeding peptic ulcers. Injection of adrenaline into the ulcer bed is often the first-line treatment; this can often raise the bleeding lesion away from the muscle layer and tamponade the blood vessel, as well as generate localized vasoconstriction. Depending on whether or not there is a visible vessel or active bleeding, clips may be applied before or after the injection of the adrenaline. Ablation with Goldprobe diathermy or APC is often used to cauterize the area, although if improperly performed it can increase the active bleeding. Haemospray is a relatively new adjunct that when sprayed on to the bleeding site, coagulates and forms an artificial clot. If available, Haemospray can often be used in emergency situations where either the endoscopist is not able to do alternative therapeutics or other modalities have been unsuccessful.

Variceal bleeding The mainstay of variceal bleeding is banding of the varices. Variceal columns begin at the GOJ and travel caudally, therefore banding at the GOJ can often help to arrest blood flow, allowing for more accurate placement of bands distally. If banding is not available, injection of sclerosant can be used, although this is generally less successful than banding. Injection of adrenaline alone is unlikely to treat variceal bleeds but can be used as an adjunct.

6. What is the management after a failed endoscopy?

After a first endoscopy, if re-bleeding occurs it is generally reasonable to perform a second endoscopy and give further endoscopic therapy. Again, management differs between variceal and non-variceal bleeding:

Non-variceal bleeding If a suitably qualified endoscopist has performed two endoscopies and the patient is still actively bleeding, consultation with the surgeons for surgery to under-run an ulcer or even a partial gastrectomy may become necessary. Although surgery for peptic ulcer disease used to be common, this is now considered as a last option due the successful outcomes from the measures that have been discussed in Question 5.

Variceal bleeding In the event that endoscopy is not able to control the bleeding, or a further re-bleed occurs, balloon tamponade with a device such as a Sengstaken or Minnesota tube can be performed, although re-bleed rates on deflation are as high as 50%. Radiological embolization could be considered, although this carries risks of ischaemia to the adjacent tissues. Finally, with variceal bleeds, transjugular intra-hepatic portosystemic shunt (TIPS) or liver transplantation could be considered if the patient is in a centre that is able to carry out these procedures. TIPS involves placing a stent from the portal vein to the hepatic vein, bypassing portal flow into the systemic circulation. This reduces the portal vein pressure and can help to reduce collateral blood flow and reduce bleeding. It can be performed radiologically, introducing a stent from the portal vein to the hepatic vein.

Further reading

Tham TCK, Collins JSA, Soetikno RM (2009) *Gastrointestinal Emergencies*, second edition. Wiley–Blackwell.

Case history 1.5: Emergency: perforated duodenal ulcer

A 22-year-old Afro-Caribbean lady presents with a 2-day history of severe epigastric pain radiating through to the back, nausea, and non-bilious vomiting. She has no past medical history apart from recently taking ibuprofen for several weeks following an injury to her knee, sustained whilst skiing. Bowels had opened normally the day before presentation, and there has been no obvious rectal bleeding, malaena, or haematemesis. She is a non-smoker, drinks a moderate amount of alcohol at university but takes no recreational drugs. On examination, heart rate is 110, BP is 128/76, and respiratory rate is 16 with oxygen saturation of 98% on air. She is apyrexial. Abdominal examination shows generalized abdominal tenderness with localized peritonitis in the epigastrium. Abdominal film is normal but erect chest X-ray confirms the presence of free air under the diaphragm. A CT is performed that suggests that the perforation is within the second part of the duodenum.

Questions

1. What are the differential diagnoses?
2. What are the common aetiological factors associated with peptic ulcer disease?
3. How does peptic ulcer disease present?
4. How do you classify peptic ulcers?
5. What is the appropriate management of a patient with suspected perforated duodenal ulcer?
6. What are the surgical options for treatment in this patient?

Answers

1. What are the differential diagnoses?

The main differential diagnoses in a patient with this history would include perforated duodenal ulcer, acute cholecystitis, gastritis and duodenitis, acute pancreatitis, and portal vein thrombosis. Other differentials include superior mesenteric artery syndrome and gastroenteritis.

2. What are the common aetiological factors associated with peptic ulcer disease?

Peptic ulcer disease comprises ulcers in the stomach or duodenum. They begin in the mucosa and extend into the underlying muscularis propia. The mucosa is potentially vulnerable to the acid and the digestive enzymes that the stomach produces in order to break down digested food so has, therefore, developed a number of protective mechanisms against them. The epithelial cells produce mucus, which forms a layer that is impermeable to acid and pepsin. They also produce bicarbonate that buffers acid that comes into close contact with the gut wall. These measures are usually sufficient to protect the underlying mucosa. Peptic ulcers occur when these measures fail to protect the mucosa, resulting in mucosal injury. Ulcer progression through the layers of the mucosa and submucosa can result in involvement of an underlying vessel causing bleeding or deeper propagation resulting in perforation.

Peptic ulcer disease can be associated with a number of factors:

- Physiological stress, especially duodenal ulcers. This can also occur in acutely sick patients on ITU (known as Curling's ulcers), and pharmacological prophylaxis (PPI or H2 antagonist) is routinely prescribed by the intensivists to prevent this.
- Non-steroidal anti-inflammatory drugs such as ibuprofen is a well-known cause of ulcers that arise as a consequent of NSAID-associated gastritis, and often the most common cause of those presenting with perforation.
- Smoking.
- Alcohol.
- Malignant ulcers tend to present in the older population, and are most commonly in the stomach. Any gastric ulcer should therefore be biopsied to rule out malignancy.

- The Gram-negative spirochaete *H. pylori* is one of the main causes of peptic ulcers. It is associated with 45% of gastric ulcers and 85% of duodenal ulcers. It colonizes the gastric and duodenal mucosa, and alkalinizes it with its urease enzyme. This can be diagnosed non-invasively on a carbon-13 urea breath test or stool antigen test, or on a CLO (campylobacter-like organism) biopsy test taken at OGD. Pharmacological eradication is usually advised. Eradication therapy comprises a 7-day course of a combination of two antibiotics and a proton pump inhibitor.

- Zollinger–Ellison syndrome, which is consequent of gastrin secretion from a pancreatic gastrinoma tumour, is a rare cause of peptic ulcer disease.

3. How does peptic ulcer disease present?

Patients may present electively at outpatient clinic with insidious symptoms in non-perforated disease or as an emergency surgical admission with bleeding or perforation.

Patients usually present with a history of ongoing epigastric pain, often a deep gnawing pain that occurs within a few hours after eating. Duodenal ulcers can commonly cause patients to wake in the night with pain. Antacids or eating may relieve the pain in duodenal ulcers but not in gastric ulcers. There may be a history of dyspepsia, heartburn, excessive belching, and bloating.

Bleeding can occur. It may be insidious and present with iron deficiency only, or it can be sudden and profuse with haematemesis or malaena. NSAID-induced gastritis progressing to UGI bleeding may be asymptomatic prior to presentation.

Patients may present with complications of ulceration, namely perforation or obstruction. Longstanding untreated duodenal ulceration becomes swollen and inflamed over time, which can result in duodenal obstruction and gastric outlet obstruction. NSAID-induced gastritis and bleeding is common, but the incidence of NSAID-induced perforated ulceration is low, reported below 1%.

Perforation presents with a sudden onset of acute abdominal pain, worse on moving or coughing, causing the patient to be very still. The patient may be vomiting. The young may not appear systemically unwell as they can physiologically compensate better. On

examination the abdomen is peritonitic, either generalized or localized to the upper abdomen, depending on the extent of spread of
peritoneal inflammation from the released gut contents.

4. How do you classify peptic ulcers?

Peptic ulcers can be classified by region (i.e. oesophageal, stomach,
or duodenal, or within a Meckel's diverticulum) or, more commonly,
using the modified Johnson classification:[*]

- Type I: ulcer along the body of the stomach, most often along the
  lesser curve.
- Type II: ulcer in the body of the stomach alongside an ulcer in the
  duodenum.
- Type III: ulcer in the pyloric channel within 3 cm of the pylorus.
- Type IV: ulcer in close proximity to the GOJ.
- Type V: ulcer anywhere in the stomach associated with chronic
  use of NSAIDS.

Type II and III ulcers are commonly associated with acid hypersecretion, whereas type I is not.

Figure 1.5.1 shows a Type III peptic ulcer.

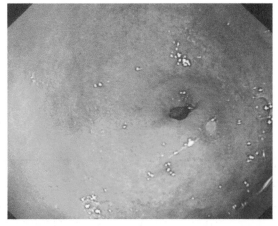

Figure 1.5.1 Photograph of a Type III peptic ulcer at the pylorus taken at OGD.
Reproduced courtesy of Corinne Owers.

5. What is the appropriate management of a patient with suspected perforated duodenal ulcer?

Initial management of patients presenting like the lady in this case scenario involves resuscitation. IV access should be obtained and IV crystalloid given. All patients should receive adequate analgesia whilst investigations are being performed and monitored for any signs of haemodynamic compromise. Anti-emetics may also help to keep the patient comfortable.

An erect chest X-ray may reveal pneumoperitoneum. However, this is not definitively diagnostic, particularly in localized perforations, so the most appropriate investigation in this case would be a CT scan, which can help to visualize free air and also localize the site of the perforation. If there is no suspicion of perforation or alternative pathology on CT, then endoscopy can be considered to rule out non-perforated peptic ulcer disease.

Once the diagnosis of perforated peptic ulcer is suspected, administration of IV proton pump inhibitor and antibiotics should be started. A nasogastric tube is placed to decompress the stomach. The patient will require immediate operative intervention, so pre-operative investigations, such as bloods and ECG, should be performed. If unwell, an arterial blood gas is advisable, alongside urinary catheterization.

6. What are the surgical options for treatment in this patient?

Surgery is indicated in peptic ulcer disease for perforation and obstruction, as well as bleeding that cannot be controlled endoscopically. This lady underwent laparotomy with under-sewing of the ulcer, followed by suture placement of a patch of omentum over the site of the perforation, which is the approach used in the majority of cases. This is usually sufficient to seal the perforation to aid healing, although in cases where the operation has been delayed, either due to late presentation or theatre issues, the tissues can become friable and more difficult to suture. Closure of the ulcer is followed by washout of the peritoneal cavity. This surgery may be performed as an open or laparoscopic procedure.

Although in the past, partial gastrectomy for definitive management of peptic ulcer disease was common, the judicious use of proton pump inhibitors and H2 antagonists have almost rendered this treatment redundant. Surgical treatment is now reserved primarily for non-healing ulcers or if endoscopic treatment of a bleeding ulcer has failed. Surgical options include:

- Vagotomy, with or without pyloroplasty.
- Antrectomy, which requires reconstruction with a gastroduodenal anastomosis (Bilroth 1).
- Gastrojejunostomy (Polya or Bilroth II).
- Roux-en-Y gastrojejunostomy.
- Subtotal gastrectomy.
- Pylorus-sparing gastrectomy.

These operations are, however, very uncommon nowadays with the successful outcomes of proton pump inhibitor therapy.

7. How should this patient be managed post-operatively?

Ward-based care is appropriate for uncomplicated cases. The NG tube is often left *in situ* overnight. IV proton pump inhibitors will continue for the next 72 hours. Enteral nutrition is started within 24–48 hours. Many advocate empirical *H. pylori* eradication therapy following a perforated peptic ulcer. This patient had an omental patch repair and received PPI therapy post-operatively. Patients who had previously been taking NSAIDs should be counselled to avoid them for life.

Further reading

Soreide K, Thorsen K, Soreide JA (2014) Strategies to improve the outcome of emergency surgery for perforated peptic ulcer. *British Journal of Surgery* **101** (1): e51–e64.

Tomtitchong P, Siribumrungwong B, Vilaichone R-K, Kasetsuwan P, Matsukura N, Chaiyakunapruk N (2012) Systematic review and meta-analysis: *Helicobacter pylori* eradication therapy after simple closure of perforated duodenal ulcer. *Helicobacter* **17** (2): 148–52.

Case history 1.6: Emergency: complications of UGI resectional surgery

A 62-year-old gentleman undergoes an Ivor–Lewis oesophagogas-trectomy for oesophageal cancer. He is otherwise fit and well with no other comorbidities, is a non-smoker, and lives at home with his wife. The operation is straightforward and he is admitted to the HDU for 2 days before returning to the ward. He develops a lower respiratory tract infection (LRTI), which is managed with antibiotics but other-wise progresses well. However, on day 6 post-operatively, he develops a tachycardia and pain in the upper abdomen, along with a pyrexia of 38.7°C. Investigation with a CT scan of his chest and abdomen dem-onstrates a leak at the anastomosis (Figure 1.6.1). This anastomotic leak is more clearly delineated on subsequent water-soluble contrast swallow (Figure 1.6.2).

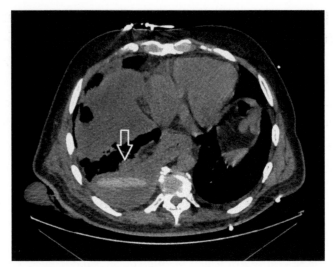

Figure 1.6.1 A CT image demonstrating accumulation of the water soluble contrast within the right pleural space (see arrow) secondary to anastomotic leak.

Reproduced courtesy of Corinne Owers.

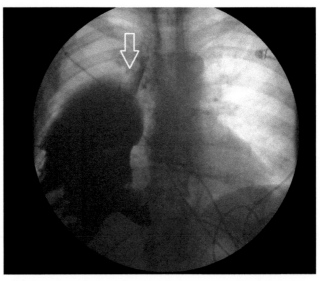

Figure 1.6.2 Image from the patient's water-soluble contrast swallow clearly shows the level of the anastomotic leak (see arrow) with contrast accumulating in the right pleural space (black).

Reproduced courtesy of Corinne Owers.

Questions

1. What are the potential complications following oesophagogastric resectional surgery?

2. How does anastomotic leak present and what are the appropriate initial investigations?

3. What ongoing management will be required in this case?

4. What are the ongoing considerations when managing complications following oesophagogastric resectional surgery?

Answers

1. What are the potential complications following oesophagogastric resectional surgery?

Oesophagogastric resections are major surgical procedures and as such have a relatively high morbidity and mortality when compared to other types of resectional surgery. Complications can be *general* or *operation-specific*, but incidence can be reduced by improved pre-operative preparation, including nutrition, good surgical technique, appropriate post-operative care, and by adopting prophylactic measures to reduce common risk factors.

General

- *Thromboembolic disease.* This is common following any type of cancer resection and also in the older population. It is, therefore, important to ensure that patients receive adequate thromboprophylaxis, both in the hospital and following discharge. Most centres prescribe 4 weeks of subcutaneous low molecular weight heparin thromboprophylaxis post-operatively for this reason.

- *Respiratory disease.* The largest number of complications following this type of surgery constitute respiratory issues. The Ivor–Lewis oesophagogastrectomy involves two painful incisions, abdominal (upper midline) and thoracic, both of which contribute to decreased ventilation and atelectasis, which can lead to lower respiratory tract infection or even respiratory failure, and mucous plugs can cause lobar collapse.

- General surgical intervention itself poses risks. These include bleeding, infection (wound, urine, intra-abdominal collection), and cardiovascular risk, including MI and stroke. The risk of mortality from cancer surgery has decreased over the years, which may be attributable to factors such as advancements in surgical technique, supra-specialization of cancer resections to high-volume centres and peri-operative patient optimization, and risk is around 2–3%. It is important to counsel patients about these risks pre-operatively and record them in the consent process.

Specific

* *Bleeding.* This is rare and when it does occur tends to present early following the operation. In most cases, this is usually from the staple/suture line, although it may be from a bleeding vessel in the area of dissection. The patient usually needs to return to theatre to treat these definitively. Bleeds arising from inside the lumen often present with haematemesis or malaena and they may be possible to manage endoscopically, although this may increase the chances of anastomotic disruption. Bleeding within the chest may result in haemothorax, which can further exacerbate respiratory complications.

* *Anastomotic leaks.* Following oesophagogastric resectional surgery, these can be catastrophic and, therefore, ensuring the principals of a good anastomosis are followed can help minimize this risk. Surgical factors that reduce the risk of anastomotic leak include:
  * Tension-free surgical repair.
  * Adequate blood supply.
  * Good surgical technique.
  * Healthy tissue.
  * Optimal nutritional status.

If any of the above factors are not optimized or present, leaks may result. Early anastomotic leaks (within 2–3 days of surgery) are generally a result of surgical failure. Those presenting later (usually around 5–10 days post-operatively) are more often the result of inadequate blood supply or tension on the anastomosis. The blood supply may be affected following a cardiovascular event following surgery, therefore optimizing cardiovascular status peri-operatively is imperative. Necrosis of the gastric conduit is a rare but major complication, the result of which can lead to significant morbidity and mortality. In this event, a further major operation is required to resect the necrotic tissue, which may necessitate the creation of an oesophagojejunal anastomosis or oesophagostomy.

- *Chylothorax.* This can result from damage to the thoracic duct during mobilization of oesophageal cancers, especially where these are advanced. This usually presents in the first week following surgery once the patient has recommenced oral feeding, particularly with fatty products. A noticeable increase in volume from the chest drain will be seen, resulting in malnutrition and immunocompromise. Surgical re-exploration is mandatory, as the thoracic duct can usually be easily identified especially if enteral fat is administered pre-operatively.

- *Recurrent laryngeal nerve palsy.* This is decreasing in incidence, and is rare where a thoracotomy is used. It may be unilateral, in which case the contralateral vocal cord may be able to compensate, and it may be transient. A tracheostomy may be required temporarily for airway protection; injection of Teflon into the cord or thyroplasty may be the required treatments.

Although the short-term complications are often more serious, long-term complications may affect quality of life and they can occasionally be difficult to manage. The main long-term issue is that of anastomotic strictures, which can occur after both stapled and hand-sewn anastomoses. In the majority of cases they can be dilated endoscopically, although this may take multiple attempts.

Severe GORD can cause significant distress to patients, particularly following Ivor–Lewis, although treatment options are limited to medical and lifestyle interventions.

2. How does anastomotic leak present and what are the appropriate initial investigations?

For any patient presenting with tachycardia, pain, and pyrexia following an anastomosis, an anastomotic leak should be high on the list of differentials.

Erect chest X-ray may serve to rule out pneumothorax and assess lung fields for signs of consolidation or lobar collapse, in cases where immediate CT scan cannot be obtained. However, the definitive investigation should be either a water-soluble contrast swallow or a CT scan of the chest and abdomen with water-soluble oral contrast.

On these investigations, contrast will be seen to extravasate from an anastomotic leak. CT will also visualize the lung parenchyma and respiratory infection. Arterial blood gas should be taken along with a full set of blood investigations and blood cultures. Both the surgical team and the critical care department should be notified of confirmed anastomotic leaks immediately and the patient worked up for theatre.

Initial management is resuscitative and requires immediate treatment of the sepsis. All patients should be given IV fluids, have a catheter inserted in order to accurately monitor fluid balance, and administered broad-spectrum antibiotics. Oxygen via mask or nasal cannulae is advisable.

It is important to communicate effectively with both the patient and their family, as the diagnosis of an anastomotic leak will mean a longer stay in the hospital with the potential for further complications.

3. What ongoing management will be required in this case?

The first principal should be control of the sepsis. Where possible this will usually necessitate a return to theatre for laparotomy +/– thoracotomy and washout. Primary repair is often not possible as the tissues will be friable and contamination can be significant. Closure of a small defect over a T-tube, creating a controlled fistula, can effectively manage a small anastomotic leak and may be the preferred option. This should be combined with feeding jejunostomy or parenteral feeding in order to optimize nutritional status and aid healing. Serial contrast swallows can demonstrate healing of the defect and guide appropriate removal of the tube.

Occasionally, the insertion of a covered stent into the lumen of the oesophagus can help to control leaks, by providing cover of the hole internally in the oesophagus and allowing the patient to take some enteral nutrition. This can help to control the fistula, but is only suitable in certain situations. Often management is predicated on both surgical and patient choice, as well as in best interests.

In cases where management with a T-tube or covered stent is not possible or in the best interests of the patient, oesophagostomy may be the best option for survival. The proximal end of the oesophagus is brought out as a stoma, with the aim of reversal once conditions are optimized. Feeding via percutaneous gastrotomy (PEG) or jejunostomy (PEJ) is mandatory.

4. What are the ongoing considerations when managing complications following oesophagogastric resectional surgery?

Optimizing nutritional status is paramount, and is often the most important aspect of ongoing management of leaks following oesophagogastric resection. Without adequate nutrition, tissue healing will be poor and definitive management in the form of further surgery will be inadvisable or impossible. Feeding is preferable enterally, which may require the use of an NJ tube, PEG, or PEJ. This is more physiological than parenteral feeding, although in situations where this is not possible or absorption of feed is limited in sick patients, total parenteral nutrition may be the only viable choice.

One of the most pertinent issues in complex cases with prolonged hospital stay is the psychological status of the patient. Thorough communication is imperative, as the patient will often want to be involved in the decisions about their management. Depression is common, and the patient may develop significant psychological needs. These can be assessed formally with the help of a psychologist, or managed by the team, depending on the severity and the needs of the patient. Quality of life in patients who remain in the hospital for long periods of time may be poor, and it is important to optimize this wherever possible.

Ensuring that continued thromboprophylaxis is provided can prevent further deterioration from thromboembolic events, which are common in these patients.

Further reading

CE Reed (2009) Technique of open ivor lewis esophagectomy. *Operative Techniques in Thoracic and Cardiovascular Surgery* 14 (3): 160–75.

Case history 1.7: Emergency: complications of metabolic surgery

A 35-year-old Caucasian lady with a BMI of 38.5 kg/m² presents to the bariatric clinic with a 3-week history of vomiting and dysphagia to solids, with significant dyspeptic symptoms. She underwent laparoscopic adjustable gastric banding 3 years previously and had lost approximately 10 kg in weight since then. She has a history of type 2 diabetes and depression, for which she is taking metformin and an anti-depressant. A barium swallow confirms the presence of a slipped gastric band, and she undergoes emergency deflation. Six weeks later a further barium swallow demonstrates that the band is still slipped, so she undergoes attempted repositioning. Unfortunately, the surgeon is unable to reposition the band and it is removed. Funding is obtained for conversion to a gastric bypass and the patient is discharged with no further problems. She represents just before her 6-month appointment complaining of further dyspeptic symptoms with an inability to eat solid foods.

Questions

1. What are the differential diagnoses for this patient?

2. What are the other complications associated with gastric banding surgery?

3. What are the appropriate initial investigations and management of this patient?

4. What are the post-operative complications associated with bariatric operations involving an anastomosis/staple line?

Answers

1. What are the differential diagnoses for this patient?

The initial presentation of dyspeptic symptoms, vomiting, dysphagia, or abdominal pain in a patient with a laparoscopic adjustable gastric band *in situ* should raise the suspicion of a slippage. The stomach herniates up through the gastric band, creating a large pouch with a small stomal opening. Non-bariatric differentials should include peptic ulcer disease, severe GORD, pancreatitis, and gastroenteritis, especially in acute presentations.

2. What are the other complications associated with gastric banding surgery?

Laparoscopic adjustable gastric banding (LAGB) surgery is associated with few short-term complications, but long-term complications can be seen in as many as 30% of LAGB patients. Apart from gastric band slippage, the gastric band can erode into the stomach. This usually presents with an increase in weight due to a lack of restriction, but may also present with dyspepsia, abdominal pain, or haematemesis.

The gastric band port and tubing can also be associated with problems. Infection of the port is troublesome and usually requires removal with replacement at a later date. Spontaneous infection of the port is often due to gastric band erosion, particularly if there has been no recent band adjustment. The port can flip, meaning that the semi-permeable membrane lies next to the abdominal wall, preventing access for band adjustments. Where access becomes impossible, the port may need to be repositioned under local anaesthetic. The tubing that connects the band and the port may either become detached or fracture; this will lead to leakage of the fluid from the band, a lack of restriction, and an inability to adjust it to optimum tightness. This will usually require further surgery once a leak is identified.

3. What are the appropriate initial investigations and management of this patient?

Initial investigations should exclude other pathology, including erect chest X-ray, blood tests, including amylase, liver function tests, and inflammatory markers. Any patient with a gastric band *in situ* presenting with these symptoms warrants urgent barium swallow to assess for signs of slippage. In the event that this cannot be done immediately, an appropriately trained professional should deflate the band. This can be done on the ward using a non-coring needle (called a Huber needle) into the subcutaneously placed port, although a standard needle can be used if necessary. In many centres, the band can be deflated at the same time as the barium swallow.

If the patient has been unable to tolerate oral fluids, IV fluid infusion should be commenced, along with analgesia. Once the band has been deflated they should be commenced on oral fluids and build up to normal diet as tolerated.

4. What are the post-operative complications associated with bariatric operations involving an anastomosis/staple line?

The gastric bypass (RYGB), sleeve gastrectomy (SG), and biliopancreatic diversion (BPD) are associated with a number of short-term and long-term complications.

Short-term

The main risks are general, such as:

- Cardiovascular or cerebrovascular events (MI, CVA).
- Thromboembolism.
- Infection.

Bariatric patients are at a high risk from these general complications. Specific risks include:

- Anastomotic bleeds and leaks. With each of these operations, anastomoses are created that can be either stapled or hand-sewn. There is, therefore, a chance of bleeding, which can be significant enough to warrant a return to theatre. Anastomoses can leak in the same way as following any type of bowel surgery, which usually presents around day 5–10 post-operatively.

Long-term

Long-term complications following these operations are rarer than those following LAGB surgery.

- Strictures at the anastomotic line can develop. As in the above case, strictures usually present with dysphagia, vomiting, or an inability to eat properly. Depending on the severity of the stricture, these are usually amenable to endoscopic or radiological dilatation. A barium swallow should be performed as a first-line investigation for patients with dysphagia, which will demonstrate any narrowing of the lumen of the bowel. These can usually be managed endoscopically, although if this fails to relieve this the patient may require dilation under radiological guidance. Advising patients to return to a sloppy diet, at least whilst waiting for dilatation, is advisable, as this means they can at least continue with oral nutrition.

- With the RYGB and BDP, the alteration in the anatomy means that a defect in the mesentery is created. Although most surgeons close these defects, occasionally an internal hernia can result as the mobile small bowel herniates through the defect. This leads to intermittent abdominal pain and may be visualized on a CT but usually requires a diagnostic laparoscopy.

- Dumping syndrome may occur after bariatric surgery, which is a condition brought about by the rapid emptying of foodstuffs into the duodenum or small bowel, where the alteration in anatomy bypasses the pylorus. Although this is more of a surgical consequence rather than a true complication, dumping syndrome can be distressing, leading to symptoms of hypotension, gastric disturbance, and hypoglycaemia. Treatment is simply by avoiding the foodstuffs that illicit dumping syndrome, usually sugars and/or carbohydrates.

- Other consequences are related to malnutrition, and include hair loss, skin, teeth and nail changes, halitosis, and lethargy.

+ Psychological issues include a change to body image, often as a result of loose skin following the weight loss, depression, or a significant change in lifestyle as a result of their changing relationship with food. Patients should be actively encouraged to seek psychological support from their GP or bariatric team.

+ Finally, following the bypass and BPD, patients may lose an excessive amount of weight, which is sometimes unexplainable. Occasionally this may necessitate feeding via TPN or even reversal of the bypasses portion of bowel.

+ Surgery can result in the development of incisional hernia, either at site of open incision or at the port site in laparoscopic surgery.

The main long-term complications following these operations involve either anastomotic or staple line strictures, malnutrition or psychological issues.

Further reading

Griffith PS, Birch DW, Sharma AM, Karmali S (2012) Managing complications associated with laparoscopic Roux-en-Y gastric bypass for morbid obesity. *Canadian Journal of Surgery* 55 (5): 329–36.

Koch TR, Finelli FC (2010) Post-operative metabolic and nutritional complications of bariatric surgery. *Gastroenterology Clinics of North America* 39 (1): 109–24.

Chapter 2

Hepatobiliary surgery

K. Raj Prasad and Imeshi Wijetunga

Case history 2.1: Elective: colorectal liver metastasis

A 55-year-old gentleman was referred to the hepatobiliary unit by the colorectal MDT. He had undergone an emergency extended right hemi-colectomy for T4 N1 M0 obstructing adenocarcinoma of the transverse colon with primary anastomosis. He had made a full recovery and had been discharged on day 5, and was treated with adjuvant chemotherapy.

On his surveillance CT 2 years following his surgery, he was found to have two lesions in segment 6/7 and one lesion in segment 4 of his liver, as well as a peritoneal deposit close to his colonic anastamosis, all suggestive of metastases on MRI and PET-CT imaging (Figure 2.1.1). He was then treated with second-line chemotherapy followed by liver resection and resection of the peritoneal deposit.

Surveillance CT imaging 1 year post-operative showed no evidence of recurrent or residual disease.

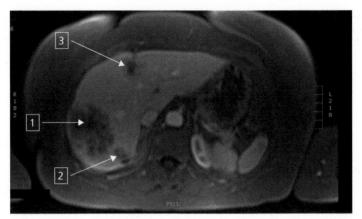

Figure 2.1.1 This MR image shows multiple liver metastases. This patient had a large segment 6/7 metastasis measuring 7cm (1) with a satellite metastasis in segment 6/7 (2). A 2-cm segment 4 metastasis (3) is also seen on this image.

Reproduced Courtesy of Imeshi Wijetunga.

Questions

1. How common are colorectal liver metastases (CRLM) and how do they develop?

2. What imaging modalities are required in the surgical workup of a patient with CRLM?

3. What factors are taken into consideration when assessing a patient for liver resection?

4. What management options are available to patients with CRLM?

5. What are the common types of liver resection?

6. Describe the risks and benefits of surgical resection that should be discussed with the patient for the purpose of obtaining informed consent?

7. How would you manage this patient following his liver resection?

8. How would you follow up patients following liver resection for CRLM?

Answers

1. How common are colorectal liver metastases (CRLM) and how do they develop?

Liver metastases from colorectal cancer occur in up to 50% of patients with colorectal cancer. Of these, approximately 25% have synchronous disease (i.e. liver metastases diagnosed simultaneously with primary colorectal malignancy) and 25% have metachronous disease (i.e. liver metastases that were not present on diagnosis of the primary disease but develop after it has been treated). Secondary deposits in the liver are most frequently caused by colorectal malignancies but other cancers, such as pancreatic, lung, neuroendocrine, and breast tumours, can lead to liver metastases, requiring thorough clinical assessment, appropriate imaging and diagnostic tests.

The spread of colorectal cancer to the liver is haematogenous via the portal circulation and is often the first site of metastatic spread. Lesions could be solitary or multiple and CRLM can also develop many years following apparent curative resection of the primary colorectal tumour as evidenced in this case.

2. What imaging modalities are required in the surgical workup of a patient with CRLM?

Mandatory imaging includes:

* Staging contrast-enhanced CT of the thorax, abdomen, and pelvis.

  This is to assess extent of disease in the liver and its relationship to major vasculature (hepatic artery, hepatic vein, portal vein, and inferior vena cava) and the biliary tract. In addition, CT would also identify other distant sites of metastatic disease that may preclude curative resection.

* MRI of the liver with liver-specific contrast.

  MRI is a more sensitive imaging modality for tumours <1 cm in diameter in the liver. MRI also helps in planning liver resection.

Optional imaging includes:

◆ PET-CT (in selected cases).

PET-CT can be a useful tool in assessment of indeterminate nodules found on other imaging and in patients at high risk of extrahepatic disease. PET-CT relies on functionalized molecules, the most commonly used one being ^{18}flurodeoxyglucose (^{18}F-FDG), which are taken up by all cells but at different rates with highly metabolically active tissues like cancerous cells showing higher intra-cellular accumulation of ^{18}F-FDG. Although PET-CT is more sensitive compared to CT and MRI, its routine use in all patients is not recommended due to limited evidence.

◆ Intra-operative ultrasound (with/without contrast).

This allows for intra-operative assessment of resectability with further assessment of metastases in relation to vasculature.

3. **What factors are taken into consideration when assessing a patient for liver resection?**

Patient factors:

◆ Suitability to undergo major surgery.

◆ Performance status.

◆ Comorbidities.

This can be determined by clinical assessment. Where there is doubt more definitive assessment can be achieved by objective tests such as cardiopulmonary exercise (CPEX) testing.

Liver-related factors:

◆ *Distribution of metastatic disease in the liver.* Widespread disease within the liver involving all segments will preclude curative resection

◆ *Relationship to major vasculature.* Involvement of major vessels that are not amenable to resection and reconstruction are contraindications to liver resection.

◆ *Quality of background liver.* Although removal of 75–80% of liver parenchyma can be achieved with low morbidity and mortality in selected cases, the presence of background liver disease reduces the functional reserve of the future liver remnant, which will preclude extensive liver resection as there is a higher likelihood of post-operative liver failure.

Contraindications to liver resection surgery:

- Poor performance status.
- Inadequate liver reserve.
- Inability to achieve margin-negative resection.
- Presence of extra-hepatic disease (except with isolated pulmonary or nodal metastases that are amenable to complete resection).

Patients with technically unresectable disease can be offered systemic chemotherapy, which may downsize the disease burden and subsequently deem them resectable. In addition, patients who would be left with a small remnant liver volume after resection may be offered portal vein embolization, occluding the portal supply to the diseased lobe to redirect blood flow and generate hypertrophy of the remnant tissue. This is performed through percutaneous access by interventional radiologists and can reduce the risk of post-operative liver failure.

4. What management options are available to patients with CRLM?

All patients with CRLM are discussed in colorectal MDTs prior to planning treatment. As surgery is the gold standard of treatment for CRLM, offering a chance for longer disease-free and overall survival, as well as definitive cure in a subset of patients, all patients who are potential surgical candidates are discussed in specialist liver MDTs. The flowchart in Figure 2.1.2 summarizes potential management strategies for patients following referral to specialist centres.

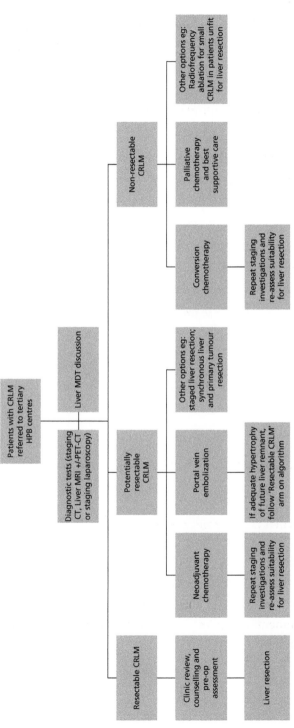

Figure 2.1.2 Management algorithm for patients referred to a hepatobiliary tertiary centre.

Reproduced Courtesy of Imeshi Wijetunga.

5. What are the common types of liver resection?

Resections have traditionally been carried out following the ana-tomical liver segmental borders (Figure 2.1.3). However, modern-day surgical treatment also incorporates non-anatomical resections or a combination of the two approaches to remove disease.

Major liver resection (four or more liver segments)

- Right hemi-hepatectomy: segments 5, 6, 7, and 8.
- Extended right hemi-hepatectomy (or right tri-sectionectomy): as above plus segment 4.
- Left hemi-hepatectomy: segments 1, 2, 3, and 4.
- Extended left hemi-hepatectomy (or left tri-sectionectomy): as above and segments 5 and 8.

Minor liver resection (less than four liver segments)

- Left lateral sectionectomy: segments 2 and 3.
- Right posterior sectionectomy: segments 6 and 7.
- Segmental liver resection: resection of any individual segment.
- Non-anatomical liver resections, e.g. metastatectomy, wedge resection.

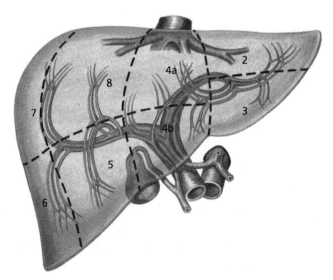

Figure 2.1.3 Pictorial representation of the Couinaud liver segment anatomy. Caudate lobe (segment 1) is not shown in the figure. Couinaud classification describes the eight independent functional liver segments, each with a branch of the portal vein, hepatic artery and bile duct as well as hepatic veins.

Reproduced Courtesy of Niaz Ahmad and Paul Brown.

6. **Describe the risks and benefits of surgical resection that should be discussed with the patient for the purpose of obtaining informed consent?**

The main benefit of surgical resection is prolonged survival and offers the only chance of cure. However, major liver resection carries risks of peri-operative mortality and morbidity, as well as the risk of disease recurrence following surgery. Surgical morbidity can be classified as early, intermediate, and late complications.

Early:

♦ Bleeding.

♦ Liver failure.

♦ Bile leak/intra-abdominal collection.

Intermediate:

♦ Infection: pneumonia, wound, intra-abdominal collection.

♦ Deep vein thrombosis/pulmonary embolus.

Late:

♦ Incisional hernia.

♦ Disease recurrence.

7. **How would you manage this patient following his liver resection?**

Post-operative management of patients following major liver resection remains variable within hepatobiliary centres. The authors adopt a routine policy of Level 2 care (high-dependency unit) following liver resection. Some centres also incorporate an enhanced recovery pathway.

Systematic assessment of the patient in the following key areas would help the junior surgeon in their approach to assessing such patients post-operatively. However, this list is not exhaustive and it is expected that any critically ill surgical patient is managed according to the Care of the Critically Ill Patient (CCrISP) guidelines.

1. Clinical assessment.

    a. Wound site, drains.

This may alert the clinician to excessive bleeding, although occult bleeding may still occur despite empty drains and dry dressings.

b. Fluid balance.

Fluid therapy should be goal-directed, guided by central venous pressure (CVP) and mean arterial pressure (MAP). It is not uncommon for patients to require more fluids post-operatively due to being maintained at low CVP intra-operatively to minimize blood loss. Human albumin solution remains a commonly used colloid following major liver resection.

2. Blood results.

a. Coagulopathy.

Deranged clotting can be a sign of liver impairment and may require correction with vitamin K or fresh-frozen plasma.

b. Liver function tests and CRP.

Alanine aminotransferase (ALT) and bilirubin tend to rise immediately post-resection and settle over time. It is not uncommon for alkaline phosphatase (ALP) to rise slowly. CRP is an acute phase protein produced by the liver and this usually rises in the presence of a functioning liver remnant. A low CRP would alert the clinical team to monitor for post-operative liver failure.

c. Haemoglobin.

It is not uncommon for patients to require transfusion post-surgery. Due to advancements in surgical (Pringle manoeuvre or portal vein clamping intra-operatively) and anaesthetic techniques (such as maintaining a low CVP intra-operatively), blood loss and requirement for transfusion in the peri-operative period have reduced in recent times.

3. Thromboprophylaxis.

Venous thromboembolism remains a major preventable cause of morbidity and mortality following major surgery. Intra-operative use of intermittent pneumatic compression, post-operative use of graduated compression stockings, subcutaneous low molecular weight heparins, and early mobilization are all helpful in reducing patients' risk.

4. Analgesia.

Most centres use epidural anaesthesia or continuous infiltration of local anaesthetic coupled with patient-controlled opiate analgesia for the first post-operative 24–72 hours, then stepping down to oral analgesia as per the WHO analgesic ladder.

5. Glycaemic control.

Intravenous insulin is usually required by diabetics, even those normally managed with oral hypoglycaemic agents.

6. Nutrition.

Oral diet and fluids are normally introduced within 24 hours but oral supplements are commonly utilized early. Nasogastric feeding or parenteral nutrition can be considered for those with inadequate oral intake under dietetic advice.

8. How would you follow up patients following liver resection for CRLM?

Follow-up protocols are variable within centres but, in general, follow-up in the first 2 years after resection is intensive, involving 3–6-monthly review of patients with surveillance imaging. Thereafter, most centres review patients annually for 5–10 years. Plasma carcinoembryonic antigen (CEA) is a glycoprotein expressed by normal mucosal cells that is overexpressed in adenocarcinoma, particularly advanced colon cancer. However, it can also be raised in other adenocarcinomas, including gastric and pancreatic adenocarcinomas, as well as non-neoplastic conditions such as inflammatory bowel disease and cigarette smoking. However, it proves useful in an established diagnosis of colorectal cancer for monitoring response to therapy and disease recurrence.

Liver recurrence is not infrequent and most patients are considered for re-resection, which increases overall survival compared to palliative therapy. Lung is the second most common site of metastatic disease. Pulmonary recurrence should be assessed in thoracic surgery MDT and considered for pulmonary resection. Patients may present with synchronous liver and pulmonary metastases. If both sites are deemed technically resectable then the patient can be offered both lung and liver resections.

Further reading

Adam R, De Gramont A, Figueras J, Guthrie A, Kokudo N, Kunstlinger F, *et al.* (2012) The oncosurgery approach to managing liver metastases from colorectal cancer: a multidisciplinary international consensus. *The Oncologist* 17 (10): 1225–39.

Case history 2.2: Elective: hepatocellular carcinoma

A 48-year-old gentleman was referred to the hepatobiliary MDT by gastroenterologists with a history of upper abdominal pain and 4-stone (25.5 kg) weight loss over 2–3 months, and a CT finding of a 20-cm lesion in the left lobe of his liver. He has no other symptoms on systemic inquiry. His past history includes hypertension. His regular medications include bisoprolol, amlodipine, and ramipril. He is a smoker of 20 cigarettes per day and drinks alcohol socially.

On examination, he is obese. There are no surgical scars. He has visible tattoos but is not icteric. His abdomen is soft but tender in the epigastrium and right-upper quadrant with a palpable firm, irregular mass. His blood results are shown in Table 2.2.1.

Table 2.2.1 Blood results

Blood results	
Hb	110
WCC	8.0
Platelets	150
Renal function	Normal
Bilirubin	22
ALT	45
ALP	320
Alb	38
PT	13
Virology screen	Negative
AFP	1,600
CEA	Normal
CA 19.9	Normal

Questions

1. What are the key differential diagnoses?

2. What are the risk factors for developing hepatocellular carcinoma? What are the sequelae of cirrhosis?

3. What management options are available for HCC?

4. What criteria does this gentleman have to fulfil to be eligible for liver transplantation in the UK?

5. How are HCC patients with positive virology for hepatitis B, C, and HIV managed?

Answers

1. What are the key differential diagnoses?

The key questions that should be addressed are:

- Is this a benign or malignant lesion?
- If malignant, is it a primary or secondary liver lesion?
- If this is a secondary deposit, where is the primary?

A serum alpha fetoprotein (AFP) of 1,600 is highly suggestive of a primary HCC in this patient. Contrast-enhanced CT and MRI using arterial, portal-venous, and delayed phases help radiologists differentiate liver lesions (see Figure 2.2.1). Early arterial phase contrast enhancement and rapid washout in the portal-venous phase are typical of HCC.

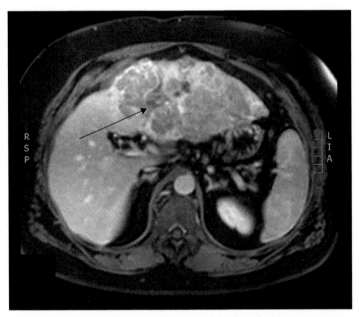

Figure 2.2.1 The contrast-enhanced MR image of the liver in this patient shows a large irregular mass occupying the entire left lobe of the liver (see arrow). There are no other intra-hepatic lesions.

Reproduced Courtesy of Imeshi Wijetunga.

2. What are the risk factors for developing hepatocellular carcinoma? What are the sequelae of cirrhosis?

The key risk factors for development of HCC are liver cirrhosis and viral hepatitis. This case highlights that HCCs can develop in non-cirrhotic livers, although this is less common. Most centres screen cirrhotic patients for HCCs routinely with ultrasound scanning (see EASL Criteria in the Further reading section for more information).

Cirrhosis is a diffuse process characterized by liver fibrosis resulting in conversion of normal liver architecture into structurally abnormal nodules and is usually an irreversible process that is the final common pathway of conditions leading to chronic liver damage.

Alcohol-related liver disease, viral hepatitis (hepatitis viruses B, C, D), non-alcoholic fatty liver disease (NAFLD), non-alcoholic steatohepatitis (NASH), or even rarer liver diseases such as haemochromatosis, autoimmune liver and biliary disease, Wilson's disease, Budd–Chiari syndrome and α-1 antri-trypsin deficiency can lead to liver cirrhosis (list not exhaustive). A large proportion of cases of cirrhosis are labelled as cryptogenic, but often this could be due to a missed diagnosis of NAFLD.

Cirrhosis leads to increased resistance to portal blood flow. This, combined with the increased blood flow in splanchnic vessels, raises the portal pressure and favours the formation of varices in the areas of porto-systemic shunting. Gastric variceal bleeding is a common complication of portal hypertension.

Ascites is another consequence of portal hypertension, which, along with other factors such as hypoalbuminaemia, vasodilatation leading to relative hypovolaemia, and activation of the renin–angiotensin–aldosterone pathway, result in Starling forces that favour the extravasation of fluid from plasma into the peritoneal cavity.

Classification of the severity of cirrhosis is important for prognostic and management purposes. The most widely used classification is the Child–Pugh classification (see Table 2.2.2). Classification into

Table 2.2.2 Child–Pugh classification of cirrhosis

Child–Pugh Score			
Score	1	2	3
Bilirubin (µmol/l)	<34	34–50	>50
Albumin (g/l)	>35	28–35	<28
Prothrombin time (seconds)	1–3	4–6	>6
Encephalopathy	None	Mild	Moderate–severe
Ascites	None	Mild	Severe (refractory to treatment)

Republished with permission of John Wiley and Sons Inc., from 'Transection of the oesophagus for bleeding oesophageal varices', Pugh, R. N. H., Murray-Lyon, I. M., Dawson, J. L., Pietroni, M. C. and Williams, R., *British Journal of Surgery*, Volume 60, pp. 646–9, Copyright © 1973, doi:10.1002/bjs.1800600817

Child–Pugh A, B, and C is based on a total score of <7, 7–9, and >9, respectively. Child–Pugh A patients have an estimated 1-year survival of 100% compared to less than 50% in Child–Pugh C.

Surgical trainees should be aware of two other severity scoring systems. First, the Modified End-stage Liver Disease or MELD scoring based on serum bilirubin, creatinine, and International Normalized Ratio (INR). Second, the UK model for End-stage Liver Disease or UKELD score, which, in addition to MELD factors, incorporates serum sodium level in the equation. UKELD is the scoring system used in the UK to aid the selection of patients for liver transplantation.

3. What management options are available for HCC?

The management options for HCC vary depending on several patient factors and features of the underlying disease, such as size, location of tumour, and quality of the background liver. The following is a summary of treatment options:

Liver resection This is the first-line treatment option for solitary lesions in patients with preserved liver function. In this patient, who has non-cirrhotic appearances of the future liver remnant (i.e. remaining liver following resection), the MDT decision was to perform a left hemi-hepatectomy.

For types of liver resections, please refer to Question 5 of Case 2.1 colorectal liver metastasis.

Liver transplantation If a cirrhotic patient with HCC is suitable for liver transplantation (see Milan criteria in Question 4), this would be the superior option, as this would treat the HCC as well as obviate the risk of disease recurrence that a cirrhotic liver would pose following other treatment modalities. In addition to the risks of major open abdominal surgery, liver transplant recipients are at risk of further complications, the main ones are summarized below:

- *Delayed graft function.* Most livers resume function immediately following transplant (i.e. primary function) with bile production observed on-table, but occasionally this can take several hours.

- *Primary non-function.* The transplanted liver never functions in the recipient. This is life-threatening and requires re-grafting as soon as possible.

- *Rejection.* Hyperacute rejection is very rare but acute cellular rejection is not uncommon. This is diagnosed on transplant liver biopsy and treated with increased immunosuppression. Chronic rejection, however, can be difficult to manage and may progress to liver failure requiring re-transplantation.

- *Biliary stenosis.* Patients usually have obstructive LFTs and dilated bile ducts on imaging. ERCP and stenting is usually the preferred option.

- *Hepatic artery thrombosis.* Can occur early in the days following transplantation and usually necessitates re-graft.

- *Hepatic artery stenosis.* Generally occurs later and is often amenable to endovascular intervention.

- *Portal vein thrombosis/stenosis.* The former requires anticoagulation and the latter is usually treated with endovascular stenting.

- *Long-term risks of immunosuppression.* Hypertension, hyperlipidaemia, diabetes (i.e. increased risk of metabolic syndrome), increased risks of lymphoma (or PTLD—post-transplant lymphoproliferative disorder) and skin cancers, drug toxicity, and renal impairment.

◆ *Disease recurrence.* Despite rigorous selection of appropriate HCC patients with information from various imaging modalities, patients are still at risk of disease recurrence. Sometimes the final histology of the explanted liver may reveal more advanced disease than predicted by pre-transplant imaging. If recurrence occurs, it usually progresses rapidly and is fatal in the immunosuppressed patient.

Trans-arterial chemoembolization (TACE) TACE involves instillation of chemotherapy-coated embolic particles directly into the hepatic artery via a transarterial catheter introduced through the femoral artery. The chemotherapeutic agents used for this purpose include doxorubicin and cisplatin, and are usually impregnated into drug-eluting beads to facilitate slow release whilst obstructing tumour blood flow. The procedure is performed by interventional radiologists under a general or local anaesthesia. The advantage of this procedure is two-fold: it allows selective disruption of arterial flow to the tumour, as well as delivering a high dose of chemotherapy directly to it, thus reducing systemic side-effects, which is often the dose-limiting factor in chemotherapy. The disadvantage, however, is that it is not a curative option. Some liver lesions can be kept under control with repeated TACE procedures. TACE can also be used as a bridging treatment for patients on the liver transplant waiting-list to keep the tumour within transplant criteria during the months on the waiting list.

Radiofrequency ablation (RFA) This is an option for selected small lesions (<3.5 cm) or inoperable tumours (such as those close to major vasculature that would preclude negative margins). The procedure is performed by interventional radiologists under a general or local anaesthesia. A needle is inserted into the tumour and then heated with a rapidly alternating current, which induces liquefactive necrosis of the surrounding cells. Like TACE, RFA can be used as an effective bridging therapy prior to liver transplantation. RFA can also be used in combination with surgery to treat multifocal disease.

Systemic therapies Sorafenib, an inhibitor of several tyrosine protein kinases, is the standard systemic therapy for unresectable HCC. Options for second-line chemotherapy are limited.

Best supportive care Patients not fit for any of the described treatment modalities should receive palliative support.

4. What criteria does this gentleman have to fulfil to be eligible for liver transplantation in the UK?

HCC is the only malignancy potentially curable by liver transplantation. However, for this to be an accepted treatment modality in the UK at present, the modified Milan criteria should be met. Any single lesion less than 5 cm or up to five lesions less than 3 cm each would be considered for liver transplantation. A lesion that is 5–7 cm may also qualify if it shows no significant progression for 6 months, during which other treatments could be administered. Extra-hepatic disease or macrovascular invasion are absolute contraindications to transplantation. In addition, the selected patients have to undergo the rigorous multidisciplinary liver transplant assessment process and be deemed fit for transplantation.

HCC patients are prioritized on the liver transplant waiting list and often receive an organ offer from a blood-group compatible donor before developing advanced chronic liver disease.

In the UK at present, only ABO-blood group compatible transplants are performed but there is emerging evidence that it is possible to pre-condition a recipient (with procedures such as plasmapheresis to deplete recipient's existing antibodies) to receive an ABO-incompatible liver transplant.

5. How are HCC patients with positive virology for hepatitis B, C, and HIV managed?

Hepatits B Antiviral treatments are an option for patients with chronic hepatitis B. Usage of hepatitis B immunoglobulin perioperatively is helpful, especially in liver transplantation for chronic hepatitis B, as it reduces reinfection rates.

Hepatits C Traditional treatment for hepatitis C involves combination therapy with interferon and ribavirin (anti-viral). Treatment course can be several months and with high rates of side-effects leading to poor compliance. Cure rates with this treatment regime can be less than 50% in hepatitis C virus Genotype 1 (one of six genotypes of the virus, each of which have several subtypes with differing virulence). New, emerging drugs, such as sofosbuvir/ledipasvir, have revolutionized treatment of hepatitis C, achieving cure rates up to 90%.

In transplant recipients, treatment is usually commenced before, and re-commenced following, transplantation. Successful eradication of the virus reduces risk of recurrent hepatitis C, which can affect the transplanted liver.

Human immunodeficiency virus (HIV) HIV is not a contraindication to resection or transplantation and patients can be managed with anti-retroviral therapy to achieve an undetectable viral load pre-transplant.

Further reading

EASL–EORTC Clinical practice guidelines: management of hepatocellular carcinoma (2012) *Journal of Hepatology* **56**: 908–43.

Case history 2.3: Elective: cholangiocarcinoma

A 71-year-old lady was referred by her GP on an urgent basis with a 4-week history of painless jaundice, pale stools, dark urine, and weight loss. Her past medical history included hypertension and arthritis. She was not known to have gallstones. Apart from antihypertensives, she was not on any other regular medications. She denied any tattoos, recent travel, or blood transfusions. She was a non-smoker who rarely consumed alcohol.

On examination, she was icteric and cachetic with visible skin excoriations. She was alert and orientated. There was no palpable Virchow's node. Her chest was clear to auscultation. Her abdomen was soft and non-tender with no palpable gallbladder or other masses. The remainder of the examination was within normal limits.

The results of her initial investigations are summarized in Table 2.3.1.

Table 2.3.1 Blood results

Hb	153
WCC	10.5
Platelets	212
Renal function	Normal
Bilirubin	252
ALT	95
ALP	368
Alb	35
PT	18
Virology screen	Negative

Questions

1. What are the key differential diagnoses?
2. What are the risk factors for developing cholangiocarcinoma?
3. What investigations are useful in planning liver resection for cholangiocarcinoma?
4. What is the benefit of pre-operative biliary drainage in patients with obstructive jaundice, what are the risks, and how can this be achieved?
5. What adjuvant therapies are recommended for cholangiocarcinoma patients undergoing resection?
6. Is liver transplantation an option for cure in cholangiocarcinoma?

Answers

1. What are the key differential diagnoses?

The distinction between benign and malignant disease is key to appropriate management. Benign biliary strictures and gallstones in the common bile duct (CBD) could present with similar symptoms. However, a malignancy arising from the biliary tree, ampulla, or pancreatic head is more likely, given this patient's history.

Biliary tract cancers are a group of malignancies arising from the biliary tree and are classified anatomically into:

- Intra-hepatic cholangiocarcinoma.
- Peri-hilar cholangiocarcinoma (Klatskin tumours).
- Distal-cholangiocarcinoma.
- Gallbladder carcinoma.

Gallbladder carcinoma represents the commonest biliary tract cancer, often diagnosed as an incidental finding following cholecystectomy for benign disease. Peri-hilar cholangiocarcinomas are those that occur at the confluence of the right and left hepatic ducts, by definition from the second-order bile ducts down to the origin of the cystic duct. This group represents up to 60% of cholangiocarcinomas undergoing surgical resection in the UK. Both peri-hilar cholangiocarcinoma and distal cholangiocarcinoma are variants of extra-hepatic cholangiocarcinoma.

2. What are the risk factors for developing cholangiocarcinoma?

Sporadic cases of cholangiocarcinoma are often idiopathic. The following list is a summary of known and potential risk factors in cholangiocarcioma:

- Biliary tract disorders such as:
  - Biliary tract anomalies, e.g. bile duct cysts.
  - Primary sclerosing cholangitis.
  - Hepatolithiasis.
- Parasitic infestations, i.e. liver fluke.

- Toxins (e.g. thorotrast contrast agent, now no longer licenced for use).
- Other associations/potential risk factors include:
  - Inflammatory bowel disease.
  - Chronic viral hepatitis (hepatitis B and C) and cirrhosis.
  - Diabetes.
  - Obesity.
  - Alcohol excess.

3. What investigations are useful in planning liver resection for cholangiocarcinoma?

Liver resection for cholangiocarcinoma is only an option for approximately 20% of patients diagnosed with cholangiocarcinoma, as it tends to present at an advanced stage with metastatic disease, which precludes curative liver resection. Routine staging CT chest, abdomen, and pelvis should be undertaken prior to planning resection, as well as contrast-enhanced MRI. Involvement of regional lymph nodes is not a contraindication to major liver resection in peri-hilar cholangiocarcinoma, as the treatment involves regional lymphadenectomy but nodal involvement is a known poor prognostic indicator.

Most centres also advocate use of PET-CT to exclude nodal and extra-hepatic disease. PET-CT relies on the high uptake and metabolism of glucose in malignant cells compared to normal cells. Fluorine-18 labelled fluorodeoxyglucose (fluorine-18 FDG) is the most common radiopharmaceutical used for PET-CT imaging. The uptake of fluorine-18 FDG is usually reported as the maximum standardized uptake value (SUVmax); the higher the value, the more avid the tumour. Generally, intra-hepatic cholangiocarcinomas show higher avidity compared to extra-hepatic cholangiocarcinomas. If the primary tumour is not FDG-avid, PET-CT cannot reliably exclude nodal or metastatic disease. Representative images are presented from CT in Figure 2.3.1, MRI in Figure 2.3.2, and PET-CT in Figure 2.3.3.

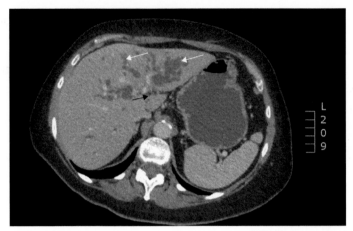

Figure 2.3.1 This contrast-enhanced CT image shows intra-hepatic ductal dilatation, mainly in the left-sided ducts (see white arrows) with a soft tissue lesion extending through the common bile duct into the cystic duct (see black arrow). No extra-hepatic disease was identified.

Reproduced Courtesy of Imeshi Wijetunga.

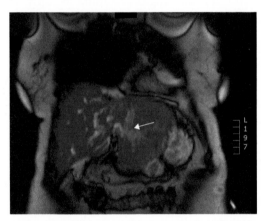

Figure 2.3.2 Coronal section MR image of the same patient showing prominent left-sided biliary duct dilatation (see white arrow) in an abnormal left lobe.

Reproduced Courtesy of Imeshi Wijetunga.

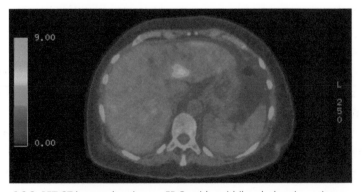

Figure 2.3.3 PET-CT image showing an FDG-avid peri-hilar cholangiocarcinoma. SUVmax 6.0.

Reproduced Courtesy of Imeshi Wijetunga.

Diagnostic laparoscopy is also an option if non-invasive imaging results are inconclusive, in order to reduce the rates of futile laparotomy.

4. What is the benefit of pre-operative biliary drainage in patients with obstructive jaundice, what are the risks, and how can this be achieved?

Long-standing biliary obstruction results in atrophy of the affected liver segments. Pre-operative biliary drainage relieves jaundice pre-operatively and is recommended to reduce the risk of post-operative liver failure following major liver resection in patients with bile duct obstruction.

Biliary drainage is ideally achieved via ERCP and stenting. This also gives the opportunity for cytology specimens to be obtained to confirm the diagnosis. ERCP can be technically challenging and percutaneous trans-hepatic cholangiogram (PTC) can be used as an alternative in patients with dilated bile ducts. Risks of biliary drainage include bleeding, cholangitis, pancreatitis, and blockage of stent. Cholangitis is rarely a presenting symptom of malignant biliary obstruction but is far more likely following biliary intervention due to iatrogenic introduction of intestinal flora into the relatively sterile biliary system.

In patients with inoperable disease, permanent metal stents can be placed as a palliative procedure, as these have a lower risk of blockage than plastic ones.

5. What adjuvant therapies are recommended for cholangiocarcinoma patients undergoing resection?

Unfortunately, there is limited Level 1 evidence for adjuvant therapies for cholangiocarcinoma. The BilCap trial, a UK multi-centre Phase III trial, is currently evaluating the efficacy of post-operative capecitabine therapy in patients who have undergone macroscopically complete resection of biliary tract cancer.

Due to their rarity, the anatomical variants of biliary tract cancer are often considered together in most clinical trials of adjuvant therapies. It is clear that biliary tract cancers represent a heterogenous group of malignancies and the benefit of adjuvant therapies need to be evaluated separately in order to identify subsets of patients who would most benefit from adjuvant treatments.

Currently, adjuvant therapy is highly recommended for patients who have had R1 resection (i.e. microscopic disease within 1 mm of a resection margin) or have positive lymph nodes. Chemotherapeutic regimens include platinum-based agents such as cisplatin coupled with gemcitabine. Currently, there are no recommended neo-adjuvant options for cholangiocarcinoma and hence only non-resectable disease is eligible for palliative chemotherapy and/or radiotherapy.

6. Is liver transplantation an option for cure in cholangiocarcinoma?

Liver transplantation is not currently a recommended treatment option for cholangiocarcinoma due to high rates of recurrence reported, which are likely precipitated by post-transplant immuno-suppression. However, in highly selected patients in specialized centres (e.g. Mayo Clinic) that utilize protocols that include neoadjuvant and adjuvant therapies, successful transplant outcomes have been reported.

The patient described in this case was deemed unfit for resection following PTC due to prolonged sepsis and poor nutrition. Unfortunately, repeat MRI imaging 6 weeks later revealed that there was disease progression involving the hepatic artery and portal vein, which was not amenable to curative surgical resection.

Further reading

Groot Koerkamp B, Fong Y (2014) Outcomes in biliary malignancy. *Journal of Surgical Oncology* 110: 585–91.

Tyson GL, El-Serag HB (2011) Risk factors for cholangiocarcinoma. *Hepatology* 54 (1): 173–84.

Case history 2.4: Emergency: symptomatic gallstones

A 42-year-old woman was admitted to hospital with an 8-hour history of right-upper quadrant and epigastric pain radiating through to the back, associated with nausea and three episodes of vomiting. She had suffered multiple episodes of similar pain in this region over the past 6 months, predominantly after meals and lasting for several hours. She had no other medical and surgical history. She does not take any regular prescription medication. She has had intentional weight loss of 3 stone (19 kg) over the last 12 months, giving her a BMI of 28 kg/m².

On examination she was alert but in pain despite 10 mg of IV morphine. Her pulse rate was 100 beats per minute, blood pressure was 135/80, respiratory rate 18 breaths per minute, and her temperature was 37.8°C. There was no clinical evidence of jaundice or chronic liver disease. She was tender in the right-upper quadrant and epigastrium on palpation, and Murphy's sign was positive. The abdomen was otherwise soft with no palpable masses. The remainder of the systemic examination was unremarkable. Her blood results are shown in Table 2.4.1.

Table 2.4.1 Blood results

Blood results	
Hb	120
WCC	13
Platelets	120
Renal function	135
Potassium	3.5
Urea	6.5
Creatinine	83
Bilirubin	21
ALT	35
ALP	120
Albumin	38
Prothrombin time	11
Amylase	40
CRP	120

Questions

1. What are the key differential diagnoses?
2. How do gallstones form?
3. What is the pathophysiology of gallstone disease?
4. What investigations should you request and how may they influence management?
5. What are the possible sequelae of gallstone disease?
6. How should this patient be managed?
7. At what stage should surgery be considered?

Answers

1. What are the key differential diagnoses?

The top differential diagnoses are biliary colic, acute cholecystitis, duodenal ulceration or perforation, and acute pancreatitis. This lady's preceding history of episodic right-upper quadrant pain increases the likelihood of gallstone disease.

2. How do gallstones form?

Bile consists of bile salts, water, cholesterol and fats, phospholipids, mucus, and inorganic salts. Bile contains salts that are important in digestion and absorption of fats, as well as fat-soluble vitamins, while it also excretes waste products such as bilirubin and cholesterol. The amphiphilic nature of the bile causes the phospholipid and cholesterol vesicles to be incorporated into mixed micelles, which maintain the cholesterol in solution. Gallstones are thought to occur where there is an imbalance of lipids and salts, with supersaturation leading to precipitation into crystals. Stones generally consist of cholesterol, calcium, or a mixture of the two. Over 80% of stones are predominantly cholesterol monohydrate stones, with 10–20% predominantly calcium. Cholesterol stones form from precipitation of disproportionately high amounts of hepatic cholesterol secretion and/or biliary stasis. Calcium stones result from calcium precipitating with unconjugated bilirubin, which can occur in the presence of high amounts of unconjugated bilirubin, as can occur in haemolysis. Bacteria can also cause calcium stones to form by hydrolysing conjugated bilirubin into unconjugated bilirubin, with subsequent precipitation into pigmented black stones through bilirubin oxidation. Bacteria can also lead to the less common brown pigment gallstones, as the fatty acid byproduct of bacterial hydrolysis of lecithin can precipitate with calcium. Mixed gallstones consist of both cholesterol and calcium bilirubinate stones, which develop in the presence of cholesterol stones colonized with bacteria.

Risk factors for the formation of gallstones include female gender, obesity, pregnancy, medications such as oesotrogen-containing compounds, and gallbladder stasis. Crohn's disease, ileal resection, and ileal disease decrease bile salt reabsorption (i.e. enterohepatic circulation), which can result in gallstone formation.

Gallstones are estimated to be present in around 15% of the population, of which a small proportion become symptomatic (estimated 1–4%).

3. What is the pathophysiology of gallstone disease?

Gallstones can produce disease within the gallbladder or as a result of stone migration out of the gallbladder into the biliary system, which can subsequently result in pain, inflammation, or infection. Within the gallbladder lumen, stones can transiently obstruct the gallbladder neck or cystic duct to give features of *biliary colic* without overt features of inflammation. This typically consists of constant right-upper quadrant to epigastric pain that is self-limiting to a period of several hours, with associated features of nausea and vomiting. Gallstones can also become impacted in Hartmann's pouch, which results in continuous secretion of mucus from the gallbladder mucosa, while the bile is resorbed by the gallbladder. The gallbladder becomes over-distended with a transparent wall called a mucocele, which may or may not be associated with generalized inflammation of the gallbladder.

Stones can also cause *acute cholecystitis*, by generating direct mechanical irritation of the gallbladder wall, particularly in the presence of biliary sludge (a mix of smaller particulate crystals precipitated from bile). Such mechanical trauma to the gallbladder wall causes release of prostaglandin I2 and E2, which result in an inflammatory response. The pain of cholecystitis is of similar nature to biliary colic but is generally described as more severe and persistent (hours to days), and typically is associated with fever. A positive Murphy's sign (pain on palpation of right-upper quadrant causing patient to catch their breath during deep inspiration, which is absent in the left-upper quadrant) is a characteristic feature of acute cholecystitis. The sign is sensitive but not specific to the condition, and can often be absent in the elderly and in acalculous cholecystitis. Cholecystitis is most commonly caused by gallstones (calculous cholecystitis) but it should be remembered that cholecystitis can also develop in the absence of gallstones (acalculous cholecystitis).

Normal gastrointestinal flora such as *E. coli* and *Klebsiella* can colonize cholesterol stones and can cause superimposed infection. Gas-producing organisms (*E. coli, Clostridia perfringens*, and *Klebsiella*) can occasionally also invade the gallbladder wall and generate gas, resulting in emphysematous cholecystitis. This occurs in 1% of cases, and more commonly in diabetic patients. There is a higher risk of perforation and gangrene in these patients, and urgent cholecystectomy is usually warranted.

Acalculous cholecystitis accounts for 5–10% of cases of cholecystitis. It commonly arises as a complication of other severe illness, such as burns or those on mechanical ventilation, but can also occur in sickle cell disease, advanced HIV disease, and a prolonged course of TPN. The pathophysiology is thought to be related to biliary stasis and increased bile viscosity, as well as hypoperfusion and consequent ischaemia of the gallbladder as a sequelae of systemic illness. Severely ill patients are predisposed to biliary stasis from dehydration and a lack of gallbladder stimulation (from cholecystokinin) where they are unable to receive enteral nutrition. A third of cases can go on to develop emphysematous cholecystitis.

4. What investigations should you request and how may they influence management?

- Blood tests should include full blood count with C-reactive protein (CRP), a full liver profile, amylase or lipase, and a clotting screen. Elevated inflammatory markers or fever in the presence of clinical signs are diagnostic criteria for acute cholecystitis. Blood cultures should be sent in pyrexial or unwell patients to seek an infective organism. Serum amylase or lipase must be used in acute cases to assess for acute pancreatitis, which can occasionally present in a similar manner, as their levels rise as they are released from the damaged pancreatic acinar cells. Amylase peaks quickly and can normalize within 24 hours, whereas lipase remains elevated for several days.

- ◆ Plain chest and abdominal radiographs are not useful diagnostic tests but can make other diagnoses or detect other complications, such as pulmonary infiltrates, ileus, bowel obstruction, and pneumoperitoneum from a perforated viscus. Calcified gallstones can occasionally be seen on abdominal radiographs, but only in about 10% of cases.

- ◆ Ultrasonography is the first-line investigation, which can reveal the presence of gallstones and identify dilatation of the biliary system from gallstones obstructing the common bile duct (CBD). It can also confirm a diagnosis of cholecystitis by revealing a thickened gallbladder wall (of over 4 mm) (Figure 2.4.1). However, sensitivity of ultrasound scanning for detecting CBD stones is low. The calibre of the CBD can also be assessed. It is

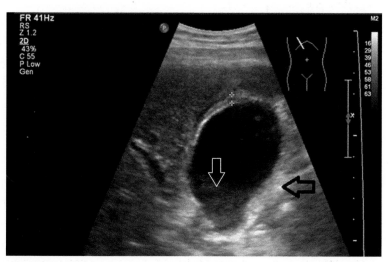

Figure 2.4.1 An ultrasound image of the gall bladder. The gall bladder wall can clearly be delineated in white around the black gall bladder lumen. It is thickened in this patient (black arrow), which correlates clinically with a diagnosis of cholecystitis. A thickened gall bladder measures 4 mm or more in diameter and is suspicious of an inflammatory process. The gall bladder appears to contain gallstones and biliary sludge (white arrow).

Reproduced Courtesy of Judith E. Ritchie.

generally considered to be dilated if it is above 10 mm in diameter, although the ductal diameter increases in older patients and those who have previously undergone cholecystectomy. Intrahepatic bile duct dilatation can also be identified.

- MRI (commonly magnetic resonance cholangiopancreatography or MRCP) may be required to further investigate any biliary dilatation seen on ultrasound or CT, as well as deranged liver function tests. This can detect bile duct stones with a high degree of accuracy.

- Endoscopic ultrasound can be used where gallstone disease is clinically suspected but where USS and MRI imaging does not reveal stones, as it can often detect microlithiasis.

- Computed tomography (CT) is occasionally used where there is diagnostic uncertainty for the abdominal pathophysiology or where more global assessment is indicated, e.g. suspected gallstone ileus. However, it should be borne in mind that CT can often fail to detect cholesterol stones, so where there is clinical suspicion of stones following CT an ultrasound should be performed.

Imaging of this lady's gallbladder revealed multiple gallstones and biliary sludge in a thick-walled gallbladder and confirmed the diagnosis of cholecystitis (Figure 2.4.1).

5. What are the potential sequelae of gallstone disease?

- *Acute cholecystitis.*

- *Acute pancreatitis.* Smaller, non-impacted stones can pass through the CBD and generate a transient increase in pressure proximally in the pancreatic duct, which can generate an acute inflammatory response. For more details about acute pancreatitis, please refer to Case 3.4 acute pancreatitis Chapter 3.

- *Ascending cholangitis.* Gallstones can lodge within the common bile duct, and bacterial colonization proximal to the level of the stone can cause ascending infection (cholangitis), a potentially lethal condition that requires prompt biliary decompression by ERCP. For more details, please see Case 2.5 acute ascending cholangitis.

- *Obstructive jaundice.* Stones can migrate into the CBD and become lodged, causing complete obstruction and resulting in biliary dilatation and obstructive jaundice. This can be imaged by MRCP or EUS and requires prompt intervention by ERCP.

- *Gallbladder empyema.* Development of sepsis within a gallbladder mucocoele can result in a gallbladder empyema. This can manifest with similar symptoms to cholecystitis but can also progress to severe sepsis with hypotension, confusion, and organ dysfunction. In the presence of severe sepsis, urgent cholecystectomy is warranted.

- *Gallbladder perforation.* Ischaemia, gangrene, and perforation arise more commonly in acalculous cholecystitis. Perforation can transiently alleviate a patient's symptoms. Free perforation will result in biliary peritonitis quite rapidly but is unusual. Localized perforation is more common, resulting in the development of a pericholecystic abscess.

- *Cholecystoenteric fistulae.* Following repeated attacks of inflammation, the gallbladder can adhere to adjacent bowel, such as the duodenum or transverse colon. Perforation will decompress the gallbladder, effectively draining the infected fluid. One should be suspicious of a perforation where pneumobilia is seen on radiological investigation (ultrasound and plain radiographs) in the absence of recent biliary intervention, and should be further investigated with CT.

- *Gallstone ileus.* Bowel obstruction (commonly small bowel) from an impacted gallstone can develop where a stone passes through a fistula. Urgent surgery is warranted to remove the stone, with primary closure of the bowel. Surgical repair of the fistula should not be carried out at the time of the initial operation and most clinicians do not perform interval biliary surgery routinely.

6. How should this patient be managed?

- Intravenous rehydration.

- Broad-spectrum antibiotics (according to local hospital anti-microbial protocol). These should be administered intravenously in the presence of a raised temperature and/or systemic upset (e.g. vomiting). Ongoing antibiotic therapy can be further guided by results of blood cultures.

- Regular analgesia.

- Urgent abdominal ultrasound to assess the gallbladder.

- In the presence of an abnormal biliary tree (such as biliary dila-tation) and/or abnormal liver function tests, an MRCP is gener-ally warranted. If this confirms ductal stones, then these must be removed promptly, either by ERCP or bile duct exploration at the time of cholecystectomy.

- Consideration for cholecystectomy. Following presentation with symptomatic gallstones there is a 50% risk of a further episode of biliary colic per year, and a 1–2% risk of developing more serious gallstone-related complications. In patients fit for surgery, chole-cystectomy is recommended. Non-surgical options are not very effective but in those unfit for surgery, oral treatment with urso-deoxycholic acid may help dissolution of stones.

7. At what stage should surgery be considered?

Urgent surgery is not clinically indicated in biliary colic, although earlier intervention does reduce readmission with further symp-toms or complications and is a cost-effective measure. Patients presenting with pancreatitis should ideally be operated in the index admission or within 2 weeks of the acute episode. Immediate cholecystectomy has been shown to be safe, with shorter length of stay and lower complication rates than delayed surgery. Urgent intervention is warranted where the patient is clinically septic from the cholecystitis and where this does not settle with appro-priate antimicrobial therapy. If the patient is too unstable or unfit to withstand surgery, then they should undergo percutaneous cholecystostomy to relieve the source of sepsis, with preparation for cholecystectomy when the episode settles. For more detailed discussion on cholecystectomy, please refer to Question 6 in Case 2.5 acute ascending cholangitis.

Further reading

Gurusamy K, Samraj K, Gludd C, Wilson E, Davidson BR. (2009) Meta-analysis of randomized controlled trials on the safety and effectiveness of early versus delayed laparoscopic cholecystectomy for acute cholecystitis. *British Journal of Surgery* **97** (2): 141–50.

Williams EJ, Green J, Beckingham I, Parks R, Martin D, Lombard M. (2008) Guidelines on the management of common bile duct stones. *Gut* **57** (7): 1004–21.

Yokoe M, Takada T, Strasberg SM, Solomkin JS, Mayumi T, Gomi H, *et al.*TG13 diagnostic criteria and severity grading of acute cholecystitis. *Journal of Hepato-Biliary-Pancreatic Sciences* **20** (1): 35–46.

Case history 2.5: Emergency: acute ascending cholangitis

A 67-year-old man presented to A&E with right-upper quadrant pain and rigors. He was known to have gallstones and has suffered occasional biliary colic. He was already on the waiting-list for a laparoscopic cholecystectomy. His past history included ischaemic heart disease and hypertension.

His observations are as follows: temperature 38.2°C, respiratory rate 23, pulse 128, blood pressure 98/72 mmHg, oxygen saturations 90% on air.

He was visibly jaundiced and he appeared distressed and dehydrated. Apart from his tachycardia and tachypnoea, his cardiorespiratory examination was unremarkable. Abdominal examination revealed tenderness in the right-upper quadrant with no rebound tenderness or guarding. His blood results are shown in Table 2.5.1.

Table 2.5.1 Blood results

Blood results	
Hb	120
WCC	27.3
Platelets	230
Sodium	135
Potassium	4.8
Urea	15
Creatinine	119
C-reactive protein	245
Bilirubin	78
ALT	101
ALP	486
Alb	38
PT	15

(continued)

Table 2.5.1 Continued

Blood results	
Arterial blood gas (on air)	
pH	7.34
PO_2	9.8
PCO_2	4.5
BE	−2.3
HCO_3	21
Lactate	3

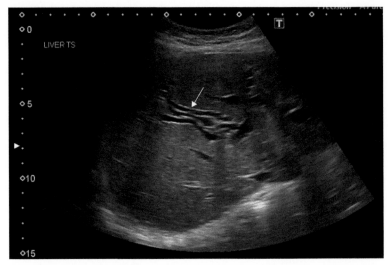

Figure 2.5.1 The sonogram shows a transverse section through this patient's liver. This shows dilated intra-hepatic bile ducts (denoted by white arrow). A few, small, mobile calculi were seen in the gall bladder. The common bile duct was not visualized in this examination and no cause of obstruction was demonstrated.

Reproduced Courtesy of Imeshi Wijetunga.

Questions

1. What triad of symptoms in this patient aids the clinical diagnosis in this patient?

2. If you were the surgical trainee assessing this patient in A&E, how would you manage this patient?

3. What bacteria are commonly implicated in ascending cholangitis?

4. The ultrasound scan reveals gallstones in the gall bladder with dilated intra-hepatic ducts but the CBD could not be visualized (Figure 2.5.1). When would you intervene with further investigations?

5. The MRCP confirms a large calculi in the CBD. What would be the next step in management?

6. What would be the definitive management for this patient?

7. What follow-up would you consider for this patient following cholecystectomy?

8. Do all patients with gall stones need cholecystectomy?

Answers

1. What triad of symptoms in this patient aids the clinical diagnosis in this patient?

Fever with rigors, right-upper quadrant pain, and jaundice is the classical triad of symptoms (Charcot's triad) that makes this gentleman's diagnosis most likely to be ascending cholangitis. In addition to these three symptoms, if the clinical presentation also includes hypotension and changes in the patient's mental status, this is known as Reynold's pentad.

2. If you were the surgical trainee assessing this patient in A&E, how would you manage this patient?

It is vital to recognize that this is a critically unwell patient. Principles of managing the critically ill surgical patient apply here with assessment and simultaneous management of the ABCs (airway, breathing, and circulation). The priorities of the initial management would be aggressive fluid resuscitation, antibiotic therapy, and oxygen supplementation.

The patient's arterial blood gas does show evidence of tissue hypoxia and metabolic acidosis, as there is a raised lactate. Supplemental oxygen should be administered along with IV fluids after establishing wide-bore IV access. IV broad-spectrum antibiotics, as per local guidelines for intra-abdominal/biliary sepsis, should be administered within 1 hour, ideally after obtaining blood for microscopy, culture, and sensitivity. Insertion of urinary catheter for monitoring fluid balance would be required given the evidence of pre-renal renal failure on this patient's biochemistry results.

Early discussion with the high-dependency unit and transfer to Level 2 care is recommended in this patient, who has evidence of organ dysfunction. If the clinical condition does not improve, an arterial line for invasive monitoring of blood pressure may be required.

There is significant risk of deterioration and close monitoring is required. Urgent ultrasound scan of the abdomen should be organized for all patients followed by urgent biliary decompression in the deteriorating patient.

3. What bacteria are commonly implicated in ascending cholangitis?

Gram-negative rods such as *Klebsiella* spp., *Escherichia coli*, and *Enterobacter* spp. are the commonest bacteria causing cholangitis. Gram-positive organisms such as enterococci and streptococci are also implicated. In endemic countries such as Thailand, cholangitis can be caused by liver flukes. Empirical antibiotic therapy will cover common organisms but it is vital that blood cultures are obtained in order to tailor subsequent antibiotic therapy according to sensitivities.

4. The ultrasound scan reveals gallstones in the gall bladder with dilated intra-hepatic ducts but the CBD could not be visualized (Figure 2.5.1). When would you intervene with further investigations?

If ultrasound scanning does not reveal a cause for dilated bile ducts, an MRCP is the next choice of investigation. The sensitivity and specificity of MRCP for detecting CBD stones is approximately 80–100%. In comparison, the sensitivity of USS for detecting CBD stones can be as low as 30%.

ERCP is reserved for therapeutic purposes and is rarely used as a diagnostic tool due to the high sensitivity of non-invasive imaging. However, in the septic, unwell patient with classical symptoms, obstructive LFTs, and dilated ducts on ultrasound imaging with confirmed gall stones in the gall bladder, urgent biliary decompression is required and an ERCP would prove both diagnostic and therapeutic. If an ERCP is not possible, or the endoscopist fails to cannulate and access the bile duct, a PTC can allow placement of a temporary stent to bypass an obstruction. If the patient improves clinically, it does suggest that the stone may have moved and may have passed spontaneously but an MRCP should be performed to determine this.

5. The MRCP confirms a large calculi in the CBD. What would be the next step in management?

Once CBD stones are confirmed, an ERCP should be performed for stone extraction. The major risks of ERCP includes bleeding, perforation, and pancreatitis. There is also a risk of technical failure, need for biliary stenting, and need for repeat procedure. All these risks should be discussed with the patient and informed consent obtained prior to proceeding with ERCP. ERCP is nearly impossible in patients who have had previous gastric bypass surgery. Patients with a history of previous upper gastrointestinal surgery should be discussed with the endoscopist. In addition, patients with duodenal diverticuli pose challenges to the endoscopist and the risk of perforation may be greater.

Under sedation, the side-viewing endoscope is manoeuvred to the ampulla of Vater, which is then cannulated and a sphincterotomy (i.e. incision of the muscles of the sphincter of Oddi) is performed. A cholangiogram can be performed at this stage to delineate the biliary tree and locate any stones. Stones can be extracted via balloon trawl or basket retrieval. Larger stones may be broken down using lithotripsy. If unable to remove stones, a plastic stent can be placed to relieve the obstruction and re-attempt removal at another ERCP at a later date. ERCP and repeated stent exchanges may be the definitive management for patients unfit for surgical CBD exploration.

Percutaneous biliary drainage is an option when ERCP is not possible or contraindicated. This involves accessing the biliary tree via percutaneous trans-hepatic cholangiography (PTC) and is possible in the presence of dilated biliary ducts. A biliary drain can be placed and can subsequently be 'internalized' during a subsequent procedure by feeding an internal stent through the external drain prior to removing the external component. This will re-establish bile flow back into the duodenum. If this is not possible, bile replacement (i.e. enteral replacement of drained bile via oral or nasogastric route) will become necessary to prevent impaired intestinal barrier function and loss of entero-hepatic circulation of bile salts.

PTC is associated with higher risks of damage to the vascular or biliary tree, as well as adjacent structures, compared to ERCP and hence ERCP is the preferred approach. In addition to the risks of ERCP, there is risk of significant bleeding and bile leak following PTC.

Laparoscopic common bile duct exploration is a potential option for managing intra-ductal stones at the same time as laparoscopic cholecystectomy. This is usually reserved for when less invasive methods have been futile or are contraindicated and when the bilirubin is only mildly raised.

6. What would be the definitive management for this patient?

To prevent any future risk of further biliary complications, this patient should be considered for a cholecystectomy once he recovers from his episode of sepsis. Ideally, this should be performed in the index admission or as soon as possible.

Laparoscopic cholecystectomy is recommended for all patients fit for surgery with symptomatic gallstone disease. The majority of elective laparoscopic cholecystectomies in the UK are performed as day-case procedures. A brief summary of the surgical steps of a conventional four-port laparoscopic cholecystectomy are as follows (this is a guide to revision of the steps involved and not intended for teaching technical skills or managing complicated cases):

1. Surgical safety. This includes theatre team briefing, which is essential to ensure all required equipment is available (including intra-operative cholangiogram equipment and radiographers, if this is indicated). In addition, the WHO safety checklist should be completed.

2. Ensure administration of prophylactic antibiotics (if indicated) and prophylaxis for deep vein thrombosis.

3. Patient preparation. With patient lying supine, skin preparation with disinfectant (usually chlorhexidine or betadine) from nipple line to inguinal ligament and laterally to anterior superior iliac spine followed by draping of the sterile field. Preparation

of laparoscopic stack, monitor, laparoscope, light cable, and diathermy is usually done by operating department practitioner/scrub nurse.

4. Induction of pneumoperitoneum. Open techniques are preferred by most surgeons via a supra-umbilical, trans-umbilical, or infra-umbilical incision and a 10 mm port. Choice of technique is guided by surgeon expertise. The abdomen is inflated with CO_2 to establish pneumoperitoneum.

5. Position patient head down (Trendelenburg position) and tilted to the left. (Check that the patient is secured to the operating table with leg straps, foot board, etc., to ensure stability when position of the table is changed.) An NG tube maybe required for decompression of the prominent stomach if it is problematic to the surgeon.

6. Identification of gall bladder followed by identification sites for further port placement.

7. Insertion of 10 mm epigastric and two 5 mm right hypochondrium ports under vision preferably after infiltration of local anaesthetic at the site prior to insertion of port.

8. A grasper is placed at the fundus of the gallbladder and the gallbladder is then retracted upwards towards the patient's right shoulder to expose the region of Calot's triangle, the anatomical space bordered by cystic duct, common hepatic duct, and cystic artery (but recent interpretation of this defines the upper border of the triangle as the inferior border of the liver).

9. Dissection to open Calot's triangle is performed using a combination of hook diathermy, blunt dissection, and suction, depending on surgeon preference, to obtain the critical view of safety. This includes exposure and delineation of Calot's triangle to identify a single duct and single artery entering the gallbladder and to completely dissect the lower part of the gall bladder off the liver bed.

10. Cystic artery and cystic duct are identified and the surrounding anatomical planes are dissected.

11. Once the surgeon is satisfied that the critical view of safety has been obtained and all structures have been correctly identified, the cystic artery is clipped with metal clips and ligated.

12. The cystic duct is then clipped prior to ligation with either metal clips or locking clips such as Hem-o-loks. If an intra-operative cholangiogram is required, it is performed at this stage.

13. The gallbladder is then dissected off the liver bed, taking care not to damage the liver parenchyma, and the surgeon remains vigilant for small accessory bile ducts (e.g. ducts of Lushka).

14. While the gallbladder remains attached to the liver by a thin layer of peritoneum, haemostasis of the liver bed is secured where required with diathermy (on spray setting) and a washout is carried out, if required.

15. Drains are not routinely used, but can be used, if required, at the surgeon's discretion.

16. The gallbladder is freed and placed in an endoscopic bag for retrieval, usually via the umbilical port under vision with the laparoscope placed in the epigastric port.

17. CO_2 is allowed to escape from the abdominal cavity prior to closure of port-sites. Usually a slowly absorbable monofilament suture on a J-shaped needle is used for closure of the rectus sheath at the umbilicus. Closure of the sheath at the epigastric port is not usually required. Skin is usually closed with absorbable subcuticular sutures.

18. The abdomen is cleaned and dressings are placed prior to recovery from anaesthetic.

7. What follow-up would you consider for this patient following cholecystectomy?

Once definitive management for gallstones (i.e. cholecystectomy) has been performed successfully, most centres do not routinely follow up patients unless there have been complications. *De novo* formation of CBD stones is rare but can occur in a small proportion of patients following cholecystectomy. Biliary obstruction due to CBD stones diagnosed within 3 years of cholecystectomy however, are likely to be retained stones, missed at the time of surgery.

8. Do all patients with gallstones need cholecystectomy?

Cholecystectomy is reserved for symptomatic gallstones. Asymptomatic patients do not require treatment unless they develop symptoms. A gallbladder empyema can be managed with a percutaneous cholecystostomy if the patient is unfit for surgery and conservative management has been unsuccessful. Fitness for cholecystectomy should be reassessed once the patient has recovered but it may be the definitive management in patients with significant comorbidities.

Further reading

National Institue for Health and Care Excellence (NICE) (2014) *Gall stone disease: Clinical Guideline [CG188]*. London: NICE.

Care of the Critically Ill Surgical Patient, third edition. Royal College of Surgeons.

Nagral S (2005) Anatomy relevant to cholecystectomy. *Journal of Minimal Access Surgery* 1 (2): 53–58.

Guidelines for the Clinical Application of Laparoscopic Biliary Tract Surgery. Society of American Gastrointestinal and Endoscopic Surgeons (SAGES) Available at: http://www.sages.org/publications/guidelines/guidelines-for-the-clinical-application-of-laparoscopic-biliary-tract-surgery/ [Accessed 28 June 2017]

Case history 2.6: Emergency: complications following laparoscopic cholecystectomy

A 37-year-old lady was admitted 2 days following an elective day-case laparoscopic cholecystectomy with abdominal pain and nausea. Apart from her history of biliary colic, she had no significant past medical history. Her operation notes indicated that she underwent a straightforward cholecystectomy with no intra-operative complications. Her immediate post-operative recovery was uncomplicated and she was discharged home the same day following her cholecystectomy.

On re-admission she was pyrexial and in considerable distress. Her heart rate was 110 beats per minute, respiratory rate 20, and blood pressure 140/90. On examination, she had rebound tenderness in her right-upper and lower quadrants, as well as epigastrium. Her blood tests revealed raised inflammatory markers. A decision was made to take her back to theatre for a diagnostic laparoscopy for suspected biliary peritonitis. A subhepatic bile collection was seen and a CBD injury was suspected. Following copious washout with warmed saline, large surgical drains were placed in the gall bladder fossa. The patient then underwent an ERCP, which showed a bile leak from an accessory duct (see Figure 2.6.1).

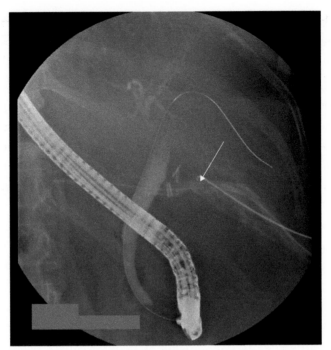

Figure 2.6.1 This ERCP image was taken following cannulation of the Ampulla of Vater, insertion of guidewire and injection of contrast into the biliary tree. This shows contrast in the biliary tree, the guide-wire in the CBD passing into the right hepatic duct, surgical clips as well as a surgical drain. The extra-hepatic biliary tree appears intact. A blush of extravasated contrast near the gall bladder fossa is clearly seen (see arrow). The appearances are in keeping with a leak from accessory bile ducts called ducts of Luschka (small bile ducts draining into the right hepatic duct or common bile duct). Injuries to these ducts are the second most common cause of bile leak next to cystic duct stump leaks.

Reproduced Courtesy of Imeshi Wijetunga.

Questions

1. What key procedure-specific risks should be discussed with all patients prior to laparoscopic cholecystectomy?

2. How are iatrogenic bile duct injuries classified?

3. How would you manage such a patient if they present during your general surgery on-call take at a district general hospital? What would be their definitive management?

4. What potential future complications could this patient suffer?

Answers

1. What key procedure-specific risks should be discussed with all patients prior to laparoscopic cholecystectomy?

- *Bile leak.* Clinically significant bile leaks are uncommon but reported incidence is between 0.5 and 2% of all cholecystectomies. These can usually be managed with ERCP and stenting with radiological drainage of the biliary collection.

- *Bile duct injury.* Laparoscopic cholecystectomy carries an approximately 1:400 risk of bile duct injury. If bile duct injury is suspected, the patient should be referred to the regional tertiary hepatopancreatobiliary unit for subsequent management.

- *Retained stone.* An intra-operative cholangiogram can be helpful in diagnosing or excluding CBD stones if there is clinical suspicion or mild derangement of liver function tests. Although it is uncommon, patients can present with CBD stones postoperatively, which can be many months following their laparoscopic cholecystectomy and which would require ERCP to remove them.

- *Vascular injury.* Due to anatomical variations, the common and right hepatic artery are at risk of damage whilst isolating the cystic artery. Any damage risks serious intra-operative arterial bleeding or ischaemic damage to the liver. Although less common, injury to the portal vein or its branches could occur. Dissecting out Calot's triangle to correctly identify anatomy is important in order to minimize risk of damage to either the arterial tree or the bile duct.

- *Bowel injury.* Laparoscopic surgery has a risk of iatrogenic damage to the bowel, usually the colon or duodenum, due to their proximity and any adhesions to the gallbladder.

- *Access injuries.* Port site-related complications, including infection and the future risk of incisional hernia that may or may not become symptomatic.

- *Post-cholecystectomy syndrome.* A constellation of symptoms that are poorly understood affecting up to 15% of patients in the months following cholecystectomy. They include indigestion, bloating, nausea, vomiting, diarrhoea, and abdominal pain. Patients should be advised that these symptoms can take up to a year to settle.

2. How are iatrogenic bile duct injuries classified?

There are several classification systems for bile duct injuries. The Bismuth classification is the oldest, described by H. Bismuth in 1982 before the era of laparoscopic cholecystectomy. Since then a number of revised classifications have been described, the most common of which is the Strasberg classification, which is similar to the Bismuth classification but with the important distinction of cystic duct and accessory duct leaks as minor injuries. Other classifications, such as the Stewart–Way and Hannover classifications, take into account associated vascular injuries, which the older classifications do not. The Strasberg classification is summarized in Table 2.6.1. According to this classification, this patient had a Class A bile duct injury, as her ERCP had shown a bile leak from an accessory duct (duct of Lushka) (Figure 2.6.1).

Table 2.6.1 Strasberg classification of bile duct injuries

Type	Description
Class A	Bile leak from cystic duct or accessory small bile duct
Class B	Occluded right posterior sectoral duct (that drains segment VI and VII of the liver)
Class C	Bile leak from divided right posterior sectoral duct with no continuity with the remainder of the biliary tree
Class D	Bile leak from common bile duct
Class E	Transected/strictured common bile duct (further sub-classified into E1–E5 variants according to distance from confluence of bile ducts)

Source: Data from Strasberg SM, Hertl M, and Soper NJ, (1995) 'An analysis of the problem of biliary injury during laparoscopic cholecystectomy', *Journal of the American College of Surgeons*, Volume 180, Issue 1, pp. 101–25.

3. How would you manage such a patient if they present during your general surgery on-call take at a district general hospital? What would be their definitive management?

The junior general surgical trainee should be familiar with assessing patients who are re-admitted following this common general surgical procedure. Often the reason for re-admission is poorly controlled pain but the possibility of iatrogenic injury should be high on the list of differential diagnoses. As with all critically ill surgical patients, the CCrISP principles of patient assessment and management should be applied here.

On clinical assessment, this patient was peritonitic, hence was scheduled for an emergency diagnostic laparoscopy after initial resuscitation with IV rehydration and appropriate antibiotics directed by local microbiology guidelines. If the patient was more stable, the investigation of choice would be an abdominal ultrasound scan to look for intra-abdominal collections, as well as dilatation of the biliary tree. A contrast-enhanced abdominal CT could also be considered as it will be useful for investigating potential vascular injuries.

In theatre, induction of pneumoperitoneum can be achieved using the same laparoscopic cholecystectomy port sites for the camera as well as the working ports. At laparoscopy, the finding of biliary peritonitis should alert the operator to suspect a major bile duct injury. A laparoscopic washout with several litres of warmed saline should be undertaken until the effluent is clear. If an injured duct of Lushka is visible in the gall bladder bed, they can be sutured laparoscopically with a non-absorbable, monofilament suture provided that the expertise exists locally. Large sub-hepatic drains (with low suction) should be placed.

The patient should be discussed with the regional hepato-pancreato-biliary (HPB) centre for transfer for assessment of injury severity and definitive management.

For suspected bile duct injury, the next step in management would be an ERCP. At ERCP, the diagnosis can be confirmed and most minor injuries can be managed by insertion of a plastic stent across the biliary sphincter to reduce the pressure in the biliary tree, which would in turn encourage healing of the injury. In the case of main bile duct injury, ERCP can be challenging and PTC may be required.

These complex injuries require assessment by a multidisciplinary team involving endoscopists, interventional radiologists, and HPB surgeons.

Once the intra-abdominal collection is drained and the bile duct has been successfully stented, a period of 8–12 weeks is allowed prior to consideration of any further surgical intervention. Outcomes of delayed reconstruction are much better compared to immediate reconstruction. If necessary, biliary reconstruction can be contemplated at this stage. This often involves a Roux-en-Y hepaticojejunostomy. For post-cholecystectomy biliary strictures, endoscopic dilatation and stenting could be the definitive management. Definitive management will depend on the extent of the original injury. Some severe injuries may require resection of the affected liver segments.

4. What potential future complications could this patient suffer?

Duct of Lushka leaks are unlikely to cause long-term complications. However, other injuries may go unrecognized initially that could result in long-term morbidity. Figure 2.6.2 is an MRI image

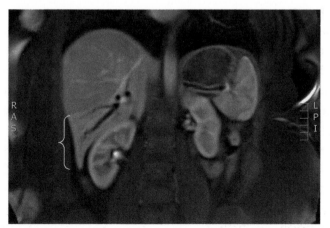

Figure 2.6.2 This is an MR image of a patient 2 years following management of a minor bile-duct injury with laparoscopic washout and ERCP. This image shows atrophic appearances of segment 6 and 7 (indicated by the white bracket) likely due to ischaemic injury. Dilated bile ducts are also seen in the affected segments.

Reproduced Courtesy of Imeshi Wijetunga.

of a patient 2 years following management of a minor bile duct injury, which illustrates this point. This illustrates that the extent of injury can be difficult to assess immediately following injury. These patients could present with biliary symptoms several months to years following their initial management of bile duct injury. This patient suffered several episodes of cholangitis and had raised liver enzymes. She proceeded on to resection of segment 6 and 7 with biliary reconstruction.

Other rare complications such as portal vein thrombosis could occur, which may be managed by portal vein stenting and anticoagulation. Portal vein thrombosis results in a risk of portal hypertension and all its associated risks.

Unsuccessful surgical repair in high bile duct injuries (Strasberg E4–E5) is an indication for consideration of liver transplantation. (Liver transplantation is discussed in more detail in Case 2.2 hepatocellular carcinoma)

Further reading

Almutairi AFMS, Hussain YAMS (2009) Triangle of safety technique: a new approach to laparoscopic cholecystectomy. *Hepato-Biliary-Pancreatic Surgery* 2009, Article ID 476159. doi:10.1155/2009/476159 Last accessed 12/11/2017.

Chun K (2014) Recent classifications of the common bile duct injury. *Korean Journal of Hepato-Biliary-Pancreatic Surgery* 18 (3): 69–72.

Strasberg SM, Hertl M, Soper NJ (1995) An analysis of the problem of biliary injury during laparoscopic cholecystectomy. *Journal of the American College of Surgeons*, Volume 180, Issue 1, pp.101–25.

Chapter 3

Pancreatic surgery

Judith Ritchie and Ahmed Al-Mukhtar

Case history 3.1: Elective: pancreatic cystic mass

A 68-year-old woman presented to her district general hospital with an episode of acute diverticulitis that was confirmed on contrast CT abdomen. This CT imaging also revealed a cystic mass in the head of the pancreas (Figure 3.1.1). Her diverticulitis was successfully managed conservatively, following which she was referred to the tertiary HPB centre for specialist input. The patient was completely asymptomatic of this lesion. The case was discussed at MDT. Subsequent endoscopic ultrasound revealed a complex 4.5 × 3 cm lesion in the head of the pancreas involving the pancreatic duct with distal pancreatic duct dilatation (Figure 3.1.2). There was no evidence of invasion into local or vascular structures. Cytology revealed some mucin vacuoles. Her blood tests and LFTs were normal. In conclusion, features were concerning for a main duct IPMN with a concern for malignant potential. She was counselled about the diagnosis and the concern for malignant potential, and she underwent a Whipple's procedure. Histology confirmed a diagnosis of main duct IPMN with some side-branch involvement with mild dysplasia of the involved branches.

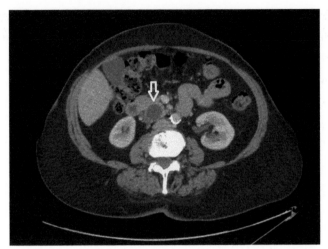

Figure 3.1.1 Image from the original abdominal CT scan showing the cystic lesion in the head of the pancreas (dark and round, denoted by the arrow).

Reproduced Courtesy of Judith Ritchie.

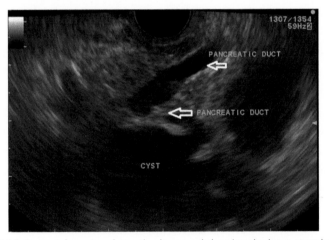

Figure 3.1.2 Image taken at endoscopic ultrasound showing the large complex cyst (marked as 'cyst') with frond-like projections on the right side, and dilatation of the distal pancreatic duct (demarcated with arrows).

Reproduced Courtesy of Judith Ritchie.

Questions

1. What are the differentials for a pancreatic lesion?
2. How are pancreatic cystic lesions classified?
3. How should you approach investigating a pancreatic mass?
4. How should pancreatic cystic lesions be managed?

Answers

1. What are the differentials for a pancreatic lesion?

A pancreatic neoplasm can be divided into three categories depending on their tissue of origin:

- Exocrine neoplasm.
- Endocrine neoplasm.
- Mesenchymal neoplasm.

Exocrine neoplasm

- Pancreatic adenocarcinoma (90–95% of lesions). Malignant.
- Metastases from other primaries. Very rare. Most commonly from renal cell carcinoma, also colonic, melanoma, breast, lung, and gastric.
- Cystic lesions. Cystic lesions can be benign or potentially malignant:
  - Benign:
    - Serous cystadenoma.
    - Pseudocyst.
  - Malignant:
    - Intrapapillary mucinous neoplasm (IPMN) (main duct, side branch, mixed variant).
    - Mucinous cystic neoplasm.
    - Solid pseudopapillary neoplasm.
    - Pancreatic adenocarcinoma with cystic degeneration (rare).

Endocrine (islet cell) neoplasm

These are either functional or non-functional. They are rare, only constituting 5% of all pancreatic lesions. Functional lesions (also known as neuroendocrine tumours) are symptomatic secondary to the pathophysiology of the tumour. The majority are sporadic but 10% are familial (multiple endocrine neoplasia 1 or MEN1).

- Functional (85% of endocrine neoplasms):

  - *Insulinomas*. Most common functional tumour. These secrete insulin. 75% are single, 10% multiple, 10% malignant. They present with Whipple's triad (abnormal behaviour, sweating, hypoglycaemia). Diagnosed on imaging and 72-hour fasting with serial serum glucose and immunoreactive insulin measurements.

  - *Gastrinomas*. Second most common. Secrete gastrin resulting in Zollinger–Ellison syndrome (peptic ulcer disease). Half are malignant. Diagnosed with serum gastrin level, identifying peptic ulcers on endoscopy and CT.

  - *Glucagonoma*. 75% malignant. Presents with diabetes mellitus and poorly defined symptoms (weight loss, diarrhoea, dermatitis). Diagnosed with glucagon level.

  - *VIPoma*. Secretes VIP resulting in profuse watery diarrhoea. 75% malignant. Diagnosed with serum VIP level and CT/MRI.

  - *Somatostatinoma*. Somatostatin production results in diabetes mellitus, gallstones, weight loss, steatorrhoea, and diarrhoea. 75% malignant. Diagnosed on somatostatin level (serum fasting, transhepatic portal vein sample).

- Non-functional (15% of endocrine neoplasms). The majority are malignant.

Mesenchymal neoplasm

2% of all pancreatic lesions:

- Lymphangioma.
- Pancreatoblastoma.
- Lipoma.
- Sarcoma.
- Schwannoma.
- Lymphoma.
- Teratoma.

2. How are pancreatic cystic lesions classified?

Cystic lesions can be classified according to whether they are benign or malignant.

Potentially malignant lesions include:

- *Intrapapillary mucinous neoplasm (IPMN)*. Main duct, side branch, mixed variant. IPMN are ductal epithelial tumours that present in older age. They arise from the main duct, side branches, or both (mixed variant). Communication with the pancreatic duct is characteristic. Main duct IPMN has the highest malignant potential. They involve the pancreatic head in 70% of cases, but can be multifocal throughout the gland in 5–10% of cases. They tend to be small. Mucin is secreted into the pancreatic duct resulting in ductal dilatation (>5 mm) at one or several points, both of which can be identified on CT. Solid mural nodules protruding into dilated ducts are suspicious of pre-existing malignancy. Tumour growth can result in chronic obstructive pancreatitis of the adjacent parenchyma, resulting in fibrosis and atrophy on imaging, which can cause diagnostic confusion where this is present along with small lesions. In side-branch IPMN the main pancreatic duct is not dilated. Side-branch dilatation is visible, as well as a lesion with multiple macro- and microcystic components, giving an appearance similar to a bunch of grapes. In mixed variant IPMN there are appearances of side-branch IPMN with a dilated pancreatic duct.

- *Mucinous cystic neoplasm (MCN)*. MCNs are rare. They present as several (<6), large (>2 cm), macrocystic, septated, mucin-producing lesions with a thick wall. They are distinguished by an ovarian-like stroma. They can calcify and rarely communicate with the pancreatic ductal system. Over 90% develop in the pancreatic tail.

- *Solid pseudopapillary neoplasm*. These are very rare pre-malignant lesions that tend to occur in young females in their second to third decade. These are large, solid lesions that degenerate and bleed, resulting in mixed solid cystic appearance. These lesions contain thin, blood-stained fluid.

Benign lesions include:

- *Serous cystadenoma.*

- *Pseudocyst.* Pseudocysts arise as the result of pancreatic duct damage and extravasation of enzymatic material, usually from acute or chronic pancreatitis or abdominal trauma. The ensuing inflammatory process walls off the fluid collection in a non-epithelialized wall of fibrous granuloma material. They are unilocular, thick-walled lesions containing non-viscous fluid with high amylase content. They may either maintain communication with the pancreatic duct or be completely walled off from it. One-third of them develop at the pancreatic head and two-thirds at the body and tail. There is usually only one, although multiple lesions can occasionally be found. Pseudocysts can be asymptomatic, but complicated pseudocysts should be treated. These present with:

  - Abdominal pain, early satiety, nausea and vomiting, and gastric outlet obstruction from compressing adjacent viscera.

  - Jaundice from CBD compression.

  - Pleural effusion from pancreatico-pleural fistula.

  - Infected cysts can present with sepsis or rupture resulting in peritonism (rare).

3. How should you approach investigating a pancreatic mass?

The widespread use of cross-sectional imaging has resulted in increased detection of pancreatic lesions, usually for imaging carried out for unrelated complaints. This has been reported in 3% of all CT scans and 20% of MRI scans. The majority of these are asymptomatic. Clinical history can still yield relevant information.

Pancreatic cystic neoplasms are also generally asymptomatic, and they may be an incidental finding on imaging carried out for other reasons, such as in this case. Intraductal papillary mucinous neoplasms (IPMNs) may present with repeated episodes of abdominal pain and may wrongly be attributed to a clinical diagnosis of chronic pancreatitis.

Investigations should seek to determine:

1. Consistency of the lesion—whether it is cystic, solid, or both.

2. Nature of the lesion—malignant or benign.

Determining consistency of the lesion:

◆ Abdominal ultrasound can differentiate cystic and solid components, but its diagnostic abilities are limited as it is not able to visualize the entire pancreas due to overlying bowel gas and abdominal fat.

◆ CT and MRI can both identify solid and cystic lesions or cystic lesions with solid components. They can detect macro- and microcystic components, septations, calcification, and nodules. MRI is the gold standard for diagnosing pancreatic pseudocysts, as it can differentiate between organized necrosis and a cystic lesion with a higher level of accuracy than CT. In addition, MRI can identify cystic lesion communication to the pancreatic duct.

Determining whether a lesion is benign or malignant:

◆ Where there is diagnostic uncertainty on imaging, EUS is a useful diagnostic adjunct to imaging in both solid and cystic lesions, as it provides opportunities to obtain high-resolution images of the lesion, particularly for small lesions below 2 cm, as well as the surrounding pancreatic parenchyma. Both cyst aspirate and tissue biopsy can be obtained for diagnostic cytology and histology at EUS or ERCP. Mucin seen to be extruding from the ampulla of Vater at EUS or ERCP is pathognomonic of main duct IPMNs. Cystic fluid can be sent for cytology, amylase, mucin, and the tumour marker carcinogenic embryonic antigen (CEA). Sensitivity for detecting mucin at cytology is poor. Measuring CEA is useful. CEA in particular has a high sensitivity and specificity between mucinous and non-mucinous cysts. It is low in pseudocysts and raised in tumours. Cytology can have a low cellular yield due to high viscosity and low yield aspirates and aspirating a microcystic region, and therefore may yield very little information. Its use is limited as it is technically challenging and not available in all hospitals. Endoscopic imaging and tissue biopsy carries risks of infection, perforation, pancreatitis, and bleeding.

- Contrast enhancement of the pancreatic ductal system at ERCP can differentiate IPMN from other cystic lesions and pseudocysts, and its excellent visualization of pancreaticobiliary anatomy will identify ductal displacement by mass or ductal obstruction and main pancreatic duct communication with cystic lesions. Filling defects in the duct from mucus or intraductal mass can be seen at ERCP but these may also cause reflux of contrast and failure to visualize.

Cross-sectional imaging can reach a diagnosis due to radiologically characteristic features and EUS can be used to carry out a more thorough assessment.

Worrying radiological features include:

- Dilated pancreatic duct between 5 and 9 mm. Main pancreatic duct obstruction is present in 60% of malignant lesions versus 2.5% of benign ones. This feature was seen in this lady's case.
- Cystic lesion over 3 cm.
- Thick or enhancing cyst wall.
- Non-enhancing mural nodule.
- Regional lymphadenopathy.

High-risk features include:

- Enhancing solid lesions.
- Pancreatic duct over 1 cm in diameter.
- Obstructive jaundice.

All cysts over 3cm without any worrying radiological features should be evaluated by EUS.

4. How should pancreatic cystic lesions be managed?

Pre-operative workup will require staging to determine the stage of disease and specialist HPB input sought through MDT. All technically resectable solid malignancies should be removed.

Investigation and management of endocrine lesions will usually involve both surgical and medical endocrinologist input. Resection is ideal for most as a high proportion of them are both symptomatic and malignant.

In terms of cystic lesions, resection is offered to all main duct IPMNs, other IPMN subtypes with any radiological features deemed high risk of malignancy, and MCNs, as a diagnostic and potentially therapeutic treatment option. Patients who are not fit for resection may be offered regional treatment, such as radiofrequency ablation at EUS.

Lesions in the pancreatic head are usually removed through the Whipple's procedure. Lesions in the body and tail are removed through distal pancreatectomy.

Other cystic lesions are monitored for any change in size or features. Six-monthly surveillance can be offered to all cysts over 3 cm with no worrying features of malignancy on imaging or EUS. Current recommendations for surveillance are:

- Side-branch IPMN with the largest cystic component of 2–3 cm can be monitored with alternating MRI and EUS.
- Side-branch IPMN with a smaller cystic component of 1–2 cm should have annual MRI, and cysts below 1 cm should be offered MRI in 2–3 years.

It is reasonable to consider surgery rather than surveillance in younger patients. If there are any changes to the cyst size or any concerning features on follow-up imaging, then resection should be considered.

If there is histological evidence of high-grade dysplasia or malignancy following resection, patients should receive surveillance MRI imaging every 2 years.

Pancreatic pseudocysts generally resolve spontaneously. They recur in 15% of cases. Complications arise in a fifth of cases, particularly those that have persistent communication with the pancreatic duct. Intervention is only warranted when they are symptomatic or when they develop complications. They are usually decompressed by drainage. Drainage can be administered either endoscopically, radiologically, or surgically (open or laparoscopic). Endoscopic approaches have a lower recurrence rate than radiological ones.

Further reading

Kim TS, Fernandez-del Castillo C (2015) Diagnosis and management of pancreatic cystic neoplasms. *Hematology/Oncology Clinics of North America* 29 (4): 655–74.

O'Grady HL, Conlon KC (2008) Pancreatic neuroendocrine tumours. *European Journal of Surgical Oncology* 34 (3): 324–32.

Tanaka M, Fernández-del Castillo C, Adsay V, Chari S, Falconi M, Jang JY et al. (2012) International consensus guidelines 2012 for the management of IPMN and MCN of the pancreas. *Pancreatology* 12: 183–97.

Zamboni GA, Ambrosetti MC, Pecori S, Manfredi R, Capelli R (2015) Solid pseudopapillary neoplasms pp. 349–72 *in* D'Onofrio M, Capelli P, Pederzoli P. *Imaging and Pathology of Pancreatic Neoplasms A Pictorial Atlas.*

Case history 3.2: Elective: pancreatic cancer

A 69-year-old gentleman is admitted to general surgery by his GP with painless jaundice. He first noticed jaundice of his sclerae 7 days ago; this has progressively worsened. He has no abdominal pain, although he has had some vague upper abdominal discomfort and reduced appetite for the past few months, and his trousers are a bit loose. Three days ago he noticed his stool has become pale and his urine has become tea-coloured. He denies nausea, vomiting, abdominal pain, and fever. He has no other past medical history and was previously in good health. He is not taking any medication. He is a lifelong smoker, smoking 10 cigarettes a day.

On examination he is comfortable. His vital signs are normal and he is afebrile. There are no masses or organomegaly on abdominal examination and other systems examinations are normal. His blood tests reveal obstructive jaundice (see Table 3.2.1).

Ultrasound reveals global intra-hepatic and extra-hepatic biliary duct dilatation. The distal CBD and pancreas could not be visualized due to overlying bowel gas. A contrast CT of the abdomen reveals a 3 cm mass in the head of the pancreas compressing the distal common bile and pancreatic ducts and encasing the superior mesenteric artery (Figure 3.2.1). He was discussed at the hepatobiliopancreatic (HPB) MDT, where his disease was deemed locally advanced and inoperable.

Table 3.2.1 Blood results

Na$^+$	145	Bili	145	Hb	140	PT	19
K+	5.2	ALP	220	WCC	9.1	APTT	55
Ur	8	AST	45	Neut	9.1	Fib	5.5
Cr	95	ALT	34	Plts	130		
GGT	110						

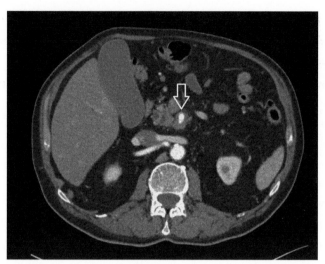

Figure 3.2.1 Image from the patient's abdominal CT showing tumour burden in the head of the pancreas. The tumour can be seen to encase the superior mesenteric artery (arrow), which is a sign of locally advanced inoperable disease.

Reproduced Courtesy of Judith Ritchie.

Questions

1. What are the possible differential diagnoses?
2. How is jaundice classified and why is this clinically important?
3. What are the complications of obstructive jaundice?
4. What is pancreatic cancer and how does it develop?
5. How does pancreatic cancer present?
6. What are the appropriate investigations in this case?
7. How should this patient be managed?
8. What is the prognosis of this disease?

Answers

1. What are the possible differential diagnoses?

This is a history of obstructive or post-hepatic jaundice. Differentials include:

- Malignancy. This may can occur with cancers arising within the ampulla or pancreatic head, compressing or invading the distal CBD, or with malignancy arising within the biliary duct (cholangiocarcinoma). This is the most likely differential in a presentation such as this. Painless obstructive jaundice and weight loss is concerning for malignancy, particularly in the older patient.

- Non-malignant biliary stricturing, which can occur in primary biliary cirrhosis and secondary to a local chronic inflammatory process, particularly in chronic pancreatitis. Usually chronic pancreatitis is associated with a longstanding history of recurrent abdominal pain with or without features of pancreatic insufficiency.

- Choledocholithiasis can occasionally present in such an atypical manner with painless jaundice or deranged liver function tests.

- Liver disease.

2. How is jaundice classified and why is this clinically important?

In order to understand the pathophysiology of jaundice, one needs to have a clear understanding of bilirubin metabolism.

Bilirubin is a breakdown product of haem catabolism released due to breakdown of old red blood cells in the spleen. This bilirubin molecule is initially water-insoluble, therefore it binds to the albumin molecule that transports it to the liver. The bilirubin molecule is taken up by the hepatocytes and is made water-soluble by conjugation with glucuronic acid via the enzyme bilirubin-UDP-glucuronosyltransferase, thus allowing it to be excreted into the bile. Once the bile is released into the gut, the gut bacteria break down the conjugated bilirubin molecule into urobilinogen and stercobilinogen. Stercobilinogen is excreted into the faeces, giving the stool its characteristic brown pigment. Urobilinogen is reabsorbed from the gut via enterohepatic circulation at the terminal ileum and then finally excreted by the kidneys into the urine.

Jaundice is commonly classified according to causes arising at the three different stages of the metabolic pathway of the bilirubin molecule:

1. Pre-hepatic.
2. Hepatic.
3. Post-hepatic.

Pre-hepatic jaundice Pre-hepatic jaundice refers to unconjugated hyperbilirubinaemia, and this may arise from:

- Increased bilirubin levels by haemolysis, e.g. glucose 6-phosphate dehydrogenase deficiency.
- Inefficient erthyropoiesis resulting in abnormal and brittle red blood cells that lyse easily, e.g. thalassaemia major, megaloblastic anaemia.
- Reduced bilirubin delivery/uptake to the liver, e.g. portosystemic shunts, low flow state of congestive heart failure, drugs that reversibly block hepatocytes from taking up bilirubin, e.g. rifampicin.
- Abnormalities in the conjugation process, e.g. Crigler–Najjar syndrome resulting in low or reduced function of the bilirubin-UGT enzyme; Gilbert's syndrome, which results in decreased bilirubin-UGT function.

Hepatic jaundice This refers to jaundice caused by pathology interfering with the liver's ability to effectively conjugate and excrete the bilirubin, resulting in a backlog of both conjugated and unconjugated bilirubin:

- Hepatitis.
- Liver infiltration with amyloidosis, sarcoidosis, TB, haemochromatosis, tumour and lymphoma.
- Wilson's disease.
- Drugs that damage the liver, e.g. isoniazid, erythromycin.

Post-hepatic jaundice This refers to jaundice resulting from biliary obstruction that prevents secretion of conjugated bilirubin, such as:

- Cancer (cholangiocarcinoma, pancreatic carcinoma such as in this case).
- Biliary duct strictures.
- Chronic pancreatitis.
- Primary sclerosing cholangitis.
- Choledocholithiasis.
- Biliary atresia in babies.

Features of the three classifications of jaundice should be sought on clinical assessment, which will help to create a list of appropriate differential diagnoses. Features are summarized in Table 3.2.2. The patient in this case clearly has post-hepatic jaundice.

Table 3.2.2 Summary of the clinical features seen in different types of jaundice

	Pre-hepatic	Hepatic	Post-hepatic
Bilirubin	Normal/↑	↑	↑
Conjugated bilirubin	Normal/↑	↑	↑
Unconjugated bilirubin	Normal/↑	↑	Normal
Conjugated urine bilirubin	Absent	Present	Present
Urobilinogen	Normal/↑	↑↓	
Alkaline phosphatase	Normal	↑	↑
Transaminases	Normal	↑	↑/normal
Stool colour	Normal	Normal/pale	Pale
Urine colour	Normal	Dark	Dark

Reproduced with permission from *Rapid Review Pathology*, 2nd ed., Goljan, Edward F., Elsevier Health Sciences, pp. 368–369, ISBN 032304414X, Copyright Elsevier (2002).

3. What are the complications of obstructive jaundice?

Jaundice is associated with:

* *Immunodeficiency.* Jaundice is associated with defective innate immunity and T cell and neutrophil dysfunction, leaving patients more vulnerable to infective organisms.

* *Risk of infection.* Cholestasis is believed to predispose to infection as it impedes reticuloendothelial cell function in the liver. Ascending cholangitis is not common in malignant biliary obstruction but may arise in immunocompromised states.

* *Fat malabsorption.* Biliary tract obstruction prevents bile release and therefore prevents emulsification and absorption of fat from the intestine. Fat passes through in the stool, causing a light clay-coloured, greasy stool that is difficult to flush (termed steatorrhoea).

* *Vitamin deficiencies, disordered clotting and increased risk of bleeding.* Lack of intestinal bile means that fat-soluble vitamins A, D, E, and K are not absorbed from the gut. Vitamin K is an essential cofactor in the production of clotting factors 10, 9, 7, and 2. This can result in prolonged prothrombin time, increased propensity to bruise, and bleeding.

* *Dehydration and renal failure.*

4. What is pancreatic cancer and how does it develop?

Around 90% of pancreatic cancers are adenocarcinomas arising from pancreatic duct epithelium. Pancreatic adenocarcinoma is the ninth most common cancer in the UK and the fifth leading cause of cancer death in the UK. Incidence increases with age: 4% of UK diagnoses are below 50 years old, 36% between 50 and 70, and 60% over 70 years of age.

Pancreatic cancer is believed to arise from a preneoplastic lesion, which progresses through a multi-step process to result in occult malignancy. Several genetic mutations and molecular aberrations have been identified in this process:

Genetic abnormalities arise with alteration in:

- Tumour suppressor genes such as p16, TP53, MADH4, and FHIT amongst others.
- Oncogene mutation such as K-ras and Her2.
- Molecular profiling has revealed upregulation of growth factor signalling, such as epidermal growth factor and vascular endothelial growth factor that fuel tumour development, as well as the tumour micro-environment, which has been found to fuel tumour development.

Around 5% of cases have familial traits. In these patients, associated germline genetic alterations that have been shown to predispose to disease development include BRCA2, Peutz–Jeghers (STK11/LKB1), familial pancreatitis (PRSS1, SPINK1), and Lynch syndrome (mismatch repair proteins).

A number of lifestyle and environmental factors have been associated with an increased risk of pancreatic cancer, including:

- High fat, nutrient-poor diet (20% of cases).
- Smoking (30% of cases).
- Physical inactivity.
- Occupational exposure to certain chemicals.
- Certain comorbidities, including diabetes mellitus and chronic pancreatitis.

5. How does pancreatic cancer present?

The nature of the presentation depends on the location of the tumour. Three-quarters of pancreatic cancers arise in the pancreatic head or neck, 10–20% in the body, and 5–10% in the tail. Clinical presentation generally arises in advanced stages of disease when the tumour invades or involves adjacent structures or organs. Consequently, half of patients present to general surgery with acute symptoms. Patients often give a retrospective history of vague complaints such as nausea, loss of appetite, malaise, abdominal discomfort, and fatigue, but there are no discernible symptoms that allow an early diagnosis to be made.

Abdominal pain is a common presenting complaint, which can be caused by either involvement of visceral afferent nerves or tumour-induced local pancreatitis. Tumours in the body or tail of the gland present with abdominal pain and generally present late. Tumours in the head compress or invade adjacent biliary drainage and present with painless jaundice in 70% of cases. They may also compress or invade into the stomach and duodenum resulting in early satiety and gastric outlet obstruction. The textbook feature of a palpable gallbladder (Courvoisier's sign) is only seen in a quarter of cases. Cachexia is an ominous feature suggestive of advanced metastatic disease. Other systemic features of metastatic disease include Virchow's (supraclavicular) node, Sister Mary Joseph's nodule, and migratory thrombophlebitis (Trousseau sign). In addition, venous thrombosis is a common consequence of advanced disease, which is treated with low molecular weight heparin.

Only 15–20% of patients present with surgically resectable disease. The remaining 80% present with unresectable locally advanced and metastatic disease. Distant metastases occurs early; first to regional lymph nodes, then the liver, and occasionally to the lungs. There may also be local invasion into the neighbouring organs such as the stomach, duodenum, colon, or peritoneum, which can present with symptoms of early satiety, gastric outlet obstruction, or colonic obstruction. Bone metastases are rare.

6. What are the appropriate investigations in this case?

- Transabdominal ultrasound is often employed first for investigation of abdominal pain. It detects gallstones and lesions in the liver, as well as biliary dilatation, which is particularly relevant in the management of the jaundiced patient. However, it can rarely identify pathology at the distal CBD or pancreas, as this area is often obscured by overlying bowel gas.

◆ Cross-sectional imaging is the first-line diagnostic approach, particularly in patients with painless jaundice, to look for organic pathology:

  ◆ CT scans are sensitive for lesions over 2 cm wide. They can also accurately determine portal vein or superior mesenteric artery involvement, and can delineate tumour compression from invasion (Figure 3.2.1).

  ◆ T1/T2 weighted MRI images in conjunction with MRCP and CT are equivalent to CT in terms of assessing the presence and resectability of primary disease, so MRI is not routinely performed for staging pancreatic malignancy. However, it is useful to delineate pancreatic and biliary duct anatomy where the CT imaging is not diagnostic. Smaller lesions and microlithiasis can also be detected using EUS.

◆ PET imaging can detect lesions at 7 mm in diameter, as well as detect metastatic deposits, but is only used in equivocal cases where other imaging modalities are not diagnostic.

◆ EUS is more invasive but allows for a more comprehensive assessment of smaller pancreatic lesions and malignant distal biliary strictures, through imaging and access for biopsy and cytology. It can also be a useful adjunct for local staging of pancreatic cancer.

◆ Tumour markers can be measured in the serum in conjunction with diagnostic imaging. These raise concerns of a malignant process. Carbohydrate antigen 19.9 (CA19.9) is raised in half to three-quarters of cases. CEA is raised in 40–45% of cases. Tumour markers may be spuriously high in jaundiced patients, so these should be measured when the jaundice has been treated.

Imaging is not reliable for detecting peritoneal metastases. These lesions can be detected below 3 mm in size at laparoscopy, which is still used in conjunction with imaging in uncertain cases or depending on surgeon preference.

A diagnosis of pancreatic cancer on a background of chronic pancreatitis can be difficult and sometimes impossible to make without a definitive surgical resection. Main duct and side duct dilatation may be present, with or without focal abnormality of the parenchyma (calcification, atrophy, and fibrosis), on both CT and MRCP in both disease states. Biopsy can be taken for histological diagnosis percutaneously or at EUS, but this may be equivocal. In this scenario, both the MDT team and the patient need to be involved in deciding the next step, which may either be close observation with serial imaging or proceeding on to a surgical resection.

7. How should this patient be managed?

Following clinical assessment, bloods should be sent for coagulation screen, full blood count, liver and renal function, and electrolytes. Patients with biliary obstruction can occasionally present with cholangitis, which is life-threatening and a surgical emergency. Charcot's triad (abdominal pain, jaundice, and fever) is suggestive of ascending cholangitis and should be treated as such while arranging urgent investigation and treatment. This constitutes broad-spectrum antibiotics that cover enteric organisms, IV fluid resuscitation, and early critical care involvement where indicated. The patient may require immediate biliary decompression to definitively treat cholangitis where it does not respond to antibiotic therapy.

Patients with mild jaundice can be investigated on an urgent outpatient basis, whereas patients with established jaundice should be admitted for medical management, which includes:

- IV access and rehydration with IV crystalloid as they are often dehydrated.
- Fluid balance recording.
- IV vitamin K should be administered to correct a deranged clotting or prophylactically where bilirubin is raised above 100 and prior to any surgical interventions or procedures. Oral vitamin K should not be used as it is poorly absorbed.

Cross-sectional imaging should be arranged to establish a diagnosis.

Management should be determined by radiologists, pancreatic surgeons, and oncologists through the cancer MDT meeting at both the treating hospital and the tertiary HPB unit. Decisions should be made with the patient at surgical consultation.

Some surgeons may proceed to resection in the presence of mild jaundice (bilirubin <200μmol/l). However, jaundice is believed to put patients at increased risk of post-operative sepsis and liver failure, and higher rates of morbidity. Therefore, many surgeons prefer to decompress the biliary system before proceeding on to resection, once the jaundice has settled. This is done using an expandable biliary stent. This is best placed at ERCP, but where this is not possible or fails, it can be placed percutaneously using PTC by interventional radiologists. Biliary stenting can be performed to treat the jaundice ahead of MDT discussion and won't affect resectability, although plastic stents are more commonly used in potentially resectable disease and metal stents are considered more permanent.

Surgery is the only potentially curative treatment modality for pancreatic cancer. Only 20% of patients are potentially resectable on presentation. Locally advanced and metastatic disease is a contraindication to resection. Radiological features of locally advanced disease include tumour encasement of the neighbouring superior mesenteric artery and coeliac axis, as well as, peripancreatic lymphadenopathy. Portal vein and superior mesenteric vein invasion does not preclude resection, as the patient can undergo cancer resection and vascular reconstruction.

The main approach to resecting a pancreatic head or neck tumour is through pancreaticoduodenectomy, Kausch–Whipple's or Long–Myer's procedure. The traditional Whipple's procedure resected the pylorus alongside the pancreatic head, duodenum, CBD, gallbladder, and adjacent lymph nodes. However, for the majority of tumours the pylorus is now preserved in this procedure, unless there is evidence of tumour invasion.

Tumours in the body and tail are resected through distal pancrea-tectomy, with resection of the spleen in distal tumours. Total pancrea-tectomy can be carried out for large or multifocal tumours. Extensive lymphadenectomy is not carried out as there is no benefit to survival and has been associated with increased morbidity. Approximately a fifth of patients have been reported to have positive microscopic resection margins (termed an R1 resection), which is a poor prog-nostic factor.

Adjuvant chemotherapy is recommended post-operatively and has shown survival advantage in R0 resections.

Symptom palliation is difficult in locally advanced disease, as pain control is very difficult in these patients. Combination analgesic and anti-emetic regimes require palliative care team input and follow-up. Oral pancreatic enzyme supplements, such as Creon, can be given to optimize nutritional status.

Interventional techniques can be used to palliate obstructions:

- Severe pain can be palliated with a coeliac block, administered by anaesthetists.

- Biliary obstruction can be relieved by placement of a permanent metal biliary stent, either at ERCP or via PTC.

- Duodenal obstruction can be stented at upper GI endoscopy.

- Single-point bowel obstruction from peritoneal disease can be bypassed at laparotomy. Multiple-point obstruction cannot.

7. What is the prognosis of this disease?

Prognosis is poor. Median survival for untreated patients is 4–6 months. Pancreatic cancer is aggressive and has the one of the highest incidence to mortality ratios of any disease, particularly as less than 20% of patients are resectable on diagnostic imaging.

An R1 resection is considered a poor prognostic factor, with a median survival of 10 months and a 2-year survival rate of 25%. Outcome is marginally better for R0 resection, with median survival of 12–19 months and 5-year survival around 20%. Better outcomes are achieved in resections for neuroendocrine and cystic pancreatic neoplasms.

Further reading

Garrido-Laguna I, Hidalgo M (2015) Pancreatic cancer: from state-of-the-art treatments to promising novel therapies. *Nature Reviews Clinical Oncology* 12: 319–34.

Jarnagin WR (2012) *Blumgart's Surgery of the Liver, Biliary Tract and Pancreas*, fifth edition. Elsevier Saunders, Philadelphia USA.

Ryan DP, Hong TS, Bardeesy N (2014) Pancreatic adenocarcinoma. *New England Journal of Medicine* 371: 1039–49.

Case history 3.3: Elective: chronic pancreatitis

A 55-year-old woman presents to the acute surgical take with a 1-day history of acute abdominal pain. This is felt in the epigastrium and radiates through to the back. This is associated with vomiting. She has a long history of recurrent acute abdominal pain over several years, which had resulted in several admissions to hospital in the last 18 months. She has recently lost 4 kg of weight. She has no other past medical history. She has smoked 20 cigarettes a day for 15 years. She no longer drinks alcohol, although prior to this she drank heavily for many years. She was a shop assistant but lost her job several years ago. On examination she looks uncomfortable and drawn. Her vital signs are normal and she is apyrexial. Her abdomen is soft, but she is very tender in her epigastric region. Her blood results are shown in Table 3.3.1.

A contrast CT abdomen was performed on this admission and revealed global pancreatic atrophy with pancreatic calcifications in the main pancreatic duct with pancreatic duct dilatation throughout (Figure 3.3.1). A diagnosis of chronic pancreatitis was made. Her acute symptoms improved with opioid analgesia and, following discharge, she was referred to the regional pancreatic surgeon.

Table 3.3.1 Blood results

Hb	130
WCC	11
Neutrophils	9.5
Platelets	340
Albumin	38
ALP	115
ALT	40
CRP	15
Amylase	105
PT	10.5

Reproduced Courtesy of Judith Ritchie.

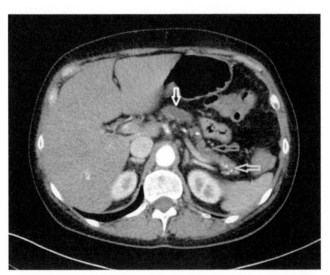

Figure 3.3.1 Image from the patient's abdominal CT scan showing atrophy of the pancreas gland (white arrow), pancreatic duct dilatation (top arrow), and pancreatic calcification in white (lower arrow).

Reproduced Courtesy of Judith Ritchie.

Questions

1. What are the relevant differential diagnoses?

2. What is chronic pancreatitis and how is it different to acute pancreatitis?

3. What is the pathophysiology of chronic pancreatitis?

4. What causes chronic pancreatitis?

5. How is chronic pancreatitis diagnosed?

6. How chronic pancreatitis managed?

Answers

1. What are the relevant differential diagnoses?

Acute pancreatitis is an important differential diagnosis to consider as this can make patients very sick; it can rapidly result in systemic illness, organ failure, and even death. Other causes of acute upper abdominal pain may present similarly, including severe gastritis, acute cholecystitis, perforated viscus, and referred pain from lower lobe pneumonia. Chronic pancreatitis is not commonly considered in the acute setting. Patients with chronic pancreatitis may present with an episode of moderate or severe acute pancreatitis. However, this may be difficult to diagnose biochemically as the disease process may have damaged the pancreas tissue to such a degree that the serum amylase may not rise in response to inflammation. Where there is doubt in these cases, treatment should be based on clinical grounds, and imaging may also be useful both for diagnosis and to rule out other pathology where there is diagnostic doubt.

Chronic pancreatitis should be borne in mind with patients presenting with a history of recurrent episodic attacks of upper abdominal pain. It is thought that many sufferers are misdiagnosed, resulting in a significant delay in time to definitive diagnosis. This is compounded by the diagnostic difficulties of this disease, which are discussed in this case. Where the condition is suspected, patients could be referred to medical gastroenterology or a pancreatic surgeon for further assessment after discharge.

2. What is chronic pancreatitis and how is it different to acute pancreatitis?

The term chronic pancreatitis describes a chronic, irretractable, fibro-inflammatory disease of the pancreas gland, which results in glandular destruction and loss of function. Loss of pancreatic tissue results in loss of:

- Exocrine function: reduced pancreatic enzyme production resulting in malabsorption of vitamins, micronutrients and fats, with the development of steatorrhoea.

- Endocrine function: reduced insulin production results in insulin-dependent diabetes

The condition initially presents with chronic abdominal pain in the majority of sufferers that is difficult to control. Patients may describe a constant, chronic abdominal pain, which can affect appetite to varying degrees, or episodic attacks of acute abdominal pain with resolution of symptoms in between attacks. Episodes of severe pain may be associated with nausea and vomiting. Chronic pain can have an ongoing impact on appetite, resulting in weight loss. Patients can also develop malnutrition through loss of pancreatic enzyme production and subsequent malabsorption of fats and vitamins, as well as reduced nutritional intake.

The chronic inflammatory process can result in a number of pathological complications in established and advanced disease:

- Damage to the pancreatic duct from the fibro-inflammatory process results in extravasation of pancreatic fluid rich in its enzymes. The ductal disruption is sealed off in two-thirds of cases by fibrosis, and inflammatory tissue walls off the extravasated fluid and inflammatory tissue to form a pseudocyst. Occasionally these collections can communicate with bodily spaces to allow passage of pancreatic fluid, such as within the pleural space (pancreatic pleural effusion) or peritoneal cavity (pancreatic ascites). This fluid typically has a very high amylase content, which can be confirmed by sending aspirate for biochemistry.

- The inflammatory process can involve the adjacent organs surrounding the pancreas. The pathogenesis is not clear but it is thought to occur secondary to pancreatic outflow obstruction and pancreatic stasis. Alcohol and smoking have been reported to contribute to an increased viscosity of the pancreatic juice, which leads to calcification and plugging within the pancreatic duct, resulting in a degree of obstruction and dilatation. Inflammatory thickening and scarring of the minor papillae can result in fibrosis and stenosis of the duodenum and distal common bile duct.

◆ Pseudoaneurysm can arise in peripancreatic arteries (commonly the splenic and gastroduodenal arteries) as a result of arterial wall involvement from nearby inflammatory processes. These can rupture causing life-threatening bleeding. Angioembolization is a preferred approach to treatment, although they can re-bleed following embolization.

◆ Splenic vein thrombosis is thought to arise due to the pro-thrombotic effect of the neighbouring inflammatory process, and can result in portal hypertension with a risk of gastric variceal bleeding.

◆ Loss of endocrine function can result in diabetes which will rapidly require insulin control.

In the long term, chronic pancreatitis is associated with a four-fold increased risk of pancreatic malignancy. Focal glandular changes can result in mass effect on imaging, which can frequently cause diagnostic confusion as inflammatory tissue and cancer can be difficult to differentiate. Biopsies may also be equivocal, and patients may need to undergo complete resections to reach a final diagnosis.

Acute and chronic pancreatitis are debated to be part of the same disease spectrum, with chronic disease manifesting after an acute attack, which the patient may or may not have been hospitalized for. Features of acute and chronic pancreatitis are compared in Table 3.3.2.

Table 3.3.2 Comparison of the clinical features of the disease process in acute and chronic pancreatitis

	Acute pancreatitis	**Chronic pancreatitis**
Age range	**Any**	**Younger patients**
Precipitating factors	**Ethanol, gallstones**, drugs, hyperlipidaemia, autoimmune, idiopathic	**Ethanol**, smoking, idiopathic
Presentation	Acute attack of abdominal pain, vomiting, haemodynamic compromise; single/multiple	Acute exacerbations of abdominal pain and vomiting; chronic abdominal pain

Table 3.3.2 Continued

	Acute pancreatitis	Chronic pancreatitis
Age range	Any	Younger patients
Inflammatory process	Acute: can develop into SIRS and result in multiple organ failure; settles and resolves in 80% with no organ damage	Chronic irretractable inflammation resulting in organ damage and failure
Complications	Acute complications: 20% develop pancreatic necrosis or collections; long-term: pseudocysts	Pseudocysts, biliary duct strictures, pancreatic pleural effusion or ascites, duodenal stenosis, steatorrhoea, diabetes, malnutrition
Hospital admissions	One or several	Multiple
Quality of life	Good where condition resolves without sequelae; affected by presence of complications	Significantly affected due to chronic severe symptoms, malnutrition, weight loss
Treatment	Supportive	Symptom palliation, nutritional supplements, insulin for diabetes

Features in bold are common and established factors.

Reproduced Courtesy of Judith Ritchie.

3. What is the pathophysiology of chronic pancreatitis?

The nature of the inflammatory process is not fully understood, however pancreatic stellate cells have been reported to play a role in initiating fibrosis, particularly in alcoholic pancreatitis. These cells reside within the pancreatic tissue. They are activated by inflammatory cytokines, transforming them into myofibroblast-like cells that instigate fibrosis. This ultimately results in glandular fibrosis, with destruction of normal anatomy and loss of function.

Pain is thought to be mediated by two channels:

◆ Chemical protease release from damaged tissue, which can activate nociceptive neurones and result in pain downstream of a number of different signalling pathways.

◆ High-pressure pancreatic duct obstruction can result in constant pain.

4. What causes chronic pancreatitis?

Chronic pancreatitis has previously been associated with a number of risk factors. The most common cause of chronic pancreatitis is alcohol. However, dose-dependent causation has not been definitively demonstrated. Only 10% of heavy drinkers develop the condition and the disease does occur in those who drink much less. This has led to the conclusion that the disease is multifactorial and a number of clinical, genetic, and pathological features interact to result in chronic pancreatitis. These are outlined in a number of classification systems, such as the M-ANNHEIM classification system: Multiple-Alcohol, Nicotine, Nutrition, Hereditary, Efferent pancreatic duct, Immunological, and Miscellaneous. This is outlined in Table 3.3.3.

Table 3.3.3 Detailed summary of the multifactorial aetiology of chronic pancreatitis

M	Multiple risk factors	
A	Alcohol consumption	Excessive (>80 g/day)
		Increased (20–80 g/day)
		Moderate (<20 g/day)
N	Nicotine consumption	
N	Nutritional factors	Hyperlipidaemia
		High fat/high protein diet
H	Hereditary	Hereditary pancreatitis
		Familial pancreatitis
		Early-onset idiopathic pancreatitis
		Late-onset idiopathic pancreatitis
		Tropical pancreatitis
		PSSR1, CFTR, SPINK1 gene mutations
E	Efferent duct factors	Pancreas divisum
		Annular pancreas, congenital abnormalities
		Pancreatic duct obstruction, e.g. malignancy
		Post-traumatic pancreatic duct scars
		Sphincter of Oddi dysfunction

Table 3.3.3 Continued

M	Multiple risk factors	
I	Immunological/autoimmune factors	Sjogrens syndrome
		Inflammatory bowel disease
		Autoimmune disease-related, e.g. primary sclerosing cholangitis, primary biliary cirrhosis
M	Miscellaneous/metabolic	Hypercalcaemia
		Hyperparathyroidism
		Chronic renal failure
		Drugs
		Toxins

Reproduced with permission from Schneider A, Lohr JM, Singer MV, 'The M-ANNHEIM classification of chronic pancreatitis: introduction of a unifying classification system based on a review of previous classifications of the disease', *Journal of Gastroenterology*, Volume 42, Issue 2, pp. 101–19, Copyright © 2007 Springer-Verlag Tokyo, DOI: 10.1007/s00535-006-1945-4

5. How is chronic pancreatitis diagnosed?

Diagnosis is achieved through a combination of imaging, functional tests, and histological confirmation from tissue biopsy.

Ultrasound and CT are commonly used for patients presenting with such symptoms, but their diagnostic capabilities are limited as they can only detect changes in advanced disease:

- Ultrasound can only detect hyperechogenic pancreatic tissue in a fibrosed, atrophic gland in established and advanced disease, and this is not commonly seen. However, it can also detect complications of the disease such as pancreatic ascites, pseudoaneurysms, and pseudocysts.

- CT can detect the same changes, as well as glandular atrophy and fibrosis, and pancreatic calcifications. It can also detect a greater range of complications, as it can image the surrounding organs more accurately, such as the bile duct, duodenum, and bowel.

- MRI is relatively more diagnostically sensitive earlier in the disease process, as loss of signal in T1 images can occur before morphological parenchymal changes develop. Use of secretin MRCP is advocated as a functional imaging test, as the amount of pancreatic secretion in response to secretin can be quantified, which can give an objective assessment of function.

◆ Endoscopic ultrasound (EUS) is the most sensitive imaging modality, which can consistently detect features such as hyperechoic foci, lobularity, and honeycombing of the gland, with main and side-branch dilatation and intraductal calculi. It also allows tissue to be taken for biopsy. EUS has superseded ERCP as a diagnostic investigation in this regard as it is associated with reduced morbidity.

◆ The gold standard functional test is 72-hour faecal fat quantification. 13C-mixed triglyceride breath test and secretin MRCP have also reported excellent sensitivities and specificities but are less widely available.

6. How is chronic pancreatitis managed?

Management is palliative. There are no targeted treatments that are effective or restorative against the disease process. Treatment aims to improve and maintain patients' quality of life. It is multidisciplinary, involving the GP, a gastroenterologist, pancreatic surgeon, dietician, and chronic pain team.

Management should incorporate:

◆ *Pain control*. This can be complex and difficult. Analgesia should be titrated to the patients' needs, working with the WHO analgesic ladder using simple and opioid preparations. In addition, pregabalin and gabapentin can be used as these are effective for nociceptive pain. Where pharmacological measures fail to control symptoms, more invasive measures may be required. Persistent pain in the presence of pancreatic duct dilatation may respond well to ductal decompression, which can be attempted endoscopically or surgically. In the absence of ductal dilatation, invasive measures can target the neural supply around the gland, e.g. coeliac nerve blocks, splanchnic nerve ablation, and nerve modulators.

◆ *Nutrition*. This should be optimized to avoid malnutrition. Patients should be started on oral enzyme replacement regimes (such as Creon), even when they do not have a history of stea-torrhoea, as a supportive measure as these patients may not be producing enough pancreatic enzymes, and enzymes can help to prevent or delay malabsorption or steatorrhoea. Ongoing dietician input and clinical follow-up is crucial. Where patients develop malnutrition despite oral enzyme and dietetic support, further intervention may be necessary such as nasogastric or PEG feeding to deliver high-calorie feed.

- *Localized complications.* Biliary and duodenal stenosis can result in jaundice and gastric outlet obstruction, respectively. These may be stented to relieve obstruction, but young patients should be offered definitive surgical management as this generally achieves a better quality of life in the long term, and avoids complications of stents such as blockage, infection, and displacement. Symptomatic pseudocysts include large cysts that compress adjacent organs, such as the stomach, causing pain and gastric outlet obstruction, and, rarely, sepsis from infection within the cyst. These are usually drained percutaneously or internally via interventional radiology through a transgastric approach.

Surgery is warranted for irretractible pain with poor quality of life and high opiate requirements.

- The dilated pancreatic duct can be decompressed by opening the duct and creating a pancreaticojejunostomy. This allows the duct to drain whilst preserving any functional residual tissue. It uses a Roux loop of jejenum that is moved to the pancreas through a mesocolic window. A lateral pancreaticojejunostomy involves opening the duct along its long axis of the gland, creating a jejunotomy along the length of the jejunal loop and creating a side-to-side anastomosis.

- Resection of fibrous tissue and ductal drainage has good reported outcomes in terms of symptomatic relief in patients with irretractible pain failing all other interventional measures. This would involve combining focal resection of the pancreatic head with longitudinal pancreaticojejunostomy (Frey's procedure) or distal pancreas with lateral pancreaticojejunostomy in those with dilated pancreatic ducts. Kausch–Whipple's procedure is used for patients with chronic pain and involvement of the duodenum and biliary system, resecting the pancreatic head and duodenum, and reconstructing the distal bile duct with a hepaticojejunostomy.

Patients should be monitored for important complications including:

- *Malignancy.* Diagnosis can be difficult, as focal fibrotic change to the gland can present a mass effect on imaging that is indistinguishable from malignancy. Malignancy and pancreatitis can often be found together, and the tumour can even induce pancreatitis. The patient may be monitored by serial imaging and proceed to resection if there are any changing features or growth, or proceed straight to resection where there are clinically concerning features. The frequency of surveillance imaging in chronic pancreatitis patients is determined by the lead clinician, usually with CT of the pancreas to detect the development of malignancy.

- *Diabetes.* These patients become insulin-dependent very quickly, as they lose significant amounts of endocrine tissue.

Further reading

Braganza JM (2011) Chronic pancreatitis. *Lancet* 377 (9772): 1184–97.

De-Madaria E, Abad-González A, Aparicio JR, Aparisi L, Boadas J, Boix E et al. (2013) The Spanish Pancreatic Club's recommendations for the diagnosis and management of chronic pancreatitis: Part 2 (treatment). *Pancreatology* 13 (1): 18–23.

Forsmark CE (2013) Management of chronic pancreatitis. *Gastroenterology* 144 (6): 1282–91; e3, doi: 10.1053/j.gastro.2013.02.008.

Gachego C, Draganov PV (2008) Pain management in chronic pancreatitis. *World Journal of Surgery* 14 (20): 3137–48.

Martinez J, Abad-González A, Aparicio JR, Aparisi L, Boadas J, Boix E et al. The Spanish Pancreatic Club's recommendations for the diagnosis and management of chronic pancreatitis: Part 1 (diagnosis). *Pancreatology* 13 (1): 8–17.

Case history 3.4: Emergency: acute pancreatitis

A 41-year-old female presents with a 6-hour history of sudden onset and worsening upper abdominal pain radiating through to her back and shoulder blades. She has vomited several times and feels very unwell. Prior to this she was well. Her bowel habit is normal and there is no history of jaundice. She has not had any previous episodes. She has had some self-limiting episodes of right-upper quadrant pain after eating over the past few months, and she is awaiting an appointment for an abdominal ultrasound ordered by her GP for this. She has no other past medical history and is not on regular medications. She is a secretary who smokes five cigarettes a day and drinks approximately eight units a week with no prior history of alcohol excess. On examination she looks acutely unwell and dehydrated. She is not jaundiced. Her blood pressure is 95/55, her pulse is regular at 110 beats a minute. Her temperature is 37.8°C. Her respiratory rate is 20 respirations per minute and her saturations are 94% on air. On examination, her abdomen is very tender in the epigastrium but there is no evidence of peritonism and no palpable masses. Table 3.4.1 shows her blood results.

A diagnosis of acute pancreatitis is made.

Table 3.4.1 Blood results

Na	145	Bili	20	PT	11.3	ABG:	
K	5	ALP	140	APTT	50	pH	7.34
Ur	5	AST	30	Fib	5	pO_2	10
Cr	95	ALT	41	Hb	140	pCO_2	5.5
Amylase	1,424	WCC	16	HCO_3	18		
CRP	5	Neut	10	Lactate	2		
Plts	230						

Reproduced courtesy of Judith Ritchie

Questions

1. What are the differentials of this presentation?
2. What is the pathophysiology of this disease?
3. List some common causative factors.
4. How does it present?
5. What are the appropriate investigations?
6. How should acute pancreatitis be managed?
7. What are the most concerning complications of acute pancreatitis?
8. What is the outcome of this disease?

Answers

1. What are the differentials of this presentation?

This case is clinically consistent with acute pancreatitis.

Other differential diagnoses that should be covered in the clinical assessment include perforated duodenal ulcer and cholecystitis. These can both also present with acute abdominal pain and a hyperamylasaemia below the diagnostic threshold of acute pancreatitis. In duodenal perforation there is often also guarding and peritonism from free intestinal contents, but this may also be present in some people with acute pancreatitis. It may also be absent if duodenal perforation is currently sealed by surrounding organs. Duodenal perforation may also have a preceding history of epigastric pain or discomfort and possibly gastrooesophageal reflux, although these can be absent, particularly where the patient has a perforated ulcer following NSAID use. Acute cholecystitis can present with upper abdominal pain with features of sepsis, although onset is relatively more insidious. The pain may be central or radiate around one or both sides of the chest wall. Upper abdominal pain can also be the presenting feature of bacterial or atypical pneumonia with referred pain, and this may or may not have a pleuritic element.

2. What is the pathophysiology of this disease?

The majority of the gland is involved in digestive enzyme production through the pancreatic acinar cell, with the remaining glandular tissue coordinating glucose homeostasis through the islet cell. Acinar cells produce and store digestive enzymes in zymogen granules in their proenzyme form, which protects the gland from autodigestion. These are released from the zymogen into the pancreatic duct in response to cholecystokinin (CCK) and vasoactive intestinal polypeptide (VIP), which are secreted as food passes through the stomach. Trypsinogen is activated once it is released into the duodenum on the intestinal brush border when it becomes trypsin, and this then activates the other 15 or so proenzymes within the small intestine.

Acute pancreatitis is inflammation of the pancreas gland. It is initiated by damage to the pancreatic acinar cell. It is thought that this is mediated by both duct obstruction from biliary stones and localized cellular toxicity from alcohol. Proenzymes are released from the damaged cell and trypsinogen is prematurely activated to trypsin within the pancreatic tissue, thereafter activating other proenzymes. These damage local tissue, generating an acute inflammatory reaction. Neutrophils and macrophages infiltrate the tissue and release a number of cytokines such as interleukin 6 and 8 and TNFα that generate local and systemic inflammatory responses. Local inflammatory response results in increased permeability of the vascular pancreatic bed, resulting in parenchymal oedema, haemorrhage, and ultimately necrosis. Systemic inflammatory response syndrome (SIRS) results in global loss of systemic vascular tone and systemic shock with renal hypoperfusion and renal failure. Pulmonary vascular permeability can arise as part of the SIRS response and can result in pulmonary oedema and infiltrates, which can progress to acute respiratory distress syndrome and acute respiratory failure.

3. List some common causative factors

The most common causes are *gallstones* and *ethanol.*

Other causes should be sought in the presenting history:

◆ *Abdominal trauma.*

◆ *Anatomical anomalies.* Pancreatic divisum occurs where dorsal and ventral pancreatic buds fail to fuse during embryological development, resulting in two pancreatic ducts. Annular pancreatitis is a developmental anomaly where pancreatic tissue surrounds the duodenum. Pancreatitis is thought to occur due to stenosis or obstruction of the pancreatic duct outflow as a result of these anatomical anomalies.

◆ *Autoimmune pancreatitis.* This is very rare, occurring in patients under 40 years of age.

◆ *Drugs.* These include azathioprine, tetracycline, 5-aminosalicylic acid, corticosteroids, oestrogens, and furosemide.

- *ERCP-induced pancreatitis.* Pancreatic duct cannulation can irritate the pancreatic duct and result in pancreatitis.
- *Genetic tendency.* SPINK1 mutation (encodes protein that inactivates trypsin); cationic trypsinogen gene (PRSS1) gain of function (catalyses trypsinogen activation to trypsin); CFTR mutation.
- *Hypertriglyceridaemia.* (NB Lipid profiles should be measured once the acute inflammation has resolved.)
- *Pancreatic tumour.* This is a rare cause.
- *Scorpion bite.* Endemic in Asia.
- *Viral illness.* Mumps, cytomegalovirus, Epstein–Barr virus, measles, and varicella zoster.
- *Idiopathic.*

4. How does it present?

This is a common cause for emergency presentation to A&E. It presents with sudden onset of severe upper abdominal pain, classically epigastric and radiating through to the back. There is often associated vomiting. Patients may be febrile if there is a systemic inflammatory response. They may also be febrile if there is biliary obstruction from gallstones and ascending infection, in which case they may be clinically jaundiced. Patients may show signs of organ dysfunction secondary to the SIRS response with reduced saturations or crepitations on auscultation and reduced urine output. Patients may be tachycardic and hypotensive, which may be due to the SIRS response causing systemic vasodilatation but this may also be compounded by dehydration.

5. What are the appropriate investigations?

Investigations include:

- Full blood count, liver and renal function, calcium, coagulation. White cell count is commonly raised.
- Serum amylase or lipase. Acute pancreatitis is diagnosed where the serum amylase is 3–4 times the normal limit units. However, it can normalize within 24 hours. Lipase is more sensitive as this

can remain elevated for 3 days. However, it is important to know that these enzymes may also be normal in established pancreatitis.

- CRP is helpful.

- Erect chest X-ray can help by ruling out pneumoperitoneum from a perforated viscus. A plain abdominal radiograph is rarely diagnostic. A sentinel loop is rarely seen (gaseous extension of the right colon stopping abruptly at the mid-transverse colon).

- CT imaging of the abdomen may be performed on admission where other differential diagnoses need to be excluded, such as perforated duodenal ulcer, or where amylase is not diagnostically high. Pancreatic inflammation may or may not be seen in acute pancreatitis. However, CT is not routinely performed for diagnostic purposes.

- Abdominal ultrasound is a routine part of diagnostic workup, as it is the radiological modality that most accurately determines the presence of gallstones. It is not useful for visualizing an inflamed pancreas gland, this is rarely visualized.

- MRCP imaging is a common investigation to request in the presence of deranged liver function tests to ensure there are no ductal stones, which may occasionally be present with deranged liver function and a non-dilated biliary system if the stones aren't causing complete obstruction.

A diagnosis of acute pancreatitis is established when two of the following criteria are present:

- Appropriate clinical history.
- Radiological evidence of pancreatitis.
- Biochemical evidence of pancreatitis.

6. How should acute pancreatitis be managed?

A full assessment of the patient's cardiovascular, respiratory, neurological and abdominal systems (using the so-called ABCDE approach) should be carried out to determine the current clinical and haemodynamic status of the patient. High flow oxygen should be administered. IV access should be obtained and IV fluid resuscitation should be administered. Strict fluid balance is mandatory. Acute pancreatitis is associated with large, rapid, third space losses, which can result in severe dehydration, and SIRS can also impact on renal function, which can deteriorate rapidly. Therefore patients should be catheterized. Arterial blood gas is a useful investigation as this gives you crucial information on the metabolic state of the patient. Evidence of acidosis (falling bicarbonate, rising lactate) indicates tissue hypoperfusion. Pyrexia occurs as part of the SIRS response and therefore does not necessarily indicate sepsis. However, in patients with jaundice and acute pancreatitis it is reasonable to assume an obstructed biliary tree, and ascending cholangitis cannot be clinically excluded. Therefore, administration of empirical broad-spectrum antibiotics may be reasonable.

SIRS can progress onto respiratory, cardiovascular, or renal failure. Hypotension refractory to over 2 litres of fluid bolus, increasing oxygen requirements and respiratory exhaustion, and oliguria are criteria for immediate escalation to critical care. Patients may require non-invasive ventilation, inotropic support, or haemofiltration in these scenarios.

Nutrition is very important. Early enteral nutrition is safe where it can be clinically tolerated. This can be instigated with oral diet, alternatively patients may tolerate feeding through a nasojejunal tube where there is delayed gastric emptying secondary to pancreatic inflammation. Enteral feeding helps to maintain the function and integrity of the bowel wall. Dietician involvement is essential and patients should be monitored for signs of malabsorption. Where enteral feeding cannot be tolerated in acute severe pancreatitis, patients should be treated with parenteral nutritional support.

7. What are the most concerning complications of acute pancreatitis?

The complications of SIRS and their subsequent morbidity and mortality are the first and foremost concern. Various scoring systems have been devised and used in different units on admission and within 48 hours of clinical presentation to identify patients with organ dysfunction and any subsequent deterioration. These include the Ranson, Imrie, and Glasgow criteria, as well as APACHE II scoring, and are useful for junior doctors in training if they understand the indication for using it. These patients can generally be identified more rapidly where SIRS is diagnosed. SIRS criteria set out by the Society of Critical Care Medicine are met with two of more of the following:

◆ Temperature over 38ºC or less than 36ºC.

◆ Heart rate above 90 beats per minute.

◆ Respiratory rate over 20 breaths per minute or $PaCO_2$ of <32 mmHg.

◆ White cell count above 12 or under $4 \times 10^9/l$.

The second concern is the risk of developing late complications as a consequence of pancreatic tissue damage. Pancreatic necrosis occurs where the inflammatory process has disrupted blood flow to the pancreas tissue and resulted in ischaemia and infarction. It predisposes to peripancreatic collections of fluid, inflammatory cells, and pancreatic enzymes. Both necrosis and peripancreatic collections may become infected. Elevated CRP levels after 48 hours of presentation suggest an ongoing inflammatory process and a higher risk of pancreatic necrosis. This patient deteriorated the day after admission, becoming tachycardic, pyrexial, and confused. She also developed type 1 respiratory failure. Her repeat CRP rose to 413. Patients with persistently elevated inflammatory markers, ongoing SIRS, or persisting clinical features should be imaged with contrast CT of the pancreas. This may show pancreatic necrosis, which can fuel further SIRS response. Her repeat CT revealed peripancreatic inflammation and evidence of patchy necrosis in the body and the head of the pancreas (Figure 3.4.1). If infected necrosis needs to be ruled out, pancreatic tissue may need to be sampled by fine-needle aspiration for culture and sensitivity. Necrosis driving ongoing SIRS through inflammation or infection may need to be debrided, which is commonly carried out by minimally invasive necrosectomy. Infected collections will require percutaneous drainage and samples sent for culture.

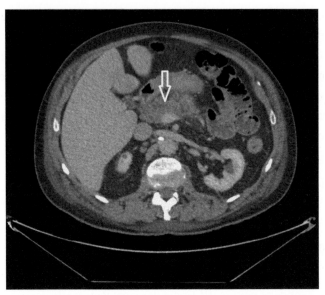

Figure 3.4.1 An image from abdominal CT following clinical deterioration a few days after admission. This shows a swollen pancreas with some peri-pancreatic fluid, confirming the diagnosis of pancreatitis. Patches of pancreatic tissue are not enhancing as the tissue normally should, appearing dark on the CT image (depicted by arrow), suggestive of pancreatic necrosis.

Reproduced Courtesy of Judith Ritchie.

Other late complications include pancreatic pseudocysts, where peripancreatic collections have been walled off with fibrous tissue. These are generally asymptomatic and resolve spontaneously over time, although large cysts can cause symptoms by compression on adjacent structures (e.g. gastric outlet obstruction or abdominal pain and mass effect). Rupture is rare but will result in peritonitis, warranting laparotomy and washout. Infection of pseudocysts is very rare and requires percutaneous drainage.

8. What is the outcome of this disease?

In 80% of cases, acute pancreatitis resolves within a week with resolution of any associated organ dysfunction within 48 hours of onset and without any long-term sequelae. In 20% of cases there may be persistent organ failure for more than 48 hours. This is termed acute severe pancreatitis. These patients require protracted inpatient treatment. Mortality is high, reported up to 50%.

Once the acute episode has settled, the cause of the pancreatitis should be sought and treated. For instance, in gallstone pancreatitis, cholecystectomy is advised within 2 weeks of the presentation of pancreatitis. Patients with alcohol-induced pancreatitis should be counselled to stop drinking. Patients with negative imaging and no obvious cause should be followed up in outpatients and imaging should be repeated along with investigations for less common causes, including hyperlipidaemia and immunoglobulins for auto-immune pancreatitis.

Further reading

Banks PA, Bollen TL, Dervenis C, Gooszen HG, Johnson CD, Sarr MG et al. (2013) Classification of acute pancreatitis-2012: revision of the Atlanta classification and definitions by international consensus. *Gut* **62**: 102–11.

Lankisch PG, Apte M, Banks PA (2015) Acute pancreatitis. *Lancet* **386**: 85–96.

Van Brunschot S, Bakker OJ, Besselink MG, Bollen TL, Fockens P, Gooszen HG et al. (2012) Treatment of necrotizing pancreatitis. *Clinical Gastroenterology Hepatology* **10**: 1190–201.

Case history 3.5: Emergency: pancreatic trauma

A 41-year-old man was taken to hospital following a road-traffic collision. He was driving his vehicle when a car pulled out in front of him and he suffered a head-on collision as he decelerated from 50 mph. He was not wearing a seatbelt and the steering wheel struck him across his abdomen. He presented with severe upper abdominal pain. His blood pressure was 105/60 and his pulse was 105 and regular. Erect chest X-ray, taken as part of the primary trauma assessment, was unremarkable. A trauma body CT scan was performed and revealed complete transection of the pancreas (Figure 3.5.1). Blood results are shown in Table 3.5.1.

He underwent an urgent laparotomy, where the proximal pancreatic stump was oversewn and the distal pancreas and spleen were removed.

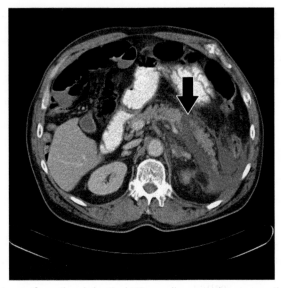

Figure 3.5.1 Image from the abdominal CT revealing complete transection of the pancreas (see arrow).

Reproduced Courtesy of Dr Anthony Blakeborough.

Table 3.5.1 Blood results

Hb	135
WCC	15
Neutrophils	11
Platelets	230
Bilirubin	15
ALP	120
ALT	45
Amylase	1,530
CRP	75

Questions

1. How common is pancreatic damage in trauma?

2. What mode of injuries result in pancreatic trauma?

3. How does pancreatic trauma present?

4. What investigations should be carried out in these patients?

5. How are pancreatic injuries managed?

6. Describe complications of pancreatic injury and their management.

This case focuses on pancreatic trauma. More detailed information about the assessment and management of abdominal trauma can be found in Case 7.6 Blunt abdominal trauma in Chapter 7.

Answers

1. How common is pancreatic damage in trauma?

Pancreatic injury is rare, occurring in less than 1% of trauma patients. It is difficult to diagnose. In the majority of cases, injury usually involves other adjacent organs and structures, in particular the duodenum (20%), the liver (50%), stomach (40%), spleen (30%), kidney (23%), and major vessels (40%). These organs are more superficial to the pancreas and, therefore, equally if not more prone to damage.

2. What mode of injuries result in pancreatic trauma?

Pancreatic damage is inflicted through both blunt and penetrating injuries.

The soft consistency of the pancreatic gland confers more protection from blunt trauma as it is retroperitoneal and cushioned by adjacent organs and overlying abdominal fat. The majority of blunt injuries are sustained through road-traffic accidents. Pancreatic injury is relatively more common in penetrating trauma.

Blunt injuries can be one or a combination of the following:

- Deceleration injuries. These occur in road-traffic accidents and falls from a significant height.

- Crushing injuries, such as steering wheel injuries in motorists or handlebars in cyclists.

These injuries can shear the pancreas against the vertebrae. A relative paucity of overlying fat in children makes the organ relatively more vulnerable to blunt trauma injury, such as a kick or fall, or through crushing injury against handlebars. Almost two-thirds of blunt injuries result in damage to the pancreatic body, with injuries to the tail and head being relatively less common. Shearing can result in pancreatic laceration, which tends to occur at the junction of the body and tail. Penetrating injuries are sustained through knife and gunshot wounds.

3. How does pancreatic trauma present?

Patients with pancreatic trauma are at risk of bleeding and pancreatic duct disruption. Patients with severe pancreatic head injury may bleed profusely from damage to major vessels running through or adjacent to the pancreatic head, presenting, at worst, in hypovolaemic and refractory shock with abdominal distension. This is a leading cause of mortality in this mode of injury. These patients require immediate laparotomy to attempt to control the bleeding. In stable patients a detailed history of the accident and the mechanisms of injury should be taken. It should be borne in mind that there may be severe vascular injury in a haemodynamically stable patient, as it may be tamponaded by the weight of the liver.

Pancreatic trauma can result in laceration or transection of pancreatic tissue, which can disrupt or even completely transect the pancreatic duct. Bile leak into the intra-abdominal cavity will cause localized peritonism and sepsis. Shoulder tip pain suggests phrenic nerve irritation from blood or bile in the subdiaphragmatic space. Bruising to the flank can suggest bleeding into the retroperitoneal space.

4. What investigations should be carried out in these patients?

Blood should be taken for haematology, coagulation, amylase, urea and electrolytes, and crossmatching. Leukocytosis is common following injury and may persist in the presence of pancreatitis.

Serum amylase can be helpful as it may be raised in pancreatic injury. The amylase level may remain persistently raised or rise over the course of a few days and is indicative of pancreatic injury. However, it is not a reliable diagnostic marker as it may be normal on first measurement, even in cases of complete transection. Levels do not correlate with severity of injury. However, it should be borne in mind that hyperamylasaemia may occur in response to other intra-abdominal pathology, such as duodenal, small bowel, and liver injury.

Plain radiographs are rarely specific but are generally carried out as part of trauma assessment as they can reveal important signs suggesting visceral trauma, such as pneumoperitoneum and extraluminal gas (Rigler's sign), as well as detecting skeletal abnormalities. Elevated right hemidiaphragm, fractured lower ribs, and loss of psoas shadow can suggest retroperitoneal bleeding. Emergency department bedside ultrasound is not commonly used in a patient presenting with polytrauma, and haemodynamically stable patients usually progress on to CT, as it rapidly generates high-resolution images.

CT is a gold standard for investigating abdominal trauma. Pancreas CT allows:

• *Delineation of the pancreatic duct.* Disruption of the pancreatic duct is an indicator for surgical intervention, as untreated rupture or stenosis of the pancreatic duct results in delayed morbidity. However, pancreatic duct disruption is not always apparent on imaging. It may, however, be inferred depending on the degree or type of parenchymal injury. Repeat imaging is reasonable where abdominal pain persists or amylase increases as subtle injuries to the duct may become more apparent.

• *Assessment of pancreatic parenchyma.* Direct signs of organ injury include focal gland enlargement or intrapancreatic haematoma. Active bleeding can be detected through active extravasation on contrast CT. Contusion can be visualized as focal or diffuse areas of low attenuation. Pancreatic fracture may be seen as glandular fragments along its long axis, but may not be visualized if fragments are not displaced. Laceration may be visualized as a hypodense line running perpendicular to the pancreas, and a higher degree of suspicion afforded where there is an adjacent (communicating) fluid collection or haematoma. Indirect features include peripancreatic and pararenal fluid collections, haemorrhage, peripancreatic fat stranding, and thickening of the left renal fascia.

Suspected pancreatic duct disruption has historically been investigated in equivocal imaging using ERCP, as duct disruption can be confirmed by contrast extravasation through the disrupted duct. However, MRCP is now used to image the pancreatic ductal system if there is concern of duct disruption that CT does not demonstrate. MRCP is much less invasive than ERCP and has the advantage of obtaining excellent views of the pancreatic parenchyma. Secretin MRCP can also be used and has been postulated to replace ERCP for determining pancreatic duct leakage, which is much less invasive with lower associated morbidity.

Angiography is an important diagnostic modality for locating occult bleeding vessels that have or have not been detected on cross-sectional imaging, which can then be subsequently embolized.

5. How are pancreatic injuries managed?

Surgical exploration is usually undertaken with gunshot or penetrating wounds where there are signs of peritonism or haemodynamic compromise, and the direct evaluation of the pancreas can be undertaken at the same time.

Parenchymal transection against the vertebral column in blunt trauma may require transection of the body with ligation of the pancreatic duct and oversewing of the distal duct, if possible. This should leave half of the gland with very low risk of glandular insufficiency. This injury is likely to have resulted in injury to the splenic vasculature, which should be sought, and a splenectomy may not be avoidable in this case. However, in most cases resection is not required after blunt trauma. Penetrating injuries can cause a range of direct and penetrating injuries to the gland. Deep, penetrating injury to the body and tail can be resected through distal pancreatectomy. Isolated injury to the pancreatic head can be drained by a Roux-en-Y pancreaticojejunostomy, whereas injury to the duodenum and pancreatic head may require a Whipple's procedure, although this is associated with a very high mortality rate. If there is evidence of bile from penetrating injuries an on-table cholangiogram and ductogram can be performed. Minor ductal damage may be amenable to stenting, either on table or at ERCP. Soft, closed suction drains can be placed around the pancreas in minor pancreatic injuries.

Pancreatic injury with an intact pancreatic duct can be managed conservatively with percutaneous drains if required. Pancreatic duct disruption is an indication for intervention, either surgical repair or pancreatic stenting at ERCP, where this is felt to be technically feasible in an otherwise stable patient.

Where there is no clinical or radiological concern of peritonism, active bleeding, visceral damage, or pancreatic duct disruption, the patient may be managed non-operatively and observed for at least 72 hours. The patient should be subjected to repeated clinical assessment, and serial amylase levels may be taken. If symptoms develop or persist, or amylase remains raised, CT imaging can be repeated or MRCP used to assess for pancreatic ductal injury.

The severity of pancreatic injury can be graded using the American Association for the Surgery of Trauma (AAST) scoring systems, which can be based on findings from radiological and/or surgical assessment (Table 3.5.2).

Table 3.5.2 The AAST pancreatic injury scoring system

Grade	Feature
I	Haematoma: minor contusion without ductal injury
	Laceration: superficial laceration without duct injury
II	Haematoma: major contusion without duct injury
	Laceration: major laceration without duct injury or tissue loss
III	Distal transection or parenchymal injury with duct injury
IV	Laceration: proximal transection or parenchymal injury involving ampulla or bile duct
V	Massive disruption of the pancreatic head

Reproduced with permission from Moore EE, Cogbill TH, Malangoni MA et al., 'Organ injury scaling, II: Pancreas, duodenum, small bowel, colon, and rectum', *The Journal of Trauma and Acute Care Surgery*, Volume 30, Issue 11, pp. 1427–9, Copyright © 1990 Wolters Kluwer.

6. **Describe the complications of pancreatic injury and their management.**

Immediate complications of pancreatic injury include:

+ *Post-trauma pancreatitis.* This can be seen on imaging as pancreatic oedema with haemorrhage and fluid accumulation in the anterior pararenal space. It is managed conservatively.

+ *Pancreatic pseudocysts.* These suggest loss of ductal integrity or leakage from a capsular tear of the pancreas gland and warrant further assessment of the pancreatic ductal system. Pancreatic pseudocysts in children are most commonly caused by trauma.

The majority of minor and isolated pancreatic injuries settle with no further sequelae. A fifth of patients develop pancreas-related morbidity. Delayed diagnosis and treatment are associated with a higher rate of morbidity and mortality. Late mortality is often from infection and subsequent organ failure.

Delayed complications from pancreatic duct injuries include:

+ Abscess formation (25% of cases). These often arise from fluid collections contaminated with Gram-negative intestinal bacteria. Management requires percutaneous or surgical drainage.

+ Fistula formation, reported in up to half of cases. Low-output fistulas may resolve spontaneously. High-output fistulas or fistulas associated with collections or infected collections require interventional management. Patients should receive supportive management, including nutritional support. Somatostatin can be used to decrease fistula output and assist closure, and collections can be drained percutaneously or endoscopically. Fistulation arising from a main pancreatic duct laceration can be treated by endoscopic stenting of the duct. Definitive surgical management in persistent fistulas depends on the region of the gland from which the fistula has formed and includes distal pancreatectomy.

◆ Delayed ductal stricture and fibrosis. This can develop in the years following the trauma, and can result in glandular atrophy. Patients may be symptomatic developing a picture of chronic pancreatitis.

Further reading

Debi U, Kaur R, Prasad KK, Sinha SK, Sinha A, Singh K (2013) Pancreatic trauma: a concise review. *World Journal of Gastroenterology* 19 (47): 9003–11.

Stawicki SP, Schwab CW (2008) Pancreatic trauma: demographics, diagnosis and management. *American Surgeon* 74 (12): 1133–45.

Chapter 4

Colorectal surgery

Peter Webster, Judith Ritchie,
and Veerabhadram Garimella

Case history 4.1: Elective: constipation

A 73-year-old female attends clinic complaining of a 1-year history of worsening constipation. She is now opening her bowels once every 5 days, despite taking regular senna. The motion is usually hard and is sometimes associated with bright red blood on wiping. She occasionally experiences 'gripey' abdominal pain and bloating. She has not lost any weight and there is no significant family history of note.

On examination she looks well. Her abdomen is distended but soft with no organomegaly or lymphadenopathy. Digital rectal examination (DRE) reveals hard faeces in the rectum but no palpable masses.

A colonoscopy performed 6 months ago was normal and blood tests performed recently by the GP were unremarkable.

Questions

1. What is constipation?

2. What are the risk factors for constipation?

3. What are the possible complications of constipation?

4. How should this patient be investigated?

5. What are the conservative treatment options for constipation?

6. What are the surgical treatment options for constipation and when should these be considered?

Answers

1. What is constipation?

The term 'constipation' has a variable definition between individuals. Medical professionals often define constipation as less than three bowel movements per week, but patients may equate constipation with stool consistency, feelings of incomplete emptying, or straining. Both constipation and chronic constipation are more clearly defined by the Rome III criteria, which is cited in the Further reading list for this case.

2. What are the risk factors for constipation?

The risk factors for constipation can be divided into extrinsic and intrinsic factors:

Extrinsic

- Low fibre intake.
- Poor hydration.
- Reduced mobility.
- Electrolyte disturbances (hypokalaemia, hypercalcaemia, hypermagnesemia).
- Endocrine disorders (hypothyroidism, hyperparathyroidism, diabetes mellitus, chronic renal failure).
- Painful anorectal conditions (haemorrhoids, anal fissure, proctalgia fugax).
- Neurological disorders (dementia, Parkinson's disease, spinal cord injury).
- Medications (opiates, anticholinergics, diuretics, iron supplements, dntidepressants).

Intrinsic

Normal defaecation requires a coordinated series of actions involving relaxation of the puborectalis muscle, descent of the pelvic floor, straightening of the anorectal angle, segmental inhibition of colonic peristalsis, abdominal wall muscle contraction, and relaxation of the anal sphincters. Any defect in this pathway can predispose to constipation. Intrinsic factors can be broadly divided into two categories: pelvic floor dysfunction and slow transit constipation.

+ *Pelvic floor dysfunction (PFD).* PFD encompasses a variety of problems, including laxity of the pelvic floor muscles, impaired rectal sensation, and reduced intraluminal pressure within the anal canal. Anatomically, the pelvic floor/anal canal unit can become distorted with rectal prolapse or perineal nerve damage (e.g. traumatic childbirth) leading to chronic constipation.

+ *Slow transit constipation (STC).* STC is characterized by reduced high-amplitude propagated contractions in the colon leading to the slow transit of faeces. Symptomatically, this results in abdominal discomfort, bloating, and infrequent defaecation. The exact mechanism underlying STC is poorly understood with several factors being implicated, including reduced cholinergic responses, enhanced adrenergic responses, and enteric neurodegeneration.

3. What are the possible complications of constipation?

Chronic constipation is an underlying factor in several anorectal conditions. Although most are benign, there are some that can be potentially life-threatening:

+ *Haemorrhoids.* The prolonged straining associated with chronic constipation and associated elevation in intra-abdominal pressure raises the pressure in the normal sub-mucosal arterio-venous vascular plexuses located in the anal canal. Resolution of constipation is essential in the treatment of haemorrhoids.

+ *Faecal incontinence.* This is the result of liquid faecal matter bypassing an obstructing solid bolus of faeces. This can lead to confusion in the diagnosis of constipation, as these patients often present complaining of diarrhoea.

◆ *Anal fissure.* Trauma to the lining of the anal canal can occur secondary to a dry, hard motions. As with haemorrhoids, the treatment of constipation is essential in helping fissures to heal.

◆ *Visceral prolapse.* Chronic constipation is a known risk factor for prolapse of the rectum, uterus, vagina, and bladder. Equally, rectal prolapse can be a causative factor for chronic constipation.

◆ *Large bowel obstruction.* The prolonged stasis of faecal matter in the rectum can lead to faecal impaction with a giant faecolith causing large bowel obstruction.

◆ *Stercoral perforation.* Prolonged faecal impaction can lead to pressure necrosis and perforation of the bowel wall culminating in stercoral peritonitis. This is associated with poor outcomes. It is very rare.

4. How should this patient be investigated?

Diagnosing constipation begins first with a detailed history to determine exactly what the patient means by the term 'constipation' and any specific risk factors for developing constipation. Physical examination includes abdominal, rectal, and gynaecological examinations.
Investigations for constipation include:

◆ *Blood tests.* Full blood count, urea and electrolytes, blood glucose, thyroid function tests. An iron-deficient anaemia may raise concern for colorectal malignancy. Hypothyroidism is associated with constipation. Elevated blood glucose may raise suspicion for undiagnosed diabetes mellitus and impaired urea and electrolytes may raise suspicion for underlying renal failure.

◆ *Colonoscopy.* This is the gold standard test if there is suspicion of colorectal malignancy causing the constipation.

◆ *Colonic transit studies.* This involves the patient swallowing a capsule that contains several small metal markers. After 5 days the patient has an abdominal X-ray and the location of the metal markers are assessed (Figure 4.1.1). If over 80% of the markers are excreted by day 5, then the colonic transit is grossly normal.

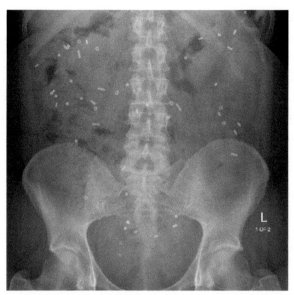

Figure 4.1.1 An X-ray image taken during colonic transit studies. A large number of metal markers can clearly be seen scattered throughout the large bowel (radio-opaque white circles and lines), suggestive in this case of colonic inertia.

Reproduced Courtesy of Judith Ritchie.

If greater than 20% of markers remain and are scattered about the colon, it is most likely due to colonic inertia. If the remaining markers are accumulated in the rectosigmoid, it is most likely due to functional outlet obstruction. Radionuclide scans are an alternative transit study that track a small amount of radioactive tracer as it progresses through the gastrointestinal tract. After ingestion of the tracer the patient attends daily to be scanned with a gamma camera. Computer analysis shows the proportion of radioactive tracer within various parts of the bowel. It is more accurate at measuring transit in differing parts of the colon, but is expensive and limited to areas that have radioisotope access.

♦ *Anorectal manometry.* This is a technique used to measure contractility in the rectum and anus. A catheter with a balloon containing a sensor is inserted into the anorectum. The patient is asked to contract and relax the sphincter muscles and try and expel the balloon whilst manometry measurements are taken.

◆ *Defaecating proctogram.* This is a form of real-time fluoroscopic imaging of a patient's defaecating mechanism. Following an enema, barium contrast is passed into the rectum and the patient is asked to defecate whilst a series of X-rays are taken. It can assess the anorectal angle, pelvic floor descent, efficiency of emptying, and size of the anal canal. It is useful for diagnosing rectocele, enterocele, sigmoidocele, internal/external rectal prolapse, and megarectum.

5. What are the conservative treatment options for constipation?

Conservative treatments can be divided into three categories: lifestyle modification, biofeedback, and pharmacological therapy.

1. Lifestyle modification.

   Patient advice regarding increased fibre intake, increased exercise, and keeping well hydrated is logical but actually lacks a formal evidence base.

2. Biofeedback.

   For PFD-type chronic constipation, biofeedback involves non-invasive retraining of the sensation and control of the pelvic floor and anorectum. Its value has been proven in improving psychological and clinical outcomes in chronic constipation.

3. Pharmacological therapy.

   There are a multitude of medical treatments available for the treatment of constipation. The correct choice of laxative agent depends upon the most likely aetiology.

◆ *Bulk-forming agents (e.g. ispaghula husks).* Bulk-forming agents are fibre supplements that expand with water to increase the bulk of stools and subsequently stimulate bowel movements. Adequate water intake is essential for this medication to work. These are considered a first-line agent in treating chronic constipation, especially in patients deficient in dietary fibre.

◆ *Stool softeners (e.g. docusate sodium).* Softens stools by having a detergent-like effect, facilitating interaction between stool and the colonic wall.

- *Osmotic agents (e.g. lactulose, polyethylene glycol 'PEG').* Osmotic agents retain water due to their hyperosmolar nature, helping the passage of stools. Studies have shown lactulose to have superior efficacy to placebo. Stool softeners should be considered in patients whom bulk-forming agents have no effect.

- *Stimulants (e.g. senna).* Stimulants act on the myenteric plexus of the colon, stimulating peristaltic contractions and resulting in a decrease in transit time.

- *Amber medications.* These are started by functional bowel specialists and include prucalopride, linaclotide, and lubiprostone.

  - Prucalopride (Resolor, Movetis) is a selective serotonin (5-HT_4) receptor agonist that stimulates colonic motility. NICE recommend prucalopride as a treatment for chronic constipation in women that have failed at least two laxatives of different classes at the highest recommended doses for 6 months and are considering invasive treatment.

  - Linaclotide (Linzess, Constella) is a guanylate cyclase 2C receptor agonist. It decreases activity of colonic sensory neurones and increases activity of colonic motor neurones. This results in reduced pain and increased smooth muscle contraction, promoting bowel movements. It is licensed for the treatment of moderate-to-severe irritable bowel syndrome with constipation.

  - Lubiprostone (Amitiza) is licensed for the treatment of chronic constipation in patients who have failed two laxatives from different classes at the maximum dose for at least 6 months. It is a bicyclic fatty acid derived from prostaglandin E1. It activates chloride channel protein 2 (CIC-2) chloride channels found on the apical aspect of gastrointestinal epithelial cells. This produces a chloride-rich secretion within the bowel lumen to aid bowel movement.

6. What are the surgical treatment options for constipation and when should these be considered?

Surgery is reserved for patients with intractable chronic constipation in STC in whom pharmacological treatments have failed.

Subtotal colectomy with ilio-rectal anastomosis is the operation of choice with patient satisfaction rates reported between 77 and 90%. Other surgical treatments include loop ileostomy, antegrade continence enema (ACE procedure), and sacral neuromodulation. The ACE procedure and sacral neuromodulation have been discussed.

◆ *Antegrade continence enema (ACE Procedure).* Also known as an antegrade appendicostomy, this involves anastomosing the appendix to the abdominal wall and fashioning a valve mechanism. The valve permits catheterization of the appendix through which an enema can be delivered, but also prevents leakage of stool. If the patient has previously had an appendicectomy, a neo-appendix can be created from the caecum.

◆ *Sacral neuromodulation.* Sacral nerve stimulators (SNSs) are implanted subcutaneously and deliver low-amplitude electrical stimulation to the sacral nerve via a lead. Often a temporary SNS is implanted initially to determine if the patient derives symptomatic benefit over several weeks. If symptoms improve this can be switched to a permanent device.

Further reading

Leung L, Riutta T, Kotecha J, Rosser W (2011) Chronic constipation: an evidence-based review. *Journal of the American Board of Family Medicine* 24(4): 436–51.

McCallum IJ, Ong S, Mercer-Jones M (2009) Chronic constipation in adults. *British Medical Journal* 338: b831.

Rome Foundation (2006) Guidelines—Rome III diagnostic criteria for functional gastrointestinal disorders. *Journal of Gastrointestinal Liver Disease* 15(3): 307–12.

Case history 4.2: Elective: anal fistula

A 29-year-old man was referred to clinic with a 4-week history of inter-mittent discharge per rectum. Approximately 1 month ago he devel-oped a perianal abscess that discharged spontaneously and he did not seek medical advice. Since that time he has opened his bowels regu-larly, but from time to time has noticed staining of his underwear with bloody and yellowish coloured discharge. He is otherwise systemically well. He has no past medical history. He smokes 10 cigarettes per day and does not drink alcohol.

On examination he looks well. His abdomen is soft with no palp-able masses, organomegaly, or lymphadenopathy. Digital rectal examination reveals evidence of a previous perianal abscess at the 7 o'clock position with a palpable non-healed tract. Proctoscopy reveals an internal opening of a fistula in the posterior midline, 4 cm from the anal verge.

Questions

1. What is a fistula?

2. What causes anal fistulas?

3. What is Goodsall's rule?

4. How are anal fistulae classified?

5. How should this patient be investigated?

6. Describe the management of anal fistulas.

Answers

1. What is a fistula?

A fistula is an abnormal communication between two epithelialized surfaces. An anal fistula consists of an inflammatory tract lined by granulation tissue between the anorectal canal and the perianal skin.

2. What causes anal fistulas?

The majority of anal fistulas are idiopathic. The cryptoglandular hypothesis follows that infection begins in the anal glands that line the dentate line in the rectum, with infection passing into the inter-sphincteric space of the anal canal. Infection spreads via the pathway of least resistance. This results in the formation of an acute anorectal abscess, which may drain spontaneously or necessitate surgical intervention. A fistula develops if the communication between the anal glands and external skin persists following drainage.

Other conditions associated with anal fistula formation include Crohn's disease, tuberculosis, hidradenitis suppurativa, HIV, foreign bodies, previous radiotherapy, and trauma.

3. What is Goodsall's rule?

Goodsall's rule is used to predict the location of the internal opening of an anal fistula based on the position of its external opening. An external opening seen posterior to a line drawn transversely across the perineum will originate from an internal opening in the posterior midline. An external opening seen anterior to the line will originate directly from the nearest crypt. Anterior fistulas, therefore, have a straight track, whereas a posterior fistula follows a more curving path.

4. How are anal fistulas classified?

There are a variety of classification systems, but the most commonly used is that described by Parks (Figure 4.2.1). This describes the relationship between the primary tract and the sphincter muscles.

A 'low' fistula describes a primary tract that passes through no, or very little, sphincter tissue and includes superficial fistulas, low intersphincteric fistulas, and low trans-sphincteric fistulas. A 'high'

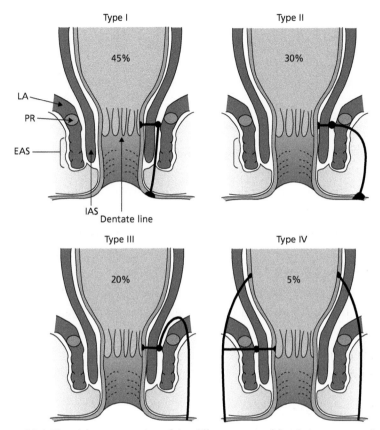

Figure 4.2.1 Pictorial representation of the different types of fistula-in-ano according to the Parks classification: Type 1 is intersphincteric; Type 2 is trans-sphincteric; Type 3 is suprasphincteric, and Type 4 is extrasphincteric.

Abbreviations: EAS—external anal sphincter; IAS—internal anal sphincter; LA—levator ani; PR—puborectalis.

Reprinted from *Surgery (Oxford)*, Volume 29, Issue 8, pp. 382–6, Tiernan JP and Brown SR, 'Benign anal conditions: haemorrhoids, fissures, perianal abscess, fistula-in-ano and pilonidal sinus', Copyright © 2011 Elsevier Ltd. All rights reserved. By permission from Elsevier, http://www.sciencedirect.com/science/article/pii/S0263931911001074

fistula describes a tract that passes through a large amount of sphincter muscle and includes high intersphincteric fistulas, high trans-sphincteric fistulas, suprasphincteric fistulas, and extrasphincteric fistulas. These are considered complex as they cannot simply be laid open like low fistulas due to the risk of sphincter damage and subsequent incontinence.

5. How should this patient be investigated?

Investigations are necessary to help identify the internal and external openings, any secondary tracts, and to help determine the underlying cause of the anal fistula. Investigations include:

- *Sigmoidoscopy.* May identify the internal opening and any underlying cause, such as proctitis.
- *Colonoscopy.* Undertaken in patients who have symptoms suggestive of IBD.
- *MRI rectum.* Considered the gold standard for fistula imaging. It provides excellent soft tissue resolution and should be used in all cases of recurrent anal fistulas and complex anal fistulas.

6. Describe the management of anal fistula.

Following investigations and confirmation of the fistula tract anatomy there are several surgical management options available. Fistula surgery aims to:

- Eliminate the fistula.
- Prevent recurrence.
- Preserve sphincter function.

A number of surgical approaches can be taken in order to achieve this:

- *Laying-open.* Fistulotomy involves division of the tissue superficial to the fistula tract allowing the wound to heal by secondary intention. It is used in low fistulas as the risk of sphincter damage is low, as are recurrence rates. Fistulotomy is not recommended for high fistulas as this can result in significant sphincter damage leading to incontinence.
- *Seton insertion.* A drainage seton is a plastic thread that is placed through the fistula tract and tied loosely (externally) to maintain patency and drainage of the tract. This prevents the re-development of any further sepsis. This is usually the initial step in high fistulas whereby laying open of the fistula is not an option due to the risk of incontinence. A cutting seton involves

sequential tightening of the seton so that it slowly cuts through muscle involved in the fistula tract and can be used safely for high fistulas.

- *Fibrin glue.* This consists of fibrinogen and thrombin and is injected into the fistula tract. This heals the tract by inducing clot formation followed by the growth of collagen fibres and new healthy tissue. Success rates of 31–85% have been described.

- *Fistula plug.* This is a biological plug manufactured from porcine small intestine mucosa. This is a sphincter-sparing procedure, with the plug being pulled through the fistula tract and being secured at the internal opening. At the external opening the plug is trimmed and left open for drainage. Over time the plug stimulates host cells to populate and eliminate the tract. The success rate of this technique is reported at 54% (excluding Crohn's patients).

- *LIFT procedure.* The ligation of intersphincteric tract (LIFT) procedure involves closure of the internal opening and excision of the infected cryptoglandular tissue through an intersphincteric approach. Success rates in complex fistulas of 40–90% have been reported.

- *Rectal advancement flap.* This procedure aims to cover the internal opening of the fistula with healthy tissue to prevent recurrence. The internal opening is identified and excised whilst the external opening is enlarged to allow drainage. A full-thickness flap of mucosa, submucosa, and part of the internal sphincter is raised. The residual internal opening is closed with an absorbable suture. The flap is then advanced 1 cm below the internal opening and sutured secure. Success rates are variable.

- *Defunctioning stoma.* A loop colostomy may be necessary in cases where perianal sepsis is difficult to control. This diverts bowel content, providing a healthier environment for sepsis to resolve. Following successful treatment of the anal fistula, the colostomy can be reversed and intestinal continuity restored.

- *Biological therapy.* Infliximab and other TNF monoclonal antibody therapies have a role in the treatment of anal fistulas associated with Crohn's disease. When used in combination with selective surgery, it leads to higher closure rates.

Further reading

Murugesan J, Mor I, Fulham S, Hitos K (2014) Systematic review of efficacy of LIFT procedure in crpytoglandular fistula-in-ano. *Journal of Coloproctology* **34** (2): 109–19.

O'Riordan JM, Datta I, Johnston C, Baxter NN (2012) A systematic review of the anal fistula plug for patients with Crohn's and non-Crohn's related fistula-in-ano. *Diseases of the Colon and Rectum* **55**: 351–835.

Sentovich SM (2001) Fibrin glue for all anal fistulas. *Journal of Gastrointestinal Surgery* **5**: 158–61.

Simpson J, Banerjea A, Scholefield JH (2012) Management of anal fistula. *Briish Medical Journal* **345**: e6705.

Tanaka S, Matsuo K, Sasaki T, Nakano M, Sakai K, Beppu R et al. (2010) Clinical advantages of combined seton placement and infliximab maintenance therapy for perianal fistulizing Crohn's disease: when and how were the seton drains removed? *Hepatogastroenterology* **57**(97): 3–7.

Case history 4.3: Elective: colorectal cancer

A 64-year-old man was referred to clinic with a 6-week history of rectal bleeding and weight loss. This was associated with several episodes of diarrhoea, loss of appetite, and fatigue. Prior to this illness he had been fit and well with no other past medical or surgical history. He drinks 20 units of alcohol a week and has smoked 15 cigarettes a day for 30 years. There is no family history of note.

On examination he is alert but looks pale, thin, and fatigued. He has a pulse rate of 90, BP of 145/85, and a respiratory rate of 18 breaths a minute. Chest examination is clear with normal heart sounds. His abdomen is soft with no palpable masses, organomegaly, or lymphadenopathy. Digital rectal examination reveals stool and red blood but no obvious masses.

The GP has performed some blood tests prior to clinic (see Table 4.3.1).

Table 4.3.1 Blood results

Hb	105
WCC	9
Platelets	120
MCV	71
Prothrombin time	11
Sodium	138
Potassium	3.9
Urea	7.5
Creatinine	90
Bilirubin	24
Alanine transferase	35
Alkaline phosphatase	120
Albumin	38

Questions

1. What are the key differential diagnoses?
2. How should this patient be investigated further?
3. What are the risk factors for colorectal cancer?
4. What screening programmes exist for colorectal cancer?
5. How is colorectal cancer staged?
6. What are the surgical management options for colorectal cancer?

Answers

1. What are the key differential diagnoses?

The top differential diagnoses are colorectal cancer, inflammatory bowel disease, and infective colitis. Rectal bleeding, a prolonged change in bowel habit, weight loss, and a microcytic anaemia is concerning for colorectal cancer.

2. How should this patient be investigated further?

+ *Colonoscopy.* This is the gold standard investigation. It allows complete investigation of the large bowel. Polyps can be excised and biopsies can be taken of any suspicious lesions.

+ *CT colonography.* This is an alternative to colonoscopy, which can be useful in certain patient groups, such as those on anticoagulation. It gives good bowel delineation (unlike standard CT) and can also provide information about local spread. However, it is not possible to take biopsies like you can at colonoscopy.

+ *CT chest/abdomen/pelvis.* Patients with confirmed colorectal cancer will have a staging CT scan to give information on any evidence of local spread and distant metastases.

+ *MRI.* This is used for pre-operative staging of rectal cancer to determine extent of invasion into the mesorectum. It can also be used to image the liver to delineate liver metastases.

+ *Trans-rectal ultrasound (TRUS).* This is used for staging rectal tumours.

3. What are the risk factors for colorectal cancer?

Although the exact cause of colorectal cancer is unknown, several factors can increase risk:

Sociodemographic factors

+ *Age.* Colorectal cancer incidence is strongly related to age. In the UK, between 2011 and 2013, 58% of colorectal cancer cases were diagnosed in patients 70 years or over.

- *Sex.* Colorectal cancer is slightly more common in men. Of the 41,581 cases diagnosed in the UK in 2011, 56% were male and 44% female.

- *Diet.* Colorectal cancer has been linked to eating red and processed meat. Colorectal cancer risk is 33% higher in people who are obese (as measured by BMI) compared to those of a healthy weight.

- *Alcohol.* An estimated 11% of colorectal cancers are linked to alcohol consumption. Risk is 21% higher in those that drink 1.6–6.2 units of alcohol per day and 52% higher in those that drink greater than 6.2 units per day compared to non-drinkers/occasional drinkers.

- *Tobacco.* Colorectal cancer risk is 20–21% higher in current cigarette smokers compared with 'never-smokers'. Risk increases with the number of cigarettes smoked per day in the order of 7–11% per 10 cigarettes per day.

Medical conditions

- *Adenomas.* A pooled analysis of 9,167 polypectomies found that multiple (>5) and larger (>20 mm) adenomas were at increased risk of developing colorectal cancer.

- *Inflammatory bowel disease.* This accounts for 1% of all cases of colorectal cancer. Risk is increased with duration of symptoms.

- *Coeliac disease.* Evidence regarding coeliac disease is conflicting,

Family history and genetic syndromes

75% of cases of colorectal cancer are sporadic. 5% are linked to genetic syndromes, including familial adenomatous polyposis (FAP) and hereditary non-polyposis colorectal cancer (HNPCC). 20% of cancers are associated with other hereditary risk factors. Bowel cancer risk is around twice as high in people with a first-degree relative with the disease compared to the general population, with an even greater risk if there are multiple or young affected relatives.

Radiation

A study in 2012 attributed 1.8% of all colorectal cancer cases in 2010 due to ionizing radiation, the majority of these being diagnostic radiation.

4. What screening programmes exist for colorectal cancer in the UK?

The NHS Bowel Cancer Screening Programme began in 2006. Men and women aged 60–69 registered with a GP are automatically sent an invitation for screening through the post every 2 years. Screening consists of a home testing kit, called a faecal occult blood test (FOBT) kit. The kit is used to collect a stool sample and is sent in a special hygienic freepost envelope to a laboratory, where it is checked for microscopic traces of blood. Patients with an abnormal result are offered an appointment with a specialist nurse to discuss further investigation, which is usually colonoscopy in the first instance.

Patients at risk of developing colon cancer may be entered into endoscopic surveillance. Guidelines have been produced by the British Society of Gastroenterology and the Association of Coloproctology of Great Britain and Ireland and endorsed by NICE. These include:

- Adenomas. Risk is stratified as:
    - Low risk: patients with 1–2 adenomas less than 1 cm in size—colonoscopy at 5 years. Negative repeat endoscopy does not warrant further surveillance.
    - Intermediate risk: patients who have had 3–4 adenomas less than 1 cm in size or one adenoma over 1 cm in size—colonoscopy at 3 years. If repeat endoscopy is negative, a further endoscopy should be performed at 3 years, but surveillance stopped if this is negative.
    - High risk: 5+ adenomas over 1 cm or 3+ adenomas, one of which was over 1 cm—colonoscopy at 1 year. If repeat endoscopy is negative, low, or intermediate risk, repeat endoscopy at 3 years.

Patients should have their risk re-stratified depending on findings at repeat endoscopy and decision made for further endoscopy based on this.

◆ Inflammatory bowel disease. Risk is stratified:

   ◆ Low risk: extensive but quiescent ulcerative colitis or Crohn's, or left-sided ulcerative colitis of similar extent—colonoscopy every 5 years.

   ◆ Intermediate risk: extensive ulcerative colitis or Crohn's with mild active inflammation, post-inflammatory polyps, or family history of colorectal cancer in first-degree relative over 50 years old—colonoscopy every 3 years.

   ◆ High risk: extensive ulcerative colitis or Crohn's with moderate or severe active inflammation, primary sclerosing cholangitis, colonic stricture, or any grade of dysplasia in the last 5 years or a family history of colorectal cancer in first-degree relative under 50 years of age—colonoscopy every 1 year.

Patients should have their risk restratified at each endoscopy.

At the time of writing, the NHS Bowel Cancer Screening Programme are piloting a new screening programme in six bowel cancer screening centres across England. This involves a one-off flexible sigmoidoscopy offered between the ages of 55 and 64. Evidence suggests that this one off examination, which includes the removal of small polyps (<10 mm) and offering colonoscopy for high-risk adenomas, reduces the incidence of colorectal cancer by 33% and mortality by 43%.

5. How is colorectal cancer staged?

There are two widely used classification systems: Duke's staging (Table 4.3.2) and the TNM classification. T denotes the degree of invasion of the local tumour, N denotes the degree of nodal invasion, and M denotes the presence of distant metastases. Duke's and TNM staging are comparable:

◆ Duke's A is equivalent to early disease with no nodal or distant metastases (T1N0M0 and T2N0M0).

◆ Duke's B is equivalent to locally advancing disease with no nodal or distant metastases (T3N0M0 and T4N0M0).

◆ Duke's C is equivalent to nodal metastases, equivalent to any T stage, N1 or N2, and M0.

◆ Duke's D denotes metastatic disease, with M1 staging, and any T, and any N stage.

TNM staging has largely superseded the Duke's staging system, however Duke's is often still reported concomitantly with TNM staging at MDTs.

Diagnosing the disease early results in improved prognoses, which is illustrated in Table 4.3.2.

Table 4.3.2 Duke's staging classification with the frequency of presentation and prognosis

Duke's stage	Extent of tumour	Frequency at presentation (%)	5-year survival (%)
A	Confined to the bowel wall	13.2	93.2
B	Through the bowel wall but no lymph node involvement	36.9	77
C	Lymph node involvement but no metastatic spread	35.9	47.7
D	Metastatic spread	14	6.6

Crown Copyright © 2009, Colorectal Cancer Survival by Stage available from http://www.ncin.org.uk/databriefings

6. What are the surgical management options for colorectal cancer?

Following MDT discussion, treatment strategy depends on a number of factors, including patient comorbidities, disease burden, and patient wishes.

For patients fit for surgery, the type of operation depends upon the location of the tumour. Generally speaking this will mean the following:

◆ Right colon: right hemicoloectomy.

- Left colon: left hemicolectomy.
- Transverse colon: extended right or left hemicolectomy.
- Sigmoid colon: sigmoid colectomy or high anterior resection.
- High rectal tumour: anterior resection.
- Low rectal tumour: abdomino-perineal excision of the rectum (APER) with end colostomy *or* ultra-low anterior resection.

There are a number of neoadjuvant treatments that are routinely used for rectal cancer:

- *Neoadjuvant chemoradiotherapy.* The only definitive indication for neoadjuvant chemoradiotherapy is the presence of a T3 or T4 tumor. Relative indications for neoadjuvant chemoradiotherapy include:
    - Presence of clinically node-positive disease in a patient with a MRI or TRUS-staged T1/2 rectal cancer.
    - A distal rectal tumour for which an APER is thought to be necessary.
    - A tumor that appears to invade the mesorectal fascia on pre-operative imaging, because of the decreased likelihood of achieving a tumor-free circumferential resection margin with upfront surgery.
- *Neoadjuvant short-course radiotherapy.* Three phase III trials have shown that neoadjuvant short course radiotherapy prior to sugery resulted in better local control than surgery alone (Dutch trial, Swedish trial, and MRC trial.) Of the trials that compared short-course radiotherapy to chemoradiotherapy, no statistical difference in local recurrence rates, disease-free survival, and overall survival were found.

Further reading

Birgisson H, Påhlman L, Gunnarsson U, Glimelius B; Swedish Rectal Cancer Trial Group (2005) Adverse effects of preoperative radiation therapy for rectal cancer: long-term follow-up of the Swedish Rectal Cancer Trial. *J Clin Oncol* 23(34): 8,697.

Botteri E, Iodice S, Bagnardi V, Raimondi S, Lowenfels AB, Maisonneuve P (2008) Smoking and colorectal cancer: a meta-analysis. *JAMA* **300**(23): 2,765–78.

Edge S, Byrd DR, Compton CC, Fritz AG, Greene FL, Trotti A (eds) (2010) *AJCC Cancer Staging Manual*, seventh edition. Springer, Philadelphia, USA.

Fearnhead NS, Wilding JL, Bodmer WF (2002) Genetics of colorectal cancer: hereditary aspects and overview of colorectal tumorigenesis. *British Medical Bulletin* **64**(1): 27–43.

Fedirko V, Tramacere I, Bagnardi V, Rota M, Scotti L, Islami F et al. (2011) Alcohol drinking and colorectal cancer risk: an overall and dose-response meta-analysis of published studies. *Annals of Oncol* **22**(9): 1,958–72.

Ma Y, Yang Y, Wang F, Zhang P, Shi C, Zou Y et al. (2013) Obesity and risk of colorectal cancer: a systematic review of prospective studies. *PLoS One* **8**(1): e53,916.

Parkin DM (2011) Cancers attributable to dietary factors in the UK in 2010. *British Journal of Cancer* **105**(s2): s24–26.

Peeters KC, Marijnen CA, Nagtegaal ID, Kranenbarg EK, Putter H, Wiggers T et al. (2007) The TME trial after a median follow-up of 6 years: increased local control but no survival benefit in irradiated patients with resectable rectal carcinoma. *Annals of Surgery* **246**(5): 693.

Sauer R, Becker H, Hohenberger W, Rödel C, Wittekind C, Rainer F et al. (2004) Preoperative versus postoperative chemoradiotherapy for rectal cancer. *New England Journal of Medecine* **351**(17): 1,731.

Case history 4.4: Elective: faecal incontinence

A 65-year-old female is referred to clinic with a 3-year history of progressive faecal incontinence. Once she develops the urge, she is unable to wait more than one minute to defaecate, which happens on an almost daily basis. She also leaks into her underwear without knowing, which has resulted in her wearing pads constantly. Her symptoms have affected her quality of life in that she rarely leaves the house and on the rare occasion she does she only visits places with easily accessible toilets. She is otherwise fit and well, with her only significant past medical history including two vaginal deliveries, the first being a forceps delivery that resulted in a tear that was repaired at the time of delivery. The GP initially recommended some pelvic floor exercises, which the patient has been undertaking with no improvement in symptoms.

On examination she looks well. Her abdomen is soft. Digital rectal examination reveals staining of the underwear, but an otherwise empty rectum with no palpable masses. She went on to undergo surgical repair of the sphincter.

Questions

1. What is faecal incontinence?
2. Describe the mechanism of faecal continence.
3. How does faecal incontinence present?
4. What are the causes of faecal incontinence?
5. How should this patient be investigated?
6. How should patients be initially managed?
7. What are the surgical options for managing faecal incontinence?

Answers

1. What is faecal incontinence?

Faecal incontinence is the inability to control faeces and expel it at an appropriate time and place. It is estimated that 1–10% of adults suffer with faecal incontinence that affects their quality of life. Patients may complain of incontinence to flatus, liquid, or solid stools.

2. Describe the mechanism of faecal continence.

The sphincter mechanism is comprised of the puborectalis muscle, and internal and external sphincter. The internal anal sphincter (IAS) is a continuation of the involuntary circular smooth muscle of the rectum. The anus is normally closed by the continuous tonic activity of the IAS. The external anal sphincter (EAS) provides voluntary control over defaecation and can reinforce the IAS by 'voluntary squeeze'. The puborectalis muscle forms a U-shaped sling around the rectum creating the recto-anal angle. At rest, the recto-anal angle is 90°. With voluntary contraction of the external anal sphincters this angle becomes more acute, whereas with defaecation it straightens out allowing the passage of faeces. The IAS has autonomic innervation and contributes 50–60% of the resting tone of the anal canal. The pudendal nerve innervates both the puborectalis and EAS, and these provide about 30% of the resting anal tone. Haemorrhoidal cushions provide the fine seal of the anal canal and can contribute to up to 25% of the overall control.

3. How does faecal incontinence present?

There are two main patterns of presentation with faecal incontinence:

- Urge incontinence: the patient feels the need to defecate, but cannot resist the urge.
- Passive incontinence: the patients defecates without warning.

4. What are the causes of faecal incontinence?

Faecal incontinence can be attributed to defects in any part of the continence mechanism, including sphincter function,

Table 4.4.1 Causes of faecal incontinence

Aetiology	Examples
Trauma	Obstetric (forceps' delivery, mediolateral episiotomy); accidental/non-accidental (penetrating trauma, sexual abuse)
Ano/colorectal diseases	Rectal prolapse, haemorrhoids, IBD, cancer, colitis, proctitis
Iatrogenic	Anorectal surgery, pelvic radiotherapy
Neurogenic	Multiple sclerosis, diabetes mellitus
Congenital	Spina bifida, Hirschprung's disease
Other	Dementia, increasing age, laxative abuse, constipation (overflow)

Reproduced with permission from 'Fecal Incontinence: Etiology, Evaluation, and Treatment', *Clinics in Colon and Rectal Surgery*, Volume 24, Issue 1, pp. 64–70, Table 2, Copyright © 2011 Georg Thieme Verlag KG.

neurological factors, rectal sensation, rectal capacity, and stool consistency. The main causes of faecal incontinence are summarized in Table 4.4.1.

Obstetric trauma is the biggest cause of faecal incontinence in women. Vaginal delivery can damage the pelvic floor and anal sphincters with direct mechanical tears of the sphincters occurring in 0.6–9% of vaginal deliveries. Faecal incontinence has been reported in up to 29% 6-months post-partum in one large cohort study. Risk is increased with forceps deliveries, prolonged labour, and high BMI.

Iatrogenic sphincter injuries from anorectal surgery are another cause of faecal incontinence. Incontinence may be inevitable after complex fistula surgery, but can occur as an unexpected complication of haemorrhoidal or anal fissure surgery. Anorectal disease itself is a significant risk for faecal incontinence, even in the absence of surgery. Mucosal and/or full-thickness rectal prolapse can stent the anal canal open and stretch the sphincters, impairing their function. Other colorectal diseases, such as inflammatory bowel disease, infective colitis, malignancy, and haemorrhoids, can all lead to faecal incontinence.

Aside from structural damage, the IAS can degenerate ultimately leading to faecal incontinence. This can be primary degeneration, most commonly seen in middle age with an equal incidence in either sexes, or secondary to something else, such as pelvic radiotherapy, systemic sclerosis, or chronic pseudo-obstruction.

Faecal incontinence is common in patients with congenital disorders. Up to 90% of patients with spina bifida report faecal incontinence and up to 80% of patients with Hirschprung's disease complain of incontinence following surgery.

5. How should this patient be investigated?

A combination of investigations are usually required in the assessment of faecal incontinence:

◆ *Flexible sigmoidoscopy.* This test can be used to identify any colorectal pathology that may be the cause of faecal incontinence.

◆ *Endoanal ultrasound.* This is used to image the sphincters and puborectalis muscle. Ultrasound can assess muscle thickness and identify scarring, areas of muscle loss and other localized pathology.

◆ *Anorectal manometry.* This assesses the neuromuscular function of the anorectum providing an objective assessment of the integrity of the internal and external anal sphincters, as well as rectal sensation. A catheter with a balloon containing a sensor is inserted into the anorectum and the sphincter function can be assessed as the patient is asked to squeeze or bear down.

6. How should patients be initially managed?

Treatment depends on the underlying cause as well as the severity of the symptoms and the effect on the patient's quality of life.

NICE recommend identifying and treating specific causes of faecal incontinence before moving on to more general management measures. Specific conditions that can be treated include:

◆ Faecal loading.

◆ Treatable causes of diarrhoea (e.g. infective diarrhoea, IBD).

- Colorectal cancer.
- Rectal prolapse.
- Haemorrhoids.
- Acute sphincter injury.
- Cauda equina syndrome.

Having eliminated any of the above causes, more general measures include:

- *Diet and fluids.* Manipulating fibre intake (increase or decrease, depending on stool consistency) benefits some patients. Changing the timing and size of meals can help patients manage the condition, but will not cure their incontinence.

- *Anti-diarrhoeal medications.* Loperamide is the first-line treatment for faecal incontinence where investigations and treatments have failed to cure the condition. Other agents that can be used include codeine phosphate and co-phenotrope.

- *Biofeedback.* This is a non-invasive technique that allows re-training of the complex muscular systems needed to maintain continence.

- *Rectal irrigation.* Irrigation is used to clean out the rectum under the assumption that the patient cannot be incontinent if the rectum is kept empty. Long-term studies have shown this to have success in managing symptoms.

7. What are the surgical options for managing faecal incontinence?

- *Sacral nerve stimulator (SNS).* This is an option for patients who fail conservative treatments that have weak but mostly intact anal sphincters and rectal function. Electrodes are inserted subcutaneously in the lower back and are connected to a pulse generator. The exact mechanism of action is not fully understood, but it is thought that electrical pulses stimulate sacral nerve roots that modulate sphincter control. A Cochrane systematic review concluded that SNS can improve faecal incontinence in some patients.

- *Sphincter repair.* Anterior overlapping sphincteroplasty is the operation of choice for patients with external sphincter defects. It involves dissecting the EAS from surrounding structures and performing a sutured overlapping repair.

- *Sphincter replacement.* Two neosphincter operations exist for faecal incontinence attributed to sphincter failure: artificial sphincter replacement and gracilis muscle transposition. Both are generally associated with high complication rates (infection, erosion, failure).

- *Antegrade colonic enema (ACE procedure).* This involves antegrade irrigation of the colon through a surgically created appendicostomy or caecostomy. It reduces incontinence by intermittently cleansing the colon.

- *Diversion colostomy.* In cases where all other medical or surgical options fail, a diversion colostomy should be considered.

Further reading

Ahmad M, McCallum IJ, Mercer-Jones M (2010) Management of faecal incontinence in adults. *British Medical Journal* **340**: c2,964.

Mowatt G, Glazener CMA, Jarrett M (2007) Sacral nerve stimulation for faecal incontinence and constipation in adults. *Cochrane Database of Systematic Reviews* 3: CD004464.

National Institute for Health and Clinical Excellence (2007) Faecal incontinence: the management of faecal incontinence in adults. Guideline number CG49.

Case history 4.5: Elective: fissure in ano

A 33-year-old man was referred to clinic with an 8-week history of bright red rectal bleeding when opening his bowels. This was associated with painful defaecation and a 'stinging' sensation for approximately 30 minutes after each bowel motion. He suffers with long-term constipation. He is otherwise fit and well. There is no history of weight loss. He is a non-smoker and drinks 10 units of alcohol per week. There is no family history of note.

On examination he looks well. He has a pulse rate of 75, BP of 130/75, and a respiratory rate of 18 breaths a minute. His abdomen is soft with no palpable masses, organomegaly, or lymphadenopathy. The patient is unable to tolerate digital rectal examination due to pain.

His GP wondered whether he had an anal fissure and started him on some rectogesic 0.4% ointment. Unfortunately, this seems to have had no benefit. The patient underwent examination under anaesthesia (EUA), which revealed a fissure at 6 o'clock. He was treated with botulinum toxin treatment, which had had good effect and the fissure subsequently healed.

Questions

1. What are the key differential diagnoses for rectal bleeding?
2. What is an anal fissure?
3. What is a sentinel pile?
4. How should this patient be investigated further?
5. What conservative treatments are available for anal fissures?
6. What surgical treatments are available for chronic anal fissure?

Answers

1. What are the key differential diagnoses for rectal bleeding?

The top differential diagnoses are an anal fissure, haemorrhoids, colorectal cancer, and IBD. Given the patient's age and persistent pain after opening his bowels, an anal fissure is the most likely diagnosis.

2. What is an anal fissure?

An anal fissure is a tear in the lining of the mucosa lining the anal canal. This is typically the result of trauma from a hard, dry bowel motion, but can also occur from persistent diarrhoea. Patients with tight anal sphincters are more prone to developing fissures. In almost 90% of cases fissures are located in the posterior midline, but can also occur in the anterior midline. Fissures that occur laterally are usually part of a disease process, such as Crohn's disease, anal carcinoma, or anal herpes infection.

3. What is sentinel pile?

A sentinel pile is a skin tag that develops at the distal fissure margin. Patients may often complain that they can feel a 'painful haemorrhoid'.

4. How should this patient be investigated further?

Typically no further investigations are needed as a patient's description of symptoms and physical examination alone are enough to make the diagnosis.

Other investigations may be requested if there is concern that the fissure is a result of another condition (e.g. Crohn's disease). This will likely involve a flexible sigmoidoscopy or colonoscopy.

5. What conservative treatments are available for anal fissures?

Spontaneous resolution of anal fissures occurs in one-third of patients and usually takes around 6 weeks. Most fissures can be successfully treated without the need for surgery.

Conservative measures include:

◆ High-fibre diet and increased fluid intake.

◆ Sitz baths.

◆ Laxatives.

◆ Topical agents. Commonly used agents include GTN (Rectogesic 0.4%) or diltiazem (Anoheal 2%). Both agents work by facilitating local vasodilatation, relaxing the anal sphincter, reducing anal pressure, and increasing blood flow to the area, encouraging the fissure to heal. Both medications should be used long-term (up to 8 weeks) and 20–30% of patients will experience headaches.

Fissures that persist for longer than 8 weeks are classified as chronic. For patients that fail medical therapy, surgical intervention in the form of botulinum toxin injections is usually the next step. Botulinum toxin binds irreversibly to pre-synaptic nerve terminals preventing the release of acetylcholine, stopping neuronal transmission. This relaxes the anal sphincter, reducing resting anal canal pressure. This effect lasts for 2–3 months until acetylcholine re-accumulates in the nerve terminals. Botulinum toxin injection into the internal anal sphincter allows healing of chronic anal fissures in 60–80% of cases. Treatments can be repeated.

6. What surgical treatments are available for chronic anal fissure?

The aim of surgery is to reduce resting anal canal tone, thereby increasing blood supply to the anoderm to improve healing. Procedures include:

◆ *Lateral internal sphincterectomy.* This procedure heals more fissures than medical management with lower recurrence rates. This technique involves an incision over the intersphincteric groove at 3 o'clock, with dissection of the internal sphincter away from the mucosa. The internal sphincter is divided for the length of the fissure, but no more than half the length of the sphincter.

◆ *Fissurectomy.* This involves excision of the fibrotic edge of the fissure, curettage of the base, and excision of the sentinel pile.

◆ *Anal advancement flap.* Also known as anoplasty, this sphincter-preserving procedure involves introduction of a healthy, well vascularized flap of skin into the fissure defect.

Further reading

Cross KLR, Massey EJD, Fowler AL, Monson JRT (2008) The management of anal fissure: ACPGBI position statement. *Colorectal Disease* 10 (Suppl. 3): 8–29.

Wald A, Bharucha AE, Cosman BC, Whitehead WE (2014) ACG clinical guideline: management of benign anorectal disorders. *American Journal of Gastroenterology* Aug; 109(8): 1,141–57.

Case history 4.6: Elective: haemorrhoids

A 30-year-old man was referred to clinic with a 1-year history of intermittent bright red rectal bleeding. His GP had previously diagnosed haemorrhoids and prescribed several different topical and suppository treatments with variable success. Recently his bleeding has been occurring more frequently. He has a poor diet and is normally constipated. His appetite and weight remain healthy. He has no medical or surgical history. He is a non-smoker and drinks a moderate amount of alcohol. He is a self-employed builder.

On examination he looks well. He has a pulse rate of 68, BP of 120/75, and a respiratory rate of 18 breaths a minute. His abdomen is soft with no palpable masses, organomegaly, or lymphadenopathy. Digital rectal examination reveals no masses and no blood. Proctoscopy reveals grade 2 haemorrhoids. These were treated successfully with banding in clinic.

Questions

1. What are haemorrhoids?
2. How are haemorrhoids classified?
3. What causes haemorrhoids?
4. Does this patient require any further investigations?
5. What conservative (non-surgical) treatments are available for haemorrhoids?
6. What are the surgical options for treating haemorrhoids?

Answers

1. What are haemorrhoids?

Haemorrhoids result from the enlargement of the normal sub-mucosal arterio-venous vascular plexuses located in the anal canal. Hemorrhoidal tissue is a normal anatomic structure located in the anal canal that plays a role in differentiating between liquids, solids, and gas, and maintaining anal continence. Haemorrhoidal disease occurs when these structures enlarge causing symptoms such as bleeding, pain, prolapse, and mucus discharge, which can irritate and result in pruritus ani.

2. How are haemorrhoids classified?

The dentate line divides haemorrhoidal tissue into internal haemorrhoids and external haemorrhoids. Internal haemorrhoids are classified into four categories:

- First-degree: confined to the anal canal. May bleed but do not prolapse.
- Second-degree: prolapse with defaecation, but spontaneously reduce.
- Third-degree: prolapse with defaecation, do not spontaneously reduce, but can be digitally reduced.
- Fourth-degree: constantly prolapsed, irreducible.

3. What causes haemorrhoids?

The exact cause of haemorrhoids is unknown. A number of factors are believed to play a role, including:

- Increased abdominal pressure (prolonged straining, obesity, pregnancy, chronic cough, ascites, pelvic malignancy).
- Constipation.
- Lack of exercise.
- Genetics.
- Ageing.

4. Does this patient require any further investigations?

Typically no further investigations are needed, as history and examination (including proctoscopy) are sufficient to confirm the diagnosis.

Other investigations should be requested if there is concern that haemorrhoids are a result of another disease process, or that symptoms (e.g. rectal bleeding) may be attributable to something else. Typically this involves a flexible sigmoidoscopy or colonoscopy.

5. What conservative (non-surgical) treatments are available for haemorrhoids?

Asymptomatic haemorrhoids do not need treatment. Initial conservative measures include:

+ *Increasing dietary fibre.*

+ *Laxatives.* These help reduce constipation and straining that can lead to haemorrhoids.

+ *Rubber band ligation.* This can be performed on grade I–III haemorrhoids. It involves placement of an elastic band on to an internal haemorrhoid to cut off its blood supply. Within 5–7 days the haemorrhoid sloughs away and falls off.

+ *Injection of sclerosant.* This involves the injection of phenol into the haemorrhoid. This causes the vessel walls to collapse and the haemorrhoid to shrivel up.

6. What are the surgical options for treating haemorrhoids?

Surgery is reserved for cases that fail conservative treatments:

+ *Open haemorrhoidectomy (Milligan–Morgan).* This involves dissection, transfixion, and excision of the haemorrhoid. A bridge of skin is preserved between each haemorrhoid to prevent post-operative anal stricture and the wounds are left open. Post-operative pain levels can be high.

+ *Stapled haemorrhoidopexy.* This is also known as the procedure for prolapsing haemorrhoids (PPH). In contrast to traditional surgery this technique does not remove the haemorrhoidal tissue.

Instead a circular stapling device is used to fashion a mucosa-to-mucosa anastomosis proximal to the dentate line. This results in relocation of the vascular cushions to a more anatomical position and disrupts their feeding arteries. As the surgery occurs proximal to the dentate line, the main advantage of this technique is significantly reduced post-operative pain levels. This technique is useful for large prolapsed piles associated with mucosal prolapse.

◆ *Haemorrhoidal artery ligation operation (HALO).* This procedure involves suture ligation of the haemorrhoidal feeder arteries above the dentate line. A Doppler probe is used to help identify these vessels. This reduces the blood flow to the haemorrhoids, thus shrinking them. NICE recommends the HALO procedure as an efficacious alternative to open haemorrhoidectomy or stapled haemorrhoidopexy in the short and medium term

Further reading

Halverson A (2007) Haemorrhoids. *Clin Colon Rectal Surg* **20**(2): 77–85.

Jayaraman S, Colquhoun PH, Malthaner RA (2006) Stapled versus conventional surgery for hemorrhoids. *Cochrane Database of Systematic Reviews* Oct 18; (4): CD005393.

National Institute for Health and Clinical Excellence (2010) Haemorrhoidal artery ligation. NICE interventional procedure guidance number 342.

Case history 4.7: Elective: hernias

A 28-year-old male mechanic was referred to clinic with a 3-month history of an intermittent lump in his right groin. He has noticed that the lump often appears on standing but disappears when lying down. When visible, the lump causes mild discomfort, but he is always able to reduce it himself. He has a normal bowel habit and has not lost any weight, and is otherwise fit and well. He has had no previous surgery. He does not smoke or drink alcohol.

On examination he looks well. He has a pulse rate of 78 beats per minute and BP of 110/74. His abdomen is soft with no palpable masses, organomegaly, or lymphadenopathy. Testicular examination is normal. On standing there is a soft non-tender palpable mass in the right groin that has a positive cough impulse. On lying down the mass is soft and completely reducible. He was diagnosed with a direct inguinal hernia and underwent open mesh repair.

Questions

1. What are the differential diagnoses of a groin lump?
2. What is a hernia?
3. Describe the anatomy of the inguinal canal.
4. Describe the anatomy of the femoral canal.
5. How do you differentiate between an indirect inguinal, direct inguinal, and femoral hernia?
6. Does this patient require any further investigations?
7. What complications can an untreated symptomatic hernia lead to?
8. What operations are available for inguinal hernia repair?
9. What are the complications of inguinal hernia surgery?

Answers

1. What are the differential diagnoses of a groin lump?

There is a long list of differential diagnoses for groin lumps, including:

- Hernia (inguinal, femoral).
- Lymphadenopathy.
- Abscess.
- Undescended testes.
- Hydrocele.
- Varicocele.
- Saphena varix.

In this case, the intermittent nature of the swelling in a young male is very suggestive of an inguinal hernia

2. What is a hernia?

A hernia is the protrusion of part of an organ through the wall of the cavity that normally contains it. In the groin this can be a direct inguinal hernia, indirect inguinal hernia, or femoral hernia.

3. Describe the anatomy of the inguinal canal.

The inguinal canal is approximately 4 cm long and is directed obliquely, infero-medially through the lower part of the antero-lateral abdominal wall. It lies approximately 2 cm superior to the medial aspect of the inguinal ligament. The anatomy is depicted in Figure 4.7.1.

The borders of the inguinal canal can be remembered by the acronym 'MALT':

- *Superior wall 'M': 2 muscles*—internal oblique muscle and trans-versus abdominis muscle.
- *Anterior wall 'A': 2 aponeuroses*—aponeurosis of internal oblique, aponeurosis of external oblique.
- *Inferior wall: 'L': 2 ligaments*—inguinal ligament, lacunar ligament.
- *Posterior wall: 'T'*—transversalis fascia, conjoint tendon.

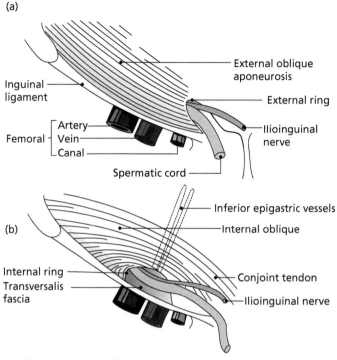

(a)

Inguinal ligament

External oblique aponeurosis

External ring

Artery
Femoral — Vein
Canal

Ilioinguinal nerve

Spermatic cord

Inferior epigastric vessels

Internal oblique

(b)

Internal ring
Transversalis fascia

Conjoint tendon

Ilioinguinal nerve

a With the external oblique aponeurosis intact
b With the aponeurosis removed

Figure 4.7.1 Pictorial representation of the right inguinal canal in a male, shown with (a) and without (b) the external oblique aponeurosis.

Reproduced with permission from Ellis H, *Clinical Anatomy*, Tenth Edition, Oxford Blackwell Science, Copyright © 2002 John Wiley and Sons Inc.

The canal has an opening (the deep or internal ring) and an exit (the superficial or external ring). The deep ring is an outpouching of the transversalis fascia and is located 1–2 cm superior to the mid-point of the inguinal ligament and lateral to the inferior epigastric vessels. The contents pass through the canal and exit through the superficial ring, a slit-like opening between the diagonal fibres of the external oblique muscle supero-lateral to the pubic tubercle.

The structures that pass through the canal differ between males and females:

- Males: spermatic cord and ilioinguinal nerve.
- Females: round ligament of the uterus and ilioinguinal nerve.

The contents of the spermatic cord can be remembered by the rule of 3s:

- *3 arteries:* artery to vas deferens, testicular artery, cremasteric artery.

- *3 fascial layers:* external spermatic (continuation of the external oblique muscle aponeurosis), cremasteric (continuation of the internal oblique muscle aponeurosis), internal spermatic (continuation of the transversalis fascia).

- *3 nerves:* genital branch of the genitofemoral nerve, sympathetic nerves, ilioinguinal nerve (travels outside the cord).

- *3 other structures:* pampiniform plexus, vas deferens, testicular lymphatics.

4. Describe the anatomy of the femoral canal.

The femoral canal forms the medial component of the femoral sheath, and is the means by which the femoral vessels pass from the abdomen into the leg. It is conical in shape, 2 cm in length, and contains the lymph node of Cloquet. Its borders include:

- Anterosuperiorly: inguinal ligament.
- Posteriorly: pectineal ligament.
- Medially: lacunar ligament and pubic bone.
- Laterally: iliopsoas muscle.

From medial to lateral it contains the femoral vein, femoral artery, and femoral vein (remembered with the mnemonic VAN, which stands for vein artery nerve). The entrance to the femoral canal is the femoral ring, through which peritoneal contents, including bowel, can herniate.

5. How do you differentiate clinically between an indirect inguinal, direct inguinal, and femoral hernia?

An indirect inguinal hernia protrudes through the deep inguinal ring into the inguinal canal, which originates lateral to the inferior epigastric vessels. It occurs as a result of failure of embryonic closure of the deep inguinal ring as the testicle passes through it. A direct inguinal hernia occurs through a weak point known as Hesselbach's triangle. The borders of this triangle are:

+ Medial border: lateral margin of rectus sheath.
+ Inferior border: inguinal ligament.
+ Superolateral border: inferior epigastric vessels.

These two hernias can be differentiated on clinical examination. After reduction of the hernia, the midpoint of the inguinal ligament is palpated and the patient is asked to cough. If the hernia is controlled, this is likely an indirect inguinal hernia. If the hernia reappears medially to where you are palpating, this is likely a direct inguinal hernia.

Inguinal hernias pass through the inguinal canal and on clinical examination these pass superomedially to the pubic tubercle. Femoral hernias pass through the femoral canal and these pass inferolaterally to the pubic tubercle.

6. Does this patient require any further investigations?

The diagnosis of an inguinal or femoral hernia is clinical. If there is diagnostic doubt, an ultrasound scan is recommended as the first-line investigation. If pain persists and ultrasound is negative, an MRI should be considered. Ultrasound should only act as a guide and the decision to operate should be based on clinical judgment.

7. What complications can an untreated symptomatic hernia lead to?

+ *Incarceration*. This is when the contents of the hernia becomes trapped and cannot be physically reduced. It may cause no additional symptoms, but may lead to more serious complications, such as bowel obstruction or strangulation.
+ *Obstruction*. If the hernia contains bowel and becomes incarcerated it may lead to bowel obstruction. Most commonly this is obstructed small bowel, but occasionally sigmoid colon can become obstructed within an inguinal hernia. Patients will

present with symptoms of bowel obstruction, including bilious vomiting, abdominal pain, distension, and obstipation.

◆ *Strangulation.* This occurs when the blood supply to the segment of incarcerated bowel is compromised. Patients will present with severe pain, vomiting, and skin changes over the hernia. They may be septic with a raised lactate on arterial blood gas. Treatment involves resuscitation and emergency hernia repair. Non-viable bowel will need to be resected.

8. What operations are available for inguinal hernia repair?

The definitive treatment for hernias, regardless of type of origin, is surgical repair. This can be performed open or laparoscopically. The ASGBI/British Hernia Society 2013 Commission Guide recommends the management strategy shown in Figure 4.7.2. Open surgical repair takes an anterior approach to the hernia and is, therefore, also referred to as anterior repair. Laparoscopic surgery takes

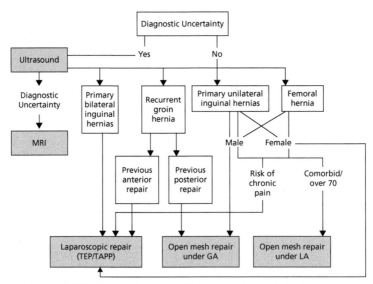

Figure 4.7.2 ASGBI/British Hernia Society 2013 Commission Guide Management strategy for groin hernias in Secondary Care.

Reproduced with permission from Sanders DL, Kurzer M and members of the Groin Hernia Surgery Guidance Development Group, 'May Association of Surgeons of Great Britain and Ireland Issues in Professional Practice', *British Hernia Society: Groin Hernia Guidelines,* Copyright © 2013 Association of Surgeons of Great Britain and Ireland, accessed at www.asgbi.org.uk

a posterior approach to the hernia, as it approaches from within the abdomen and is, therefore, also referred to as posterior repair.

Within the guideline, primary unilateral groin hernias in females are recommended for laparoscopic repair over open repair. This is based on evidence from the Swedish Hernia Registry, which prospectively followed over 6,000 women following an inguinal hernia repair. In patients that experienced a recurrence, multivariate analysis revealed the risk of re-operation was reduced when TAPP (trans-abdominal pre-peritoneal) laparoscopic repair was performed at the time of primary repair.

Two different techniques of laparoscopic inguinal hernia surgery are commonly performed: TAPP and TEP (totally extra-peritoneal). Currently, there is no evidence suggesting TAPP ahead of TEP or vice versa.

9. What are the complications of inguinal hernia surgery?

- *Seroma/haematoma*. This is due to the collection of fluid or blood in the dead space that remains once a hernia sac has been reduced. They are relatively common, occurring in around 5% of operations. Most collections resolve spontaneously without intervention.

- *Chronic pain*. Pain after hernia repair is common and reported to occur in up to 50% of operations. Systematic reviews and meta-analyses of laparoscopic versus open surgery for inguinal hernia repair have generally reported that the laparoscopic group suffered less acute pain, less chronic pain, less severe chronic pain, and less post-surgery paraesthesia in the groin. The incidence of chronic pain following inguinal hernia surgery is 5% (1 in 20).

- *Recurrence*. Hernia recurrence occurs in up to 15% of patients, depending upon the type of hernia repair initially performed, patient comorbidities, and time since the original repair. Recurrence rates of 2–3% are observed in tension-free mesh repairs. Systematic reviews and meta-analyses of laparoscopic versus open surgery for inguinal hernia have generally reported similar recurrence rates.

- *Mesh infection.* The incidence of mesh infection is similar between laparoscopic and open hernia repairs occurring in 0.1–0.2% of cases. It can occur acutely in first few post-operative weeks or much later (months to years after surgery). Mesh infections can be diagnosed clinically but ultrasound or CT may be employed to aid diagnosis.

- *Testicular complications.* Interference with the blood supply to the testicle can lead to testicular pain, ischaemic orchitis, and testicular atrophy. Long-term testicular complications are reported in 2.2% of open mesh repairs and 1.9% of laparoscopic mesh repairs.

Further reading

British Hernia Society (2013) *Groin Hernia Guidelines.* Association of Surgeons of Great Britain and Ireland.

Grant AM and **EUHT** (2002) Collaboration. Laparoscopic versus open groin hernia repair: meta-analysis of randomised trials based on individual patient data. *Hernia* 6(1): 2–10.

Koch A, Edwards A, Haapaniemi S, Nordin P, Kald A (2005) Prospective evaluation of 6895 groin hernia repairs in women. British Journal of Surgery 92(12): 1,553–8.

McCormack K, Scott NW, Go PM, Ross S, Grant AM; EU Hernia Trialists Collaboration (2003) Laparoscopic techniques versus open techniques for inguinal hernia repair. *Cochrane Database of Systematic Reviews* 1: CD001785.

Neumayer L, Giobbie-Hurder A, Jonasson O, Fitzgibbons R Jr, Dunlop D et al. (2004) Open mesh versus laparoscopic mesh repair of inguinal hernia. *New England Journal of Medicine* 350(18): 1,819–27.

Case history 4.8: Elective: inflammatory bowel disease

A 28-year-old male was referred to clinic with a 6-month history of diarrhoea, abdominal pain, and weight loss. The diarrhoea was intermittent and occasionally contained blood. This was associated with colicky abdominal pain. He had lost 10 kg over the last 6 months despite having a healthy appetite. There is no history of foreign travel. There is no significant family history. He smokes 15 cigarettes per day and drinks 10 units of alcohol per week.

On examination he looks pale and thin. Abdominal examination reveals generalized tenderness, but no organomegaly or lymphadenopathy. Rectal examination revealed soft stool only with no blood or mucus. Several stool cultures were taken and all were negative. The GP suspected a diagnosis of inflammatory bowel disease (IBD).

Questions

1. What are the differential diagnoses?

2. What is inflammatory bowel disease?

3. What are the extra-intestinal manifestations of IBD?

4. How should this patient be investigated?

5. What are the surgical management options for ulcerative colitis?

6. What are the surgical management options for Crohn's disease?

Answers

1. What are the differential diagnoses?

The key differential diagnoses are IBD (Crohn's disease and ulcerative colitis), infective colitis and coeliac disease, gastrointestinal malignancy, and irritable bowel syndrome. Malignancy is less common in the younger patient groups but cannot be clinically excluded with such a presentation. However, bleeding is less suggestive of irritable bowel disease and coeliac disease.

2. What is inflammatory bowel disease?

IBD comprises a group of idiopathic, chronic inflammatory intestinal conditions, the main two being ulcerative colitis (UC) and Crohn's disease. The aetiology of both UC and Crohn's disease is unknown, although they are both treated as autoimmune diseases.

Both UC and Crohn's disease cause symptoms of abdominal pain, diarrhoea, and weight loss. Crohn's disease can affect any part of the gastrointestinal tract from mouth to anus. Inflammation of the bowel wall is transmural and there are often 'skip lesions' with intervening normal mucosa. UC affects the colon only, with inflammation confined to the mucosa and submucosa, and is continuous from the rectum travelling proximally. UC has a higher incidence than Crohn's disease. Oral aphthous ulcers are more common in Crohn's disease than ulcerative colitis and reflect disease activity.

3. What are the extra-intestinal manifestations of IBD?

Aside from gastrointestinal symptoms, several other systems of the body can be affected by IBD:

◆ *Musculoskeletal.* Up to 50% of patients treated for IBD will develop osteopenia and up to 15% will develop osteoporosis (partly due to steroid use). Arthropathies are seen in up to 30% of IBD patients. Peripheral arthropathies affect multiple small joints and have little relation to gastrointestinal disease severity. Ankylosing spondylitis is seen in approximately 5% of IBD patients and is related to disease activity.

- *Hepatobiliary.* Primary sclerosing cholangitis (PSC) is present in 3% of Crohn's disease and UC patients. It can present independent of intestinal disease activity. In UC the presence of PSC increases the risk of malignancy of both the colon and hepatobiliary system.

- *Opthalmological.* Iritis, uveitis, and episcleritis can occur in up to 8% of IBD patients. They are unrelated to disease activity.

- *Cutaneous.* Pyoderma gangrenosum and erythema nodosum occur in up to 5% of IBD patients. Conversely, up to 50% of patients with pyoderma gangrenosum will have IBD.

4. How should this patient be investigated?

The diagnosis of IBD is made using a combination of endoscopic, radiological, histological, and haematological investigations.

Colonoscopy Colonoscopy with at least two biopsies is the investigation of choice for diagnosing colitis. It permits classification of disease based on endoscopic appearance, severity of mucosal disease, and histological features.

Radiology Imaging can be helpful in making a diagnosis and assessing disease extent:

- *MRI.* MRI has the advantage of no ionizing radiation and has excellent capabilities of imaging the small bowel. This is particularly important in Crohn's patients who are young and often need repeated imaging. It has a high sensitivity for detecting complications such as abscess formation and fistulation. Pelvic MRI is also employed for the evaluation of perianal Crohn's disease.

- *CT abdomen/pelvis.* CT provides similar information to MRI. It is the 'gold standard' for extraluminal complications. Compared to MRI it is readily available, provides rapid image acquisition, and has superior spatial resolution. However, it does carry a significant radiation burden.

- *Barium fluoroscopy.* High-quality barium studies have superior sensitivity over cross-sectional imaging techniques for detecting subtle, early mucosal disease. In established disease, CT and MRI are equivalent. Barium fluoroscopy imparts a radiation dose, but not as significant as CT.

- Abdominal *X-ray.* The abdominal X-ray is important in acute assessment of patients with suspected severe IBD to rule out toxic megacolon.

- *Capsule endoscopy.* This involves ingestion of a capsule that takes pictures as it passes through the small bowel. It provides imaging of the small bowel, which cannot be visualized by endoscopy between the third part of the duodenum and the terminal ileum.

Haematological. Several blood tests can be performed to help diagnose and assess the severity of IBD:

- *Perinuclear ANCA (pANCA).* pANCA is an autoantibody found in the serum of up to 70% of UC patients, but only 30% of Crohn's disease patients.

- *Nutritional markers.* Albumin, B12, and ferritin levels can be used to assess the consequence of acute and subacute disease in IBD.

- *Inflammatory markers.* White cell count and CRP can be measured serially to monitor levels of inflammation.

5. What are the surgical management options for ulcerative colitis?

Up to 30% of patients ultimately require surgery for the treatment of UC. The operative indications include an acute flare unresponsive to intensive medical therapy, poorly controlled disease, acute complications (such as megacolon or perforation), and risk of malignancy (presence of dysplasia). The decision to operate is often made in conjunction with a gastroenterologist, colorectal surgeon, and the patient. The type of operation performed depends upon whether it is an elective or acute setting, but options include:

♦ *Subtotal colectomy and end ileostomy.* This is the operation of choice in patients with a severe acute flare not responsive to intense medical therapy. The entire colon is excised and the rectal stump is preserved. It can be oversewn and left in the peritoneal cavity or delivered as a mucous fistula.

♦ *Panproctocolectomy and end ileostomy.* This is an option for patients in the elective setting. The entire colon and rectum are excised and an end ileostomy is created.

♦ *Ileal pouch-anal anastomosis (IPAA).* This procedure is performed after the colon and rectum have been removed. Two or more loops of small bowel are sutured/stapled together to form a reservoir. This is then anastomosed to the anus to re-establish intestinal continuity. An upstream defunctioning ileostomy is usually created to protect the IPAA, which is then reversed at a later date. This operation has the benefit of no permanent stoma, continence, and defaecation via the normal route.

6. What are the surgical management options for Crohn's disease?

Up to 75% of patients with Crohn's disease will require surgery after 10 years of disease. Crohn's disease is incurable and disease can recur following surgery. Elective surgery may involve:

♦ *Bowel resection.* Diseased segments of bowel can be resected and a primary anastomosis performed or defunctioning stoma created.

♦ *Strictuloplasty.* This is a more conservative approach for patients with multiple strictures of the small bowel as opposed to performing several resections. An incision is made lengthways along the narrowed segment of bowel. The two ends of the incision are then pushed together and sutured widthways.

Further reading

Mowat C, Cole A, Windsor A, Ahmad T, Arnott I, Driscoll R et al. (2011) Guidelines for the management of inflammatory bowel disease in adults. *Gut* **60**: 571–607.

Case history 4.9: Emergency: pilonidal abscesses

A 42-year-old male lorry driver presents with a painful swelling in his natal cleft. This has developed gradually over 4 days. Today he is barely able to sit down. He has a medical history of type II diabetes for which he is on metformin. On examination the patient is hirsute and has a BMI of 29. He has a 3 × 3 cm raised swelling with a punctum with some ooze at the top of the natal cleft with some surrounding cellulitis. His temperature is 37.5°C, his pulse is 90 beats per minute, and blood pressure 142/65. The patient was given oral antibiotics and underwent surgical incision and drainage of the abscess under general anaesthetic the next day on the emergency theatre list. He made an uneventful recovery.

Questions

1. What is the diagnosis and what are the appropriate differential diagnoses?
2. What is pilonidal disease?
3. How does pilonidal disease present?
4. How is pilonidal disease managed?

Answers

1. What is the diagnosis and what are the appropriate differential diagnoses?

The case is highly suggestive of a pilonidal abscess.

Clinically relevant differential diagnoses include:

- Anorectal sepsis extending into the natal cleft.
- Abscess secondary to hidradenitis suppurativa.
- Complex fistula disease in the presence of IBD.

2. What is pilonidal disease?

Pilonidal disease is the pathological consequence of chronic infection of a hair follicle in the natal cleft. This can be due to obstruction of the follicle or an ingrowing hair creating a foreign-body reaction. Inflammation of the follicle (folliculitis) develops leading to rupture of the follicle and extension of the inflammation into the surrounding subcutaneous tissue, resulting in chronic inflammation and fibrosis. This can result in the formation of one or multiple sinus tracts within the subcutaneous plane, which may be interlinked. This is an acquired condition, commonly developing in the hirsute and it is associated with sweating, sitting, local buttock friction or trauma, and obesity. It occurs in 26 per 100,000 patients and occurs twice as commonly in men than in women.

3. How does pilonidal disease present?

Pilonidal disease can present acutely with an *abscess* or with the chronic features of pilonidal *sinus*:

- *Acute pilonidal abscess.* Half of cases of pilonidal disease present acutely with an abscess within the natal cleft. This is caused by skin organisms, usually staphylococcus. There is usually an acutely tender swelling in the natal cleft and, occasionally, surrounding cellulitis. Midline pits may be visible representing the opening of the underlying tract. The sinus tract runs cephalad in 90% of cases, presenting with abscess higher than those with sinus tracts running caudally.

◆ *Chronic pilonidal sinus.* This presents as a sinus tract from the follicle that opens on the skin in the natal cleft, which can be visualized as a small hole. It is often chronically painful and inflamed, and discharges bloody fluid or pus. However, it can also be asymptomatic. Occasionally, a complex network of sinus tracts can form. This is generally referred electively to outpatients, although they can occasionally present on the acute take if they are symptomatic.

4. How is pilonidal disease managed?

Acute pilonidal abscess should be drained immediately, to prevent further spread of infection and to give symptomatic relief to the patient. An underlying pilonidal sinus tract is not commonly identified at the time of presentation in the presence of inflammation and infection, but may manifest after the abscess has been drained as midline pits may subsequently become visible. The incision to drain the abscess should be made off the midline away from any potential underlying sinus with curettage of the abscess cavity. The abscess cavity should be left open to heal through granulation. Excision of an identifiable pilonidal tract at the time of draining the abscess is technically difficult in the presence of active infection and has been associated with recurrence in over half of such patients as well as delayed healing, and is generally not undertaken at the same time of draining the abscess. The sinus can be definitively managed once the infection and inflammation has settled. However, most cases settle once the abscess has drained and do not require further intervention.

Management of pilonidal sinus disease is generally done on an elective basis and is, therefore, only briefly outlined here. Treatment of a pilonidal sinus employs both medical and surgical interventions. Medical approaches generally employ cleaning the tract and the surrounding area. Use of shaving and laser hair removal may be advocated in the first instance to keep the area around the sinus tract free of hairs that may propagate ongoing inflammation. These are particularly useful measures to recommend after definitive treatment to reduce the risk of recurrence. Minimally invasive approaches include irrigation and curettage of the sinus tract before closing the tract with products such as fibrin glue and phenol. Curettage is rarely used alone, as it is associated with a high rate of recurrent symptoms.

Surgical excision involves removal of the entire tract with an ellipse of surrounding skin. The approach to excision may be either midline or off-midline. Any inflammatory fibrous tissue should be removed by curettage. Any side tracks should be sought by gentle exploration with a probe, and identified tracks should also be excised. There are a number of ways to handle the resulting defect and wound, which will depend on the size of the defect that is created by the excision:

- The wound may be left open to heal through granulation. This can be difficult for many patients to tolerate and will impact on quality of life.

- Primary closure can be attempted, either immediately or as a delayed procedure to allow the wound chance to drain first. Closure can result in quicker wound healing but it is believed to be associated with a higher rate of infection and its associated morbidity. Surgical approaches include:

  - *Marsupialization*. The sinus is incised and the cavity is curetted, and the skin borders are raised and sutured to the presacral fascia, suturing the wound open whilst forming a closed pouch. The wound can then be packed and dressed. This produces a smaller wound that is more tolerable to the patient with reduced risk of infection.

  - *Flap closure*. Alternatively the entire sinus is excised and the defect closed with a flap. There are a number of flaps and procedures that can be used for this, depending on the size of the defect and surgeons' preference:

    - *Bascom's procedure*. The sinus is excised through an off-midline incision and a skin flap created by undercutting the skin from the opposite side of the natal cleft, drawing this over to recontour the cleft and close the defect. A drain is sited deep to this to aid drainage.

- *Karyakis procedure.* The sinus is excised through a midline elliptical incision and the incision is undercut to free enough skin and superficial tissue to appose and suture across the defect to obtain wound closure.
- *Lateral surgical flaps* such as X–Y fasciocutaneous advancement or rhomboid flaps can be used for larger defects.

Patient consent should cover both immediate surgical risks, such as bleeding, pain, and anaesthetic risks, and delayed risks (surgical site infection, sinus recurrence, and unsatisfactory cosmetic result, including scar and cavity formation). Deploying a tissue flap often requires a drain to allow drainage and prevent serous fluid collecting beneath the reconstruction, and this should be covered in the consenting process. Higher recurrence risks have been reported where a midline approach to excision is taken versus an off-midline approach, cited as 9% versus 2%.

Further reading

Steele SR, Perry WB, Mills S, Buie WD (2013) Practice parameters for the management of pilonidal disease. *Diseases of the Colon and Rectum* **56** (9): 1,021–7.

Case history 4.10: Emergency: anorectal sepsis

A 30-year-old man presents to the emergency department with abdominal pain, fever, and malaise. He gives a 2-day history of anal pain, which has been increasing despite regular use of simple analgesia, and it has now become difficult to tolerate. Today he has noticed some swelling around the anal verge. He feels hot, nauseous, and unwell. This is his first presentation. He has no past medical history and is not taking any medications. He is an accountant who smokes 10 cigarettes a day.

On examination he appeared flushed and uncomfortable. His temperature was 37.8°C, pulse rate was 95 beats per minute, and blood pressure was 142/76. On rectal examination he has a tender fluctuant swelling at 3 o'clock, protruding superficially lateral to the anal verge. Digital rectal examination was poorly tolerated due to pain. A diagnosis of perianal abscess was made. He proceeded to EUA under general anaesthetic, where the abscess was incised and drained. Examination did not reveal any fistulous tracts to the anorectal abscess.

Questions

1. List some causes of acute perianal pain.
2. What is the pathophysiology of anorectal sepsis?
3. How do patients present?
4. How should patients be assessed?
5. How should perianal abscess be treated?
6. When is post-operative imaging required?
7. What is the role of rigid sigmoidoscopy in general surgery?

Answers

1. List some causes of acute perianal pain.

- Prolapsed or acutely thrombosed haemorrhoids. Prolapsed haemorrhoids may become sore from irritation and rubbing. Thrombosed haemorrhoids are acutely painful due to ischaemia.
- Fissure-in-ano results in severe anal pain initiated by passing stool, followed by a period of throbbing pain due to pelvic floor spasm.
- External skin lesions, e.g. herpes simplex warts.
- Perianal sepsis. Formation of an abscess within the superficial or deep perianal tissue. This can arise externally within hair follicles in the skin. Alternatively, they can arise internally, which is termed anorectal sepsis.
- Perianal haematoma.

2. What is the pathophysiology of anorectal sepsis?

In 90% of cases of anorectal sepsis, infection is thought to manifest within the anal glands and then passes into adjacent tissue. This is referred to as sepsis of cryptoglandular origin. The anus contains 4–10 anal glands at the level of the dentate line, which demarcates the distal squamous epithelium of the distal two-thirds of the anus from the proximal columnar epithelium of the proximal third. These glands penetrate the internal sphincter and end at the intersphincteric groove. Sepsis is believed to establish when these glands become obstructed and are unable to secrete, giving any organisms within these glands the opportunity to proliferate and to extend into the anal wall, and to penetrate the intersphincteric groove. In 10% of cases, abscess formation can be associated with other causative factors such as IBD, trauma, HIV, and radiation therapy. It may also arise secondary to dehiscence of a surgical bowel anastomosis performed as part of a rectal resection. Anorectal abscess may be associated with fistula formation, an abnormal communication between two epithelialized surfaces. Fistulae are covered in detail in Case 4.2 in this chapter.

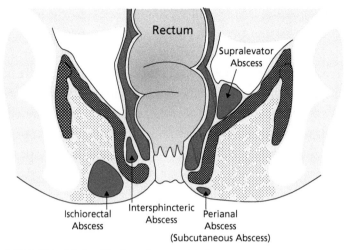

Figure 4.10.1 Pictorial classification of anorectal abscesses.

Reproduced with permission from Lewis RT and Bleier JI, 'Surgical treatment of anorectal crohn disease', *Clinics in Colon and Rectal Surgery*, Volume 26, Issue 2, pp. 90–9, Copyright © 2013 Georg Thieme Verlag KG, DOI: 10.1055/s-0033-1348047.

Suppurative infection tracks distally in the vertical plane in 50% of cases to result in the formation of a perianal abscess. It can also track laterally across the external sphincter to give rise to an ischiorectal abscess, or track proximally in the vertical plane to generate a deeper supralevator abscess. The most common site for abscess formation is perianal, followed by ischiorectal, intersphincteric, supralevator, and submucosal sites (Figure 4.10.1).

Causative organisms may arise from skin such as staphylococcus and streptococcus species, as well as gut organisms such as *Escherichia coli*, bacteroides, bacillus, and *Klebsiella* spp. The presence of gut organisms has been associated with a higher rate of fistula formation.

Anorectal sepsis affects patients between 20 and 60 years of age, and is more prevalent in males.

3. How do patients present?

Presentation depends on the level and extent of anorectal sepsis that the patient is suffering from.

In perianal and ischiorectal abscess, patients present with a painful swelling around the back passage that has generally been developing over the course of several days. Perianal abscesses form at the anal margin, whereas ischiorectal abscesses are a little more lateral, pointing or bulging on the inner buttock cheek. These patients may have difficulty sitting due to acute discomfort from the abscess. Patients with deeper abscesses within the intersphincteric or supralevator planes may present with deep anal pain that may be exacerbated by bowel movement. Patients with associated fistulae may also report leakage of pus or blood from the anal canal in between bowel movements. Patients may also be pyrexial or septic.

4. How should patients be assessed?

A full clinical history and examination is essential, as this can yield a lot of relevant information. Clinical assessment should seek information on:

- The duration of the problem.
- Presence of sepsis: temperature, tachycardia, hypotension, serum lactate level, malaise, and systemic upset.
- Associated gastrointestinal symptoms, such as perianal bleeding, discharge, or change in bowel habit.
- Preceding gastrointestinal history should be sought to determine prior diagnosis and/or clinical features of IBD, including diarrhoea, abdominal pain, weight loss, and a positive family history of IBD.
- Past medical history: conditions that can lead to an immunocompromised state, such as diabetes, malignancy, current chemotherapy, HIV, or previous organ transplant; recent pelvic surgery.
- Drug history: any immunosuppressants or long-term steroid therapy.

Examination should comprise external examination, digital rectal examination (DRE), rigid sigmoidoscopy, and proctoscopy.

- External examination can reveal an abscess at or near the anal margin in patients with perianal or ischiorectal abscess. However, patients with intersphincteric or supralevator abscesses may have no discernible features on clinical examination other than deep tenderness on rectal examination.

♦ DRE can yield useful signs. Areas of induration palpable on DRE are suggestive of an underlying fistula, which may be visualized at rigid sigmoidoscopy.

♦ Rigid sigmoidoscopy can visualize fistulous openings and also identify inflamed mucosa, which may indicate active IBD and which may be associated with the abscess. Focal fullness may be visualized on examination in patients with abscesses that do not extend superficially.

Patients may be in too much pain to tolerate DRE or rigid sigmoidoscopy, and these patients will, therefore, need to be booked for EUA to facilitate a thorough examination.

Bloods should be sent, including full blood count, urea and electrolytes, CRP, and clotting. White cell count and CRP are often raised in the presence of infection or inflammation but may also be normal, particularly in recurrent anorectal sepsis.

Cross-sectional imaging, such as CT or MRI, may be used in patients with anorectal pain and negative findings on clinical examination and EUA, or in those with a complicated and protracted history of ongoing or recurrent anorectal sepsis.

5. How should anorectal sepsis be treated?

Drainage is often achieved at the time of the EUA. There is generally clinical suspicion of sepsis underlying the patient's presentation, therefore patients should be consented for drainage of sepsis, as well as EUA.

Perianal and ischiorectal sepsis is drained externally through the perianal skin. A cruciate incision is made into the abscess cavity with excision of the cruciate skin edges to deroof it. A pus swab should be sent for microbiology, which can help to direct antibiotic treatment in progressive or persistent sepsis. The walls of the abscess should be curettaged, with a finger in the anus to ensure that curettage does not extend near to or through the anal wall. The cavity is irrigated and packed with an absorbent dressing, such as sorbsan, to help it to drain. Intersphincteric and suprasphincteric abscesses should be drained internally into the anorectal canal.

Fistulas associated with an abscess should also be managed, as these can lead to persistent and recurrent infection with its associated morbidity. The approach depends on the location of the fistula in relation to the anal sphincter. Approaches to the surgical management of fistulae are covered in Case 4.2 in this chapter.

Antibiotic therapy is only indicated if there is adjacent cellulitis or in an immunocompromised state such as diabetics, as these patients are at higher risk of developing necrotizing soft tissue infection. Prophylactic antibiotics should be administered to those with prosthetic heart valves, congenital heart disease, or a history of bacterial endocarditis. Where indicated, antibiotics should be broad spectrum with anaerobic and Gram-negative cover.

In patients presenting with sepsis secondary to perianal Crohn's, medical treatment of the underlying Crohn's should also be addressed promptly. This is important as up to 50% of Crohn's patients develop fistula formation and recurrent sepsis. Treatment is usually initiated by gastroenterologists whose input should be sought before discharge.

6. When is post-operative imaging required?

Fistula formation leads to recurrent anorectal sepsis, and has been estimated to develop in up two-thirds of patients. Therefore, patients presenting with a second episode of anorectal sepsis should be imaged on an outpatient basis 6–8 weeks later, once the sepsis has been treated and acute inflammation has settled, to determine whether the patient has an underlying fistula. MRI is considered gold standard as it can map the fistulae and identify the location of the opening tract, which allows surgical planning and management. Endoscopic ultrasound, with or without hydrogen peroxide injection, can also help to identify and delineate tracts of complex fistulae.

7. What is the role of rigid sigmoidoscopy in general surgery?

The rigid sigmoidoscope is an instrument that facilitates examination of the anorectum to identify any intraluminal pathology. It is

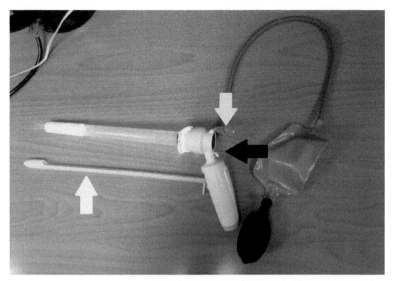

Figure 4.10.2 Photograph of the rigid sigmoidoscope. The tube is introduced into the rectum using a plastic introducer (lower arrow) inserted through the window (middle arrow), which is removed once it is in place. Closure of the window (top arrow) results in a closed tube through which air can be passed using the black pump to insufflate the rectum.

Reproduced Courtesy of Judith Ritchie.

a rigid, plastic tube measuring 20 cm in length with a light source. A hand-operated pump is attached and used to insufflate the anorectum with air, which allows circumferential assessment of the anorectal lumen and its mucosa for any abnormalities (Figure 4.10.2).

The main advantage of rigid sigmoidoscopy is that it does not need any bowel preparation prior to use and is generally well tolerated by patients, therefore making it a useful adjunct to clinical assessment in a variety of different settings, such as theatre, colorectal outpatient clinics, and surgical admission wards.

Specific indications for rigid sigmoidoscopy include:

- *Rectal bleeding.* Use of a rigid sigmoidoscope and proctoscope can identify an anorectal source, such as haemorrhoids, mucosal inflammation, or a rectal tumour. It is avoided where the patient is presenting with both bleeding and abdominal pain, in case there is active inflammation of the distal large bowel and rectum (e.g. locally advanced diverticulitis, ischaemia, infective colitis) to which instrumentation and air insufflation may result in damage or perforation of the rectal wall.

- *Alterations in bowel habit.* A distal rectosigmoid tumour may be identified.
- *Anorectal pain and sepsis.*
- *Sigmoid volvulus.* Rigid sigmoidoscopy is used to safely place a flatus tube under visualization to decompress the volvulus, an important procedure that can prevent the patient from developing bowel ischaemia. Passage of the scope is therapeutic and can result in rapid passage of proximal faecal matter and gas, therefore the clinician should prepare themselves prior to the procedure with incontinence sheets, apron, and cautious positioning and technique at the bedside.

Rigid sigmoidoscopy is contraindicated in:

- Clinical or radiological suspicion of perforated bowel.
- Suspected or confirmed peritonitis.
- Toxic megacolon.
- Acute diverticulitis.
- Haematological disorders that predispose to bleeding.

Further reading

Goldberg SM, Tawadros PS (2014) Anal sepsis: anatomy, pathophysiology and presentation *in* Cohen R, Windsor A, *Anus: Surgical Treatment and Pathology*, pp.221–29. Springer Publishing, London.

Case history 4.11: Emergency: acute diverticulitis

A 79-year-old woman presented with a 5-day history of pain in the left iliac fossa region. It started as an ache and has been getting progressively worse. Today she feels hot, lethargic, anorexic, and unwell. She has been passing loose stools, but these did not contain blood or mucus. She had no urinary symptoms. She has had several bouts of left-lower quadrant pain over the last year for which she has not sought medical attention and that have been self-limiting in nature over a few days. She was diagnosed with diverticulosis 2 years ago on investigations for altered bowel habit. She also suffers from hypertension, COPD, and osteoarthritis, for which she has had both hips replaced. On examination she looked flushed and unwell. Her temperature was 38.4°C, her pulse was regular running at 105 beats per minute, and blood pressure is 105/71. On abdominal examination she was very tender in the left iliac fossa, and there was a fullness on palpation to this region. She was not peritonitic. Bowel sounds were present. Blood tests reveal a marked leukocytosis, an elevated CRP, and acute renal impairment (see Table 4.11.1).

Plain chest and abdominal films showed gas throughout the bowel with no evidence of free air. CT scan revealed an inflammatory mass at the sigmoid colon with a communicating collection in the presacral space (Figure 4.11.1). A diagnosis of perforated sigmoid diverticulitis was made. The patient was started on antibiotics and the collection was drained percutaneously under radiological guidance. She improved clinically.

Table 4.11.1 Blood results

Hb	140
WCC	21.2
Neutrophils	16.1
Platelets	380
Na	140
K	5
Ur	10
Cr	140
CRP	150

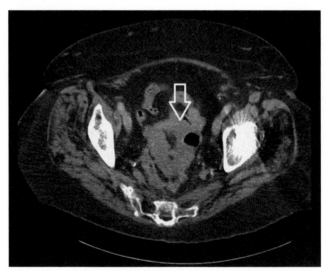

Figure 4.11.1 Image from the patient's abdominal CT scan, which showed an inflammatory mass (see arrow) at the level of the sigmoid colon.

Reproduced Courtesy of Judith Ritchie.

Questions

1. What is diverticular disease?

2. How does acute diverticulitis present?

3. What is the pathophysiology of acute diverticulitis?

4. What are the complications of acute diverticulitis and how do they present?

5. How should diverticulitis be investigated and managed?

6. The patient responds well to management and is ready for discharge. She asks about follow-up and her chances of recurrent attacks. What should you tell her?

Answers

1. What is diverticular disease?

Diverticulae are outpouches of colon wall that form from the gastro-intestinal lumen. They are generally very small, measuring only a couple of millimetres in diameter. They can form anywhere within the intestinal tract, from the duodenum to the distal sigmoid. However, colonic diverticulae are much more common and are the focus of this case discussion. The incidence of diverticulae rises with increasing age—they are present in 2.5% of those below 40 years of age, in 5–10% of those over 45 years, and in 80% in those over 85 years old.

Diverticulae have been associated with a low-fibre diet, lack of exercise, and obesity. These factors disrupt coordinated colonic motility, which can result in an increased colonic intraluminal pressure. This in turn can result in weakening of the abdominal wall at vulnerable points, usually at the sites where the vasae rectae (blood vessels) penetrate the bowel wall on the anti-mesenteric border. They do not develop in the rectum.

Diverticulae can form throughout the colon, but are most commonly found in the transverse, descending, and sigmoid colon. They can be classified as true or false:

- True diverticulae contain all layers of the bowel wall (mucosa, muscularis propria, and adventitia). They tend to more commonly form at the caecum and in the ascending colon.

- False diverticulae contain mucosa and submucosa only. They develop in the descending and sigmoid colon.

Diverticulae are often diagnosed on investigations for abdominal pain and altered bowel habit, as they can be readily visualized intraluminally on colonoscopy, on barium enema and also on CT imaging (Figure 4.11.2).

The presence of multiple diverticulae is termed diverticulosis. Diverticulosis is asymptomatic in three-quarters of cases. Symptomatic presentation is due to acute inflammation within the diverticula, termed acute diverticulitis. There is some evidence in

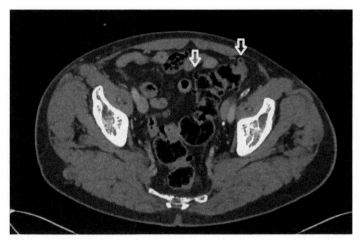

Figure 4.11.2 An abdominal CT image that shows simple diverticulae (see arrows). These can be seen on the scan as outpouchings containing air on the side of the colon wall.

Reproduced Courtesy of Judith Ritchie.

the literature that low-grade mucosal inflammation can co-exist adjacent to the diverticulae, referred to as diverticular colitis or segmental colitis, which may explain why some patients are chronically symptomatic of their diverticular disease in the absence of acute inflammation.

Patients may often confuse the terms diverticulosis and diverticulitis, but good history-taking can often help to differentiate between the two.

2. How does acute diverticulitis present?

Diverticulitis can be classified as:

- Simple or uncomplicated diverticulitis, where there is simple inflammation. It is a mild and self-resolving inflammatory process.

- Complicated diverticulitis, where patients develop complications such as sepsis or obstruction.

In uncomplicated disease, patients develop localized diverticular inflammation that is self-limiting and resolves without sequelae with clinical resolution of symptoms within a few days. Patients classically report left-lower quadrant pain and tenderness, feeling unwell with poor appetite, and fever. Nausea and vomiting are common features, and patients may report constipation or diarrhoea at the time of the attack. Urinary symptoms can sometimes be present due to pressure effects from inflammation around the sigmoid pressing on to the bladder. Patients can be febrile at presentation.

3. What is the pathophysiology of acute diverticulitis?

Acute diverticulitis is believed to develop as a consequence of obstruction within the diverticular neck, most commonly through faecal impaction. This can also entrap gut microbes into the diverticular pocket. The obstructed diverticula will swell due to ongoing mucosal secretion. Mucosal inflammation arises within the diverticulum, giving rise to acute diverticulitis, and can spread to involve the adjacent pericolic fat and mesentery. Gut microbes can proliferate and establish infection, which can track beneath the submucosa to create a pericolic abscess or infection further into the mesentery. An abscess can be walled off within the pelvic peritoneum generating localized tenderness, but where it cannot be contained it will result in abdominal peritoneal contamination with consequent peritonitis. In severe cases, perforated diverticulitis may be large enough to allow passage of faeces into the peritoneum, resulting in faecal peritonitis.

Occasionally the inflammatory process can compromise the blood supply to the diverticula and the resultant ischaemia results in mucosal ulceration and necrosis with subsequent micro- or macro-perforation. Involvement of the adjacent colonic wall and its mesentery can result in an inflammatory mass called a phlegmon, generally following a rupture of the diverticulum.

4. What are the complications of diverticulitis and how do they present?

The term complicated diverticulitis encompasses a spectrum of complications that arise when the inflammatory process progresses. These include:

- *Obstruction.* This can occasionally arise in an acute attack due to bowel oedema and spasm secondary to the inflammatory process.

It may also develop due to pressure effects from an adjacent phlegmon or abscess developing within and adjacent to the colonic wall. Persistent inflammatory attacks can also result in fibrosis, which can lead to obstruction. A fibrosed phlegmon appears as a solid mass on CT imaging and fibrosis of the bowel can result in stricturing. Both of these features can be difficult to distinguish from malignancy. Complete obstruction is rare, partial obstruction is more common.

- *Pericolic abscess.* This can develop as an infective complication of an acute attack or as a complication of recurrent attacks of diverticulitis. Patients are tachycardic, pyrexial, or frankly septic.

- *Peritonitis* from peritoneal contamination with infection or faeces following diverticular perforation. Patients are extremely sick, appearing pale and shocked. They have signs of peritonism on abdominal examination or a rigid abdomen. They are hypotensive, tachycardic, and often pyrexic. They may have signs of severe sepsis and be peripherally shut down. This is a surgical emergency and should be recognized early, as prompt surgical intervention is warranted.

- *Colonic fistulation* to adjacent organs. This develops in 2% of complicated disease, in the presence of chronic inflammation involving adjacent organs, such as the bladder (colovesical fistula) and vagina (colovaginal fistula), and very rarely to the skin (colocutaneous fistula). These patients are not commonly septic and often present electively. Colovesical fistula presents with passage of faecal matter in the urine (faecaluria) or the sensation of passing flatus through the urinary tract (pneumaturia). Colovaginal fistula presents with passage of faeces from the vagina. These fistulas are complex and should be investigated thoroughly, sometimes requiring both CT and MRI imaging. Patients should be referred to consultant colorectal surgeons who specialize in dealing with colonic fistulas, and input may also be needed from gynaecological and urology specialists, depending on the nature of the fistula.

5. How should diverticulitis be investigated and managed?

Patients may present with mild cases to their GP, who may make the diagnosis based on the patient's past medical history or on clinical suspicion. The GP may instigate outpatient management in patients with mild symptoms without fever, vomiting, or peritonism, prescribing analgesia, oral antibiotics, and gut rest. Patients diagnosed on clinical suspicion may be referred later, on an outpatient basis once the attack has subsided, for colonoscopy or barium enema, which can visualize the diverticulae intraluminally. More symptomatic or complicated cases will present or be referred to hospital for inpatient management.

Thorough assessment of the patient will generate a clinical history consistent with acute diverticulitis, but it cannot always be distinguished from other differentials, including bowel obstruction, gut ischaemia, or bowel perforation, particularly in complicated disease. Septic and peritonitic patients require immediate investigation and intervention, and prompt action is crucial. These patients should receive immediate resuscitation with high flow oxygen, intravenous crystalloids, intravenous antibiotics, and analgesia (the sepsis six). A urinary catheter should be passed and frequent observations taken. Haemodynamically stable patients should receive analgesia, intravenous fluids, and antibiotics. Blood cultures should be sent on septic patients. Choice of antibiotic must cover gut organisms, generally Gram-negative rods and anaerobic bacteria, and is guided by local antibiotic policy. Patients with suspected localized disease can be allowed clear fluids orally. Stable patients are usually imaged, within the first 24 hours of admission, with abdominal CT. This is commonly diagnostic for acute diverticulitis, as well as its complications. Both CT and clinical findings govern management. Barium enema is not often given in such acute presentations, as contrast extravasation through a perforated diverticulum can result in chemical peritonitis, beside it being an uncomfortable and unpleasant test in an acutely unwell patient. Colonoscopy is rarely performed in the acute setting as bowel insufflation and passing a scope in inflamed bowel can risk perforating the bowel.

The Hinchey classification system allows the surgical and radiological team to classify patients based on their complications (Table 4.11.2).

Table 4.11.2 The Hinchey classification

	Hinchey classification		Modified Hinchey classification	Management
I	Pericolic phlegmon or abscess	Ia	Confined pericolic inflammation (phlegmon)	Antibiotics
		Ib	Confined pericolic abscess	Antibiotics/drain
II	Pelvic, intra-abdominal, or retroperitoneal abscess	II	Pelvic, distant intra-abdominal, or retroperitoneal abscess	Drain
III	Generalized purulent peritonitis	III	Generalized purulent peritonitis	Surgery*
IV	Generalized faecal peritonitis	IV	Faecal peritonitis	Surgery
		Fistula	Colovesical, colovaginal, coloenteric, colocutaneous	
		Obstruction	Large or small bowel obstruction	

*There is debate about the form of surgery here.

Adapted from *The American Journal of Gastroenterology*, Volume 100, Issue 4, pp. 910–17, Andreas M Kaiser, Jeng-Kae Jiang, Jeffrey P Lake, Glenn Ault, Avo Artinyan et al., 'The Management of Complicated Diverticulitis and the Role of Computed Tomography', Copyright © 2005, by permission of Macmillan Publishers Ltd.

Localized and pelvic abscesses may require percutaneous drainage alongside antibiotics, facilitating attainment of pus for microbiological culture and sensitivity to identify any causative organisms. Percutaneous drainage is appropriate for those that are technically accessible with abscesses around 4 cm or greater in size, whilst antibiotic therapy and close observation is generally effective first-line for smaller abscesses in stable patients.

Emergency surgical intervention is warranted for patients with:

◆ Peritonitis.

◆ Bowel obstruction.

◆ Abscess that cannot be accessed percutaneously for drainage.

◆ Sepsis that fails to be managed by a percutaneous drain.

Surgery may require laparotomy or laparoscopy, depending on the exact indication and circumstance. Laparotomy is usually carried out for obstruction, sepsis, and macroperforation with faecal contamination for surgical management and copious washout. Hartmann's procedure and colostomy is advocated by many surgeons, with total sigmoid colectomy minimizing the chance of diverticular recurrence in any remnant sigmoid.

With the advent of laparoscopic surgery, there may be a role for laparoscopy and washout, and placement of drains. However, this is not standard practice across the UK at present.

Elective resection is carried out for:

+ Fistulating disease.

+ Perforated diverticulitis that has settled clinically but that cannot be distinguished from a perforated carcinoma on imaging, requiring resection for a definitive histological diagnosis.

+ Persistent attacks. This is controversial and is usually taken on a case-by-case basis.

6. The patient responds well to management and is ready for discharge. She asks about follow-up and her chances of recurrent attacks. What should you tell her?

The patient should receive outpatient endoscopy to rule out any underlying malignancy.

Published recurrence rates vary quite widely, generally up to a third of cases, with complicated disease occurring in 4% of cases. Recurrence is more common in younger patients. She should also be advised to eat a high-fibre diet, avoid constipation, and maintain an active lifestyle to combat known risk factors.

Further reading

Morris AM, Regenbogen SE, Hardiman KM, Hendren S (2014) Sigmoid diverticulitis: a systematic review. *JAMA* 311(3): 287–97.

Case history 4.12: Emergency: ischaemic bowel (acute mesenteric ischaemia)

A 72-year-old woman presents with a 6-hour history of sudden onset severe, constant, central abdominal pain, which has been getting progressively worse. She feels unwell and has vomited several times. She has a history of hypertension treated with an ACE inhibitor and mild arthritis for which she takes simple opioid analgesia. She has no gastrointestinal history. She is an ex-smoker, having smoked 20 cigarettes a day for 40 years in the past.

On examination she looks pale and unwell. Her pulse is irregular running at 98 beats per minute. Her blood pressure is 105/60, saturations are 95% on air, and her respiratory rate is 26 breaths per minute. Her abdomen is generally very tender but with no clinical evidence of peritonism or guarding. Bowel sounds are reduced. CT angiogram showed a thromboembolus within the proximal superior mesenteric artery (SMA) (Figure 4.12.1). The lady underwent emergency laparotomy and embolectomy. The bowel was predominantly viable, requiring only localized resection of non-viable bowel with primary anastomosis.

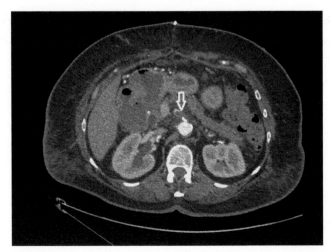

Figure 4.12.1 Image from the patient's CT showing a thrombus (see arrow) occluding blood flow (which is depicted as white from the contrast proximal to the occluding thrombus) from the aorta through the proximal superior mesenteric artery.

Reproduced Courtesy of Judith Ritchie.

Questions

1. What are the key differentials in such a presentation?
2. What is mesenteric ischaemia and how can it be classified?
3. What are the causes of acute mesenteric ischaemia?
4. What is the pathophysiology of mesenteric ischaemia?
5. How does acute mesenteric ischaemia present?
6. What are the appropriate investigations?
7. How should acute mesenteric ischaemia be managed?
8. What is the prognosis?

Answers

1. What are the key differentials in such a presentation?

Acute intestinal ischaemia is a key differential here. This fits a clinical picture of sudden onset of constant, acute, and severe abdominal pain with a severity that is incongruent with examination findings. Acute pancreatitis, intra-abdominal sepsis, including diverticulitis and cholecystitis, and perforated viscus may also present with a similar picture. Perforated viscus generally manifests with signs of peritonism on clinical examination where there is peritoneal contamination, but may be occult if the perforation is localized and walled off by adjacent viscera without peritoneal spill.

This is not a typical presentation for bowel obstruction but history and investigations should seek to rule this out.

2. What is mesenteric ischaemia and how can it be classified?

Mesenteric ischaemia refers to the clinicopathological sequelae of inadequate blood flow through the coeliac axis and superior mesenteric artery to the small bowel.

Mesenteric ischaemia can either be acute or chronic in nature:

♦ Acute mesenteric ischaemia results in ischaemia, infarction, and necrosis of the bowel wall. It has an acute and systemic presentation and is a life-threatening condition.

♦ Chronic mesenteric ischaemia arises where there is non-occlusive ischaemia within the mesenteric vasculature, such as with diffuse and severe atherosclerosis. It has a more indolent presentation, with chronic post-prandial abdominal pain ('mesenteric angina') and weight loss, although these patients can develop an acute-on-chronic presentation if they proceed to develop a complete occlusion.

This case focuses on acute mesenteric ischaemia.

3. What are the causes of acute mesenteric ischaemia?

Mesenteric ischaemia is either occlusive (complete) or non-occlusive (incomplete) in nature. Occlusive ischaemia is caused by any pathology preventing arterial supply to the bowel, which can be intrinsic or extrinsic to the artery.

Intrinsic pathology includes:

• *Embolus*. An embolus constitutes any material causing an obstruction in the vascular system, such as atheroma, tumour, gas, fat, and amniotic fluid.

• *Thrombus*. This is a solid mass of blood constituents. It can form on a ruptured atherosclerotic plaque. This may occur on plaques within the aorta and occlude the origin of the coeliac axis or mesenteric arteries. Alternatively, it may break off from one to form a thromboembolism. In addition, thrombi can occur in hypercoagulable states such as protein C or S deficiency or factor V leiden. They can also form from venous stasis, such as with a deep vein thrombosis (DVT), and within the ventricles of the heart in the presence of uncoordinated cardiac activity, such as atrial fibrillation. Fragments of thrombus can embolize and travel through the systemic circulation. The smaller calibre mesenteric arteries are susceptible to occlusion from such thrombi.

• *Arterial spasm*. The colonic vessels are particularly sensitive to low flow states and vasoconstriction.

• *Arterial injury* or dissection secondary to blunt trauma, angiography, or ligation following aortic surgery may give rise to arterial ischaemia.

Extrinsic pathology includes:

• Compression from adjacent pathology, such as severe colitis.

• Venous congestion from mesenteric venous thrombosis. This been reported to account for 10% of cases of acute mesenteric ischaemia. Thrombus formation within the intramural vessels results in haemorrhagic infarctions with mucosal sloughing, oedema, and haemorrhage. The establishment of ischaemic bowel is more gradual in onset in mesenteric venous thrombosis than arterial ischaemia.

◆ Bowel intussusception or volvulus, which can mechanically occlude the blood supply.

Non-occlusive ischaemia can arise in low flow states, such as cardiac failure, sepsis, and hypovolaemia. It also occurs in those with diffuse atherosclerotic disease who can, therefore, not compensate for a hypovolaemic insult. It generally occurs in the elderly, those with multiple comorbidities, or the critically ill.

Acute mesenteric ischaemia is most commonly thromboembolic in nature. Emboli are in the majority of cases cardiac in origin, in the presence of atrial fibrillation or following a myocardial infarction. Thrombosis can occur at atherosclerotic plaques at the site of origin of the SMA from the aorta, whereas emboli usually lodge distal to the SMA origin. The level of occlusion, and consequently the extent of ischaemia, depends on the size of the emboli, with larger emboli occluding the entire SMA and smaller emboli lodging more distally to give a segmental occlusion. SMA occlusion usually results in infarction, due to the lack of collateral circulation to the small bowel.

4. What is the pathophysiology of mesenteric ischaemia?

Ischaemia is the effect of insufficient oxygen supply to a tissue relative to its demand, which occurs as a result of a reduction in the blood supply to it. It may be reversible if the cause is identified and removed in sufficient time. Infarction describes the consequent tissue death, which occurs as a result of irreversible ischaemia. Necrosis describes the consequent tissue death on a cellular level that results from cellular injury, as opposed to programmed cell death or apoptosis, and is synonymous with infarction.

Persistent ischaemia results in tissue infarction and necrosis, in a process that progresses through a number of stages:

1. *Mucosal infarction* involves the mucosa only. This results in release of proteolytic enzymes, which can lead to mural and transmural infarction, making the mucosa more permeable to bacteria, toxins, and vasoactive substances. Translocation of these organisms through the bowel wall into the systemic circulation can result in septic shock or multi-organ dysfunction. Infarcted mucosa can

regenerate without any consequence in the long term, if the cause of ischaemia is treated or removed.

2. *Mural infarction* involves both mucosa and submucosa and extends into the underlying muscularis propria. The mucosa becomes haemorrhagic and swollen due to underlying submucosal oedema and may ulcerate. Serosanguinous fluid may be released into the peritoneal cavity. Removal of the cause of ischaemia leads to a lengthy healing process involving granulation tissue, which can result in fibrous stricture formation.

3. *Transmural infarction* occurs when infarction extends throughout the entire bowel wall through the muscularis propria. Tissue necrosis has established by this stage. The bowel dilates and becomes gangrenous, the serosa becomes congested and coated in white fibrin. The gangrenous bowel tissue is prone to perforation. Patients are severely systemically compromised by this stage and resection of the affected bowel is required. Ongoing necrosis is ultimately fatal to the patient.

Occlusive ischaemia results in hypoxia, the extent of which is dependent on:

◆ The level of occlusion in the arterial tree, which in the case of the small bowel can determine how much bowel is affected.

◆ The adequacy of collateral blood supply to maintain blood flow and perfusion in the presence of an occlusion. The collateral supply for the superior mesenteric artery is poor, unlike that of the inferior mesenteric artery.

◆ Anatomical variation of the arterial blood supply, which can arise due to variation in the process of embryological fusion of the ventral visceral segmental branches of the dorsal aorta.

There may be restoration of the gut blood supply in non-occlusive ischaemia, however this can still result in tissue damage as a consequence of hypoxic-reperfusion injury, which generates free radicals that cause mucosal damage.

5. How does acute mesenteric ischaemia present?

Occlusive mesenteric arterial ischaemia presents with sudden onset of acute and severe abdominal pain. Patients often start vomiting and may also experience diarrhoea, as the resultant hypoxia and a build-up of tissue metabolites result in bowel spasm, which precipitates gut emptying. Patients become rapidly dehydrated due to third space losses, leading to tachycardia, tachypnoea, and circulatory failure. Suspicion should be raised in older patients with atrial fibrillation, recent arterial embolic phenomena, or congestive cardiac failure with severe pain that does not fit physical examination findings.

Patients with non-occlusive mesenteric ischaemia are generally already very sick. Ischaemia is usually precipitated by a hypovolaemic insult. This may be difficult to detect in critically ill or intubated patients, who may simply develop a worsening clinical state. Mesenteric ischaemia should, therefore, be borne in mind in such patients.

Mesenteric venous thrombosis has a more indolent presentation, with a couple of weeks of abdominal pain, nausea, and diarrhoea, but where acute ischaemia develops these patients will have similar symptoms and features to arterial ischaemia.

As the tissue infarcts, the patient will develop peritonism. The infarcted tissue propagates systemic inflammatory response syndrome with multi-organ failure and ultimately death.

6. What are the appropriate investigations?

Acute mesenteric ischaemia is a difficult diagnosis to make, requiring a high degree of clinical suspicion. A thorough history is extremely helpful. Patients should undergo regular observations and recordings of vital signs. Basic investigations include:

- ECG tracing to look for arrhythmias.
- Arterial blood gas and serum lactate, to assess for metabolic acidosis, which often arises as a result of tissue ischaemia.
- Full blood count and CRP. White cell count is commonly raised.

- Serum electrolytes, renal and liver function tests.

- Serum amylase.

- Plain abdominal radiographs may be performed during initial assessment to rule out obstruction or perforation, but they are not diagnostically helpful in many cases. Features of ischaemia include thumb-printing due to mucosal oedema, intramural gas (pneumatosis coli), or free intraperitoneal gas following rupture. Features of ischaemia on plain film are present in less than 40% of cases.

- CT abdomen with intravenous contrast can rule out other causes of an acute abdomen, such as acute pancreatitis, intussusception, and volvulus. Some radiological features of intestinal ischaemia can be discerned on contrast CT, including thickened bowel wall, mural haematoma and gas, mesenteric vessel congestion, intra-peritoneal air, or gas in the mesenteric or portal system. Signs are often non-specific, which is why the diagnosis is driven predominantly on clinical grounds. Air in the portal tract is a late sign and is, therefore, associated with a poor prognosis.

- CT angiogram is readily available in many centres now and employs multi-slice technology with contrast enhanced scanning, which has significantly improved the diagnostic capabilities for detecting thromboembolism causing mesenteric ischaemia.

- Mesenteric angiography is gold standard and can be used if CT angiography is not available or if its findings are equivocal.

7. How should acute mesenteric ischaemia be managed?

Management includes ABCDE assessment and resuscitation. High flow oxygen should be administered. Patients should be maintained nil by mouth and given intravenous fluid resuscitation, as patients rapidly become dehydrated. Patients should be catheterized and staff should maintain careful fluid-balance recordings. Opiate analgesia should be titrated to give symptomatic relief. Empirical broad-spectrum intravenous antibiotics covering enteric organisms should be given to cover the risk of systemic sepsis from bacterial translocation through ischaemic gut. Patients should undergo contrast CT angiogram or mesenteric angiography, where possible, as this can locate the level of any obstructing thromboembolism and aid with pre-operative planning.

Occlusive ischaemia is a surgical emergency and warrants immediate surgical exploration. In the presence of peritonitis, radiological or laboratory evidence of infarction or perforation, or strong clinical suspicion, urgent surgical exploration is warranted.

Management requires:

+ Identifying the site and cause of ischaemia.

+ Restoration of blood flow. This should be done at the time of surgery. This may involve general and vascular surgeons and vascular interventional radiologists. The technical approach to restoring vascular patency differs according to the cause, and pre-operative vascular imaging can be very important. Proximal SMA thromboembolus is treated by arteriotomy and embolectomy, whereas SMA thrombosis in the presence of widespread atherosclerotic disease requires aorto-mesenteric bypass.

+ Assessment of bowel viability. Non-viable ischaemic or infarcted bowel should be resected. Mesenteric arterial cascades can be digitally assessed for the presence or absence of arterial pulsation. Potential viability is suggested where mesenteric arterial pulsation to vessels can be palpated by the surgeon within the mesentery of affected small bowel, as well as bowel peristalsis stimulated by touch. Colour changes (dusky to blue to black) and loss of sheen is suggestive of infarction. Ischaemic and necrotic bowel should be completely resected to leave bowel with adequate vascular supply. The surgeon ensures that the resected ends of bowel are well perfused prior to anastomosing. If there is concern for the anastomosis, for instance in the presence of infarction and systemic compromise, the primary anastomosis may also be protected with a proximal double-barrel (loop) stoma or, alternatively, an end stoma should be created with a distal mucous fistula.

- Patients should be anticoagulated, which has traditionally been achieved with heparin infusions, starting intra-operatively (following restoration of blood flow and any resection) and continued post-operatively.

Some centres may use papaverine to reduce arterial spasm and improve blood flow in both non-occlusive mesenteric ischaemia and peri-operatively following treatment of occlusive mesenteric ischaemia.

Patients who survive the initial insult and surgery may have typically lost a large length of bowel. They will require a multidisciplinary approach to manage their nutrition, commonly with long-term TPN. They may also have a very proximal high output stoma, such as a jejunostomy. Some patients may be considered for intestinal transplant.

8. What is the prognosis?

The prognosis of this condition remains poor. Outcome is dependent on the level of occlusion, the degree of organ dysfunction at presentation, and comorbidities. The mortality rate is reported to reach 50% for those diagnosed within 24 hours of the onset of symptoms and less than 30% thereafter.

Further reading

Khan T, Smith FCT (2016) Mesenteric ischaemia. *Surgery (Oxford)* 34 (4): 203–10.

Case history 4.13: Emergency: large bowel obstruction

An 84-year-old woman presented with a 5-day history of being unable to open her bowels. She had not passed wind for 3 days (obstipation). Her abdomen has felt generally bloated for the last week, and it has become progressively distended over the last 4 days. She has felt unwell and nauseous for 2 days. Her past medical history included hypertension and one myocardial infarction 6 years ago, following which she required cardiac stents. She was an ex-smoker with 10 pack years and rarely drank alcohol. Over the last few months she had experienced constipation, passing thin, narrow stools upon effort once every other day. On examination she looked clinically dry. Her pulse was regular at 90 beats per minute and her blood pressure was 140/75. Her respiratory rate was 22 respirations per minute and saturations 96% on air. She was afebrile. Her abdomen was markedly distended and tympanic. On examination she was generally uncomfortable but there was no peritonism. Plain abdominal X-ray revealed marked dilation of the colon to the point of the sigmoid colon, beyond which no air was present. Abdominal CT revealed an annular constricting sigmoid tumour (Figure 4.13.1). The ileocaecal valve appeared competent on imaging and the small bowel was collapsed.

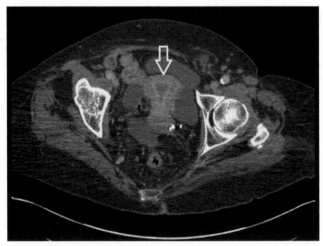

Figure 4.13.1 An image from the patient's CT abdomen pelvis, which shows a constricting tumour around the sigmoid colon (see arrow).

Reproduced Courtesy of Judith Ritchie.

Questions

1. What is the diagnosis and what are the potential differentials?
2. What is the pathophysiology of large bowel obstruction?
3. What is the difference between complete and partial large bowel obstruction?
4. How is pseudo-obstruction diagnosed?
5. How does large bowel obstruction present?
6. List some characteristic and concerning features on imaging.
7. How would you manage this patient?

Answers

1. What is the diagnosis and what are the potential differentials?

This case is consistent with large bowel obstruction. This is less common than small bowel obstruction, comprising 20% of all bowel obstructions. The aetiology is also very different, and appropriate differentials are:

- Intraluminal obstruction caused by:
  - Malignancy.
  - Complicated diverticulitis (abscess/phlegmon).
  - Strictures due to recurrent diverticular inflammation or as a consequence of healing from previous colonic ischaemia.
- Colonic volvulus.
- Incarceration and strangulation of a large bowel loop in a hernia, e.g. sigmoid colon incarcerated in an indirect inguinal hernia, comprising a closed-loop obstruction.
- Pseudo-obstruction that may be:
  - Acute.
  - Chronic.

2. What is the pathophysiology of large bowel obstruction?

Mechanical obstruction prevents passage of stool and flatus. Swallowed air and fermented gas, faecal matter, and fluid secreted by the small bowel continue to accumulate in the large bowel proximal to the obstruction. This results in bowel dilatation and mucosal oedema, both of which can impair arteriovenous supply. Depending on the degree of resultant ischaemia, bacterial translocation, dehydration, and electrolyte abnormalities can result and the bowel can perforate.

Volvulus results from bowel twisting on its mesentery. Chronic faecal loading of the sigmoid is thought to increase the weight on its elongated mesentery, putting it at increased risk of torsion. True caecal volvulus is the result of incomplete embryological development of the dorsal mesentery, predisposing the terminal ileum, caecum, and ascending colon to twist around themselves. Sigmoid volvulus is covered in Case 7.3 in Chapter 7. Volvulus can result in rapid obstruction to the blood vessels within the mesentery resulting in ischaemia, as well as an acute, closed-loop obstruction to the twisted bowel. Both of these constitute surgical emergencies.

3. What is the difference between complete and partial large bowel obstruction?

Complete (acute) obstruction describes complete occlusion of the bowel lumen preventing passage of gas, fluid, and faecal matter. This results in abdominal distension, discomfort, and failure to pass flatus or stool. There is reduced or absent bowel sounds. The onset of nausea and vomiting occurs once the pathophysiology is established, although it is less common in obstruction of the descending sigmoid. Complete obstruction occurs with mechanical obstruction and acute pseudo-obstruction.

Partial obstruction of the large intestine describes a narrowing or incomplete obstruction of the bowel lumen, thereby generating a degree of obstruction but ultimately allowing faecal passage. It is less common and presents with recurrent episodes of colicky abdominal pain, distension, and alternating bowel habit. There may be hyperactive bowel sounds. The exact nature of the obstruction should be determined through careful and comprehensive history-taking, and thorough clinical examination and appropriate investigations. Both strictures and malignancy can cause partial obstruction of the bowel.

4. How is pseudo-obstruction diagnosed?

Acute pseudo-obstruction is bowel obstruction in the absence of a mechanical obstruction. It cannot be clinically differentiated from mechanical bowel obstruction on history or examination. The disease most commonly affects the right side of the colon, with patients developing colicky abdominal pain, constipation, nausea, and vomiting. On examination patients have a distended, tympanic, and tender abdomen with hyperactive or hypoactive bowel sounds. It commonly develops secondary to a number of precipitating factors, including:

◆ Pneumonia.

◆ Electrolyte imbalance (particularly low potassium).

◆ Myocardial infarct.

◆ Stroke.

◆ Acute renal impairment.

◆ Retroperitoneal malignancy.

Diagnosis of pseudo-obstruction is determined on imaging where no mechanical obstruction can be found. Plain abdominal radiograph will commonly reveal massively distended loops of large bowel with cut-off points at the hepatic or splenic flexure or rectosigmoid junction, but without gas-fluid levels. Abdominal CT will fail to reveal any mechanical obstruction also. In indeterminate or prolonged cases, contrast enema is considered diagnostic. Clinically, a distended rectum on rectal examination may raise suspicions of this presentation.

Pseudo-obstruction is distinct from ileus as pseudo-obstruction affects the large bowel whereas ileus affects both small and large bowel. Ileus is associated with vague abdominal pain, constipation, nausea, and vomiting, with a silent, distended, tympanic abdomen. Abdominal plain radiograph reveals small and large bowel dilatation with no distinct cut-off and gas throughout the colon.

5. How does large bowel obstruction present?

The presentation of large bowel obstruction is largely dependent on the underling pathology:

1. *Colon cancer.* Only 4% of colon cancer presents with obstruction, yet 85% of acute obstructions are malignant, of which a quarter are found to have synchronous liver metastases on imaging. Caecal and ascending colon tumours are rarely clinically symptomatic prior to presentation, although there may be iron-deficiency anaemia from chronic bleeding into the stool. The onset of obstruction is often associated with the rapid onset of central colicky abdominal pain and vomiting. Tumours arising between the descending colon and the rectum often have a preceding clinical

history. Descending colon/sigmoid cancers may have a history of dark blood mixed with the stool as well as mucus, and altered bowel habit. Stool frequency may be increased and loose. Rectal tumours may have a preceding history of constipation, pain on passing a bowel motion, and sensation of incomplete passage of stool (termed tenesmus). Obstructing descending and rectosigmoid tumours are rarely painful and vomiting is less common.

2. *Diverticulitis.* This is very rare, occurring in less than 10% of all cases of diverticular disease. In the acute setting, obstruction may result from a peridiverticular abscess. Patients may present with obstruction and signs of sepsis (pyrexia, tachycardia, and dehydration). The region of the abscess will be very tender, and a palpable mass may be felt. More commonly, recurrent attacks of diverticulitis result in colonic wall thickening due to pericolic annular fibrosis or kinking of the bowel due to inflammatory adhesions. This will more likely result in a picture of partial obstruction, as previously discussed.

3. *Colonic volvulus.* Volvulus results from axial twisting of bowel on its mesentery and constitutes 5% of large bowel obstructions. Sigmoid volvulus is most common and is discussed in detail in Case 7.3 in Chapter 7. Volvulus also occurs at the caecum in 22% of cases of volvulus and 2% at the transverse colon. There is an acute onset of cramping abdominal pain, abdominal distension, nausea, and vomiting. Ischaemia will result in rapid metabolic disturbance and raised serum lactate, and the patient may become hypotensive and tachycardic as their clinical condition worsens.

6. List some characteristic and concerning features on imaging.

In the presence of large bowel obstruction, concerning features are:

◆ Radiological features consistent with large bowel obstruction in the presence of a competent (closed) ileocaecal valve. This constitutes closed-loop obstruction, as the large bowel cannot be decompressed by passage of bowel contents back into the small bowel, resulting in obstruction at two points. This puts the patient at high risk of rapid onset of bowel ischaemia and subsequent perforation. The caecum is relatively thin-walled and has the largest diameter of the colon. It thereby requires less pressure to distend, which will rapidly compromise its blood flow with resultant ischaemia and necrosis. The serosal wall splits, with herniation of mucosa and caecal perforation resulting in peritonitis.

◆ Mural and intraperitoneal gas are concerning for perforation.

7. How would you manage this patient?

Appropriate first-line investigations:

◆ Bloods should be sent for haematology, coagulation and clinical chemistry, amylase, CRP, and crossmatch.

◆ Plain erect chest and supine abdominal radiographs are useful to identify obstruction and visceral perforation. Plain abdominal film may not always demonstrate dilated bowel, particularly when there is a history of previous colonic resections or abdominal surgeries.

◆ An urgent contrast CT of the abdomen and pelvis will be required. Colonoscopy is not a first-line investigation in an emergency presentation with complete obstruction.

◆ An arterial blood gas is useful to determine the metabolic status of the patient, and a raised serum lactate will alert to hypoperfusion caused by severe dehydration and ischaemia.

◆ Broad-spectrum antibiotics should be given in the presence of sepsis or where there has been a prolonged history of obstruction, as bacterial translocation is more likely to have occurred.

Patients with clinically suspected bowel obstruction should be kept nil by mouth and started on intravenous fluids. A nasogastric (NG) tube should be passed to decompress the stomach, to prevent vomiting of gut contents, and risk of pulmonary aspiration. Strict fluid balance should be maintained, with ongoing replacement of fluid lost through NG tube.

Subsequent management will depend on the underlying pathology. Colonic stents can be deployed to relieve partial obstruction from tumours in complete obstruction where there are no signs of perforation and systemic illness. They can be used both for palliative decompression of the bowel in patients with unresectable disease or significant comorbidity, or for temporary decompression ahead of elective resection. This is deemed safer, as emergency surgery for malignant bowel obstruction is associated with much higher rates of morbidity and mortality than in elective resections, generally from anastomotic leak. However, there have also been some concerns that micro-perforations at the time of stenting can worsen oncologic outcomes with higher rates of loco-regional recurrence. Consent to bowel stenting includes counselling to the risk of bowel perforation (4%), stent migration (12%), and re-obstruction (7%). It is important to have a plan for a patient should their stent fail or perforate. Emergency surgery in these circumstances generally requires laparotomy. Distended bowel proximal to the obstruction will be tense and should be decompressed with suction. If there is any peritoneal contamination or concerns about the potential for anastomotic leak (where there has been oedema or ischaemia), the patient could have an emergency resection and an end ileostomy or colostomy, which could be re-anastomosed a few months later.

Curative resection requires wide excision of the tumour and any local advancement. Advocated surgical approaches to obstructing tumours are:

- Right hemicolectomy, with or without primary anastomosis for right-sided tumours.
- Extended right hemicolectomy for transverse colon tumours.
- Left hemicolectomy and primary anastomosis or Hartmann's (resection, colostomy, and rectal closure) in left-sided tumours.

Complete large bowel obstruction in diverticular disease requires an immediate laparotomy and resection of the affected bowel. In the absence of perforation or diffuse inflammation, the bowel can be anastomosed, although a loop ileostomy may be placed, depending on the patient's clinical condition and surgeon's preference, as this will protect the distal anastomosis and allow it good opportunity to heal. Benign strictures are not very easily relieved with stents.

Acute pseudo-obstruction and ileus are both treated conservatively in the first instance. Acute pseudo-obstruction is associated with a 5% risk of perforation, usually at the caecum, therefore repeated

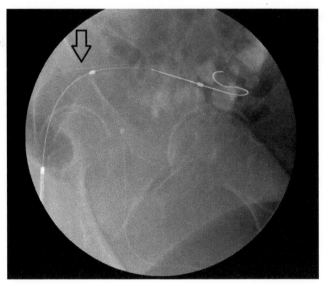

Figure 4.13.2 Image taken at stenting showing deployment of the stent across the tumour. The stent can be seen with a mesh appearance (see arrow) being deployed over the white guide wire.

Reproduced Courtesy of Judith Ritchie.

clinical and radiological examinations are warranted until symptoms resolve. In protracted cases with a caecum below 10 cm in diameter, colonoscopy can be performed, which can be both diagnostic and therapeutic, as it aids decompression through the procedure or placement of a decompression tube. Caecal distension of more than 10 cm, or radiological or clinical signs concerning of impending perforation, warrants surgical intervention and resection.

Occasionally, acute pseudo-obstruction and ileus can follow a prolonged course. Where patients have not eaten for over 5 days, involvement of the dietetic and nutrition teams should be sought, as the patient will require parenteral nutritional support.

This patient's obstruction was successfully treated with a colonic stent (Figure 4.13.2). Her disease was considered inoperable and she was palliated.

Further reading

Glancy DG *(2014) Intestinal obstruction. Surgery (Oxford)* **32** *(4): 204–11.*

Sawai RS (2012) Management of colonic obstruction: a review. *Clinics in Colon and Rectal Surgery* **25** (4): 200–3.

Case history 4.14: Emergency: rectal bleeding

A 71-year-old woman presents with a 10-hour history of frank rectal bleeding. This started after an urge to defecate, at which point she passed loose brown stool with fresh red blood. She has opened her bowels six times since, passing less stool with each motion and now reports only passing fresh blood. She is anxious but otherwise has no other associated symptoms. This is her first episode of rectal bleeding. There has been no altered bowel habit or weight loss preceding this episode. She is otherwise in good health and maintains an active lifestyle. She is not taking any medications. On examination she appears well, with no clinical signs of anaemia. Her pulse is 80 beats per minute and regular, her blood pressure 125/65, her saturations 98% on air, and respiratory rate of 16 breaths a minute. On examination her abdomen is soft and non-tender with no palpable masses. Digital rectal examination and proctoscopy are both normal. Rigid sigmoidoscope is passed to 10 cm and reveals blood-streaked mucosa only, with no visible lesions. Haematology is normal (see Table 4.14.1).

The patient was managed conservatively with close observation. The bleeding settled overnight and she was discharged. Colonoscopy was carried out 5 weeks later and revealed diverticulosis. A retrospective diagnosis of diverticular bleeding was made.

Table 4.14.1 Blood results

Haemoglobin	140	PT	10.9
WCC	9.1	APTT	54
Neutrophils	6.5	Fibrinogen	3.3
Platelets	245	Renal function	Normal
Liver function	Normal		

Questions

1. What features distinguish the site of the intestinal bleeding?
2. What are the common causes of lower gastrointestinal bleeding?
3. How is rectal bleeding investigated and managed?
4. When is emergency intervention warranted for lower gastrointestinal bleeding?

Answers

1. What features distinguish the site of the intestinal bleeding?

Upper gastrointestinal bleeding arises from a source proximal to the ligament of Treitz, and lower gastrointestinal bleeding arises from below this level. The colour of the blood passed per rectum can help towards focusing appropriate investigations for diagnosis, as this can be affected by the anatomical source of the bleeding. The history should determine how dark the bleeding is.

Malaena is black tarry, sticky foul-smelling stool that results from bleeding in the proximal intestines. It is a product of the digestive process on blood that has been passed into the stomach or small intestine anywhere proximal to the level of the caecum. Alteration of the haemoglobin by digestive enzymes and intestinal bacteria results in the characteristic black colour. It is distinguishable from stools of patients on iron supplements, which are grey-black in colour and occasionally loose but lack the odour or sticky consistency of malaena.

Lower intestinal bleeding is red. Maroon/port-coloured blood suggests bleeding from the right side of the colon. Bright red blood suggests bleeding from the left side of the colon.

However, despite these general rules of thumb, the clinician should be cautious. Passage of fresh red blood can occur in brisk upper gastrointestinal bleeding with rapid intestinal transit. Blood is altered to form malaena as it makes a relatively slow passage through the intestinal tract over a period of 6–24 hours, therefore such brisk bright red bleeding from an upper GI source will be significant and may potentially result in haemodynamic compromise. This is not uncommon, as 15% of patients presenting with massive rectal bleeding will have an upper gastrointestinal source.

2. What are the common causes of lower gastrointestinal bleeding?

Upper gastrointestinal bleeding is covered in Case 1.4 in Chapter 1.

Aetiology of lower gastrointestinal bleeding can be broken down thus:

- *Bleeding from anatomical structures.*
  - Diverticular bleeding in the presence of diverticulosis. The diverticulae generally arise at the site where the vasae rectae penetrate the bowel wall and muscular layers to supply the mucosa. The protruding diverticulum is thought to tent or abut the blood vessel. Chronic trauma and inflammation are believed to erode and damage it, causing bleeding into the colon lumen. Bleeding occurs in 20% of diverticular disease and can be profuse, occasionally requiring transfusion. However, 80% of cases are self-limiting and rarely require intervention.
  - Meckel's diverticulum. This is a congenital abnormality arising from incomplete closure of the vitellointestinal duct during embryonic development, arising 2 ft (60 cm) proximal to the ileocaecal valve. It is a true diverticulum containing all layers of bowel wall, and can contain ectopic pancreatic, gastric, or duodenal mucosa, as well as colonic mucosa that arises from the pluripotent cells that line it. Complications of persistent Meckel's diverticulum include haemorrhage, perforation, and bowel obstruction. It should be suspected in any patient with massive painless gastrointestinal haemorrhage, particularly in children. The diverticulum should be resected. This can be achieved laparoscopically in the elective setting or with a segmental ileal resection if it is for prolonged bleeding.
  - Haemorrhoids. These develop when the vascular cushions within the anal wall swell and stretch the suspensory muscles, eventually leading to prolapse down through the anal canal. They can thrombose, which is an acutely painful event that can result in erosion or trauma to the skin and subsequent bleeding. Bleeding can also occur in painless haemorrhoids due to trauma to the skin during wiping at toilet, with bright red blood on the paper or in the toilet bowl without mixing in the stool. These are discussed in Case 4.6 in this chapter.
  - Bleeding from colonic ischaemia. This is an acute phenomenon occurring as a result of tissue ischaemia to the mucosa and submucosa. This can result from vascular occlusion, such as a

thromboembolism to the blood supply to the colon. The blood supply to the large colon typically has an excellent collateral blood supply that prevents bowel infarction. However, it can also occur where the collateral supply is lost or where there is localized ischaemia in colonic inflammation secondary to infective or inflammatory bowel disease. Ischaemic colitis causes mucosal wall sloughing, oedema, and bleeding, and it will present with abdominal pain, bleeding per rectum, and dehydration. Patients will be sick with abdominal pain, dehydration, fever, and diarrhoea in inflammatory and infective colitis.

+ Radiation damage to the colon. The small bowel, colon, and rectum are also prone to damage from radiation therapy for abdominal and pelvic malignancies. Radiation-induced telangiectasia can develop within the small intestine, colon, and rectum. Some patients present months and years after radiation treatment with bleeding, diarrhoea, and incontinence due to radiation damage to the colon. These have been reported to respond well to argon beam coagulation therapy at endoscopy and sucralfate enemas in rectal lesions.

+ Malignant lesions can bleed due to mucosal infiltration as well as tumour ischaemia. Gastrointestinal stromal tumours (GIST) arise in the small bowel in a third of cases, and can present with abdominal pain and malaena. Bleeding from colon cancers is more insidious. Frank blood is not always visible in stool but detectable on laboratory examination, a feature that is now used for faecal occult blood screening for colorectal cancers. However, large lesions in the descending colon and rectum can become ischaemic, ulcerate, and bleed, with mild and intermittent episodes.

+ *Vascular sources.* Angiodysplasia is a vascular lesion arising as a consequence of degeneration of previously healthy submucosal veins in the colon wall. Although the pathophysiology has not been well described, it is thought to result from chronic venous obstruction occurring in episodes of colonic dysmotility and dilatation over time. Three-quarters develop at the caecum and ascending colon, and 15% in the jejenum and ileum. There may be a single or multiple lesions. It can present with abdominal pain and malaena. Angiodysplasia in the stomach, duodenum, and the large bowel can be treated with endoscopic obliteration.

Most common causes of lower gastrointestinal bleeding are diverticulae. Small bowel lesions are more commonly vascular in nature and account for 10% of bleeding per rectum. However, aetiology can also differ by age: in younger patients, tumours, Meckel's diverticulum, and Crohn's disease are common causes of small bowel bleeding. Vascular lesions and NSAID-related bleeding is commoner in older patients.

3. How is rectal bleeding investigated and managed?

Initial assessment should determine how significant the bleed is and whether the patient is haemodynamically compromised. This requires a comprehensive history of the event, detailing volume and frequency of episodes of bleeding, and whether this is mixed with stool. Past medical history and relevant systemic enquiry should be sought. Recent or current anticoagulant use should be specifically enquired about in the drug history.

High flow oxygen should be administered to sick patients particularly those with significant haemorrhage and haemodynamic compromise. Two large-bore intravenous cannulae should be sited for resuscitation and potential transfusion, which may be required in those with a history of massive or ongoing bleeding, or where there is concern of upper gastrointestinal bleeding with fast transit. Bloods should be sent for haematology, coagulation, liver and renal function, and blood grouping and crossmatch. Urgent haematologist advice should be sought for patients on anticoagulation, as this should be reversed to help stop the bleeding. Haemoglobin measurement on a venous blood gas may be useful in those who are acutely compromised. However, it should be borne in mind that haemoglobin levels often take hours to accurately represent the actual level following blood loss, and the decision to transfuse should be based on volume loss, clinical status, and oxygen requirement. In massive haemorrhage, with or without haemo-dynamic compromise, patients will require other products such as platelets, and in acute settings this can be provided in a massive transfusion pack.

Perform volume assessment, and instigate fluid balance and intra-venous fluid resuscitation. Transfusion is indicated where 40% of circulating volume has been lost, but may be required with 30–40% loss or in symptomatic or high-risk patients with cardiovascular dis-ease, in whom reduction of the oxygen-binding capacity in anaemia can precipitate myocardial ischaemia and infarction. Keep actively bleeding patients nil by mouth while they are observed. Instigate strict stool charting to measure volume and consistency of blood and stool, and the nature of any blood.

An urgent diagnostic and therapeutic upper GI endoscopy should be carried out where there is concern of upper gastrointestinal bleeding with fast transit, as this warrants urgent rule-out. Lower gastrointestinal bleeding is self-limiting in the majority of cases, so patients are commonly given supportive therapy and observation, without any acute investigation, monitoring blood loss and serum haemoglobin and coagulation, and administering transfusions. Investigations are performed at a later date to determine the source of the bleeding. Where the bleeding settles within 12–24 hours, these investigations can be done on an outpatient basis. First-line investi-gation is a colonoscopy, and capsule endoscopy for investigations of the small bowel where no colonic pathology is found.

4. When is emergency intervention warranted for lower gastrointestinal bleeding?

Urgent investigation and intervention is warranted for those with ongoing and heavy bleeding that does not settle or those who display haemodynamic compromise and tissue ischaemia from hypoperfu-sion despite resuscitation.

* In a sick patient with massive rectal bleeding, an urgent upper gastrointestinal endoscopy should first be performed to rule out an upper GI bleeding source.

- Colonoscopy has also traditionally been a first-line approach in the emergency setting. It is relatively safe, facilitates diagnosis, biopsy, and treatment to any bleeding vessel with sclerotherapy, epinephrine injection, clips, laser, or thermocoagulation. It can also be used on the table at emergency surgery to help visualize the luminal aspect of the large bowel. However, it cannot investigate the small bowel. In addition, endoscopic views may be obscured in an emergency procedure from faeces or ongoing haemorrhage, making this technically difficult or impossible to reach diagnosis or provide treatment.

- CT angiography with contrast is becoming increasingly common as radiological facilities for these are now becoming more available. CT imaging is minimally invasive, and technological advances have improved diagnostic capability in localizing bleeding vessels at rates as low as 0.3 ml/min on helical scans. It also has greater diagnostic capabilities, as it can detect underlying pathology, such as tumours and colitis.

- Interventional radiography can employ a number of minimally invasive treatments to stop bleeding with the benefit of avoiding surgery, particularly advantageous in high-risk surgical patients. Transcatheter embolization is most commonly used in the lower GI tract, which can employ a single embolic agent or a combination of them, such as coils, gel foam, glue, and polyvinyl alcohol particles, to embolize small, bleeding vessels. It has 80–90% success rates. However, it is not without risk, and procedural complications include arterial thromboembolism, catheter site bleeding, and contrast nephropathy, which may result in acute renal failure, particularly where there has been preceding hypoperfusion from hypovolaemia. Depending on the anatomical location of the vessel, there is a risk of regional ischaemia secondary to the embolization.

- Intra-arterial vasopressin infusions can be used to stave bleeding until intervention can be made, but is not suitable for a definitive treatment due to high rates of re-bleeding and is not commonly used.

Surgical intervention is only deployed where bleeding is ongoing and medical, endoscopic, or angiographic measures have failed to stop it, which is thankfully very rare. Resection may also be indicated for the underlying cause irrelevant of the bleeding; for instance, resection of ischaemic colitis, where there are concerning features of pending or established bowel perforation and peritoneal inflammation.

Surgery for irretractable lower intestinal bleeding is associated with a high risk of morbidity and mortality. Wherever possible, the site or level of bleeding should be identified before surgery. On-table colonoscopy can be used for this purpose. Surgical exploration should localize the source for targeted resection. Where the level of the bleeding has not been identified pre-operatively, segments of bowel can be isolated with non-crushing bowel clamps to identify the segment that bleeds and fills with blood. Localized segmental bowel resection should be carried out at the level of bleeding. Where the site cannot be located, a subtotal colectomy and end ileostomy can be carried out. Blind segmental resection is not advised as re-bleeding, morbidity, and mortality are unacceptably high. In the case of a bleeding tumour, emergency surgical resection of resectable lesions provides definitive treatment for the bleeding.

Surgical patients will be nursed on critical care post-operatively, as hypovolaemic shock and surgical trauma can precipitate multiorgan failure.

Further reading

Ghassemi KA, Jensen DM (2013) Lower GI bleeding: epidemiology and management. *Current Gastroenterology Reports* 15 (7): 10.1007/s11894-013-0333-5.

Sharma RK, Kain VJ (2008) Emergency surgery for Meckel's diverticulum. *World Journal of Emergency Surgery* 3 (27). Doi: 10.1186/1749-7922-3-27.

Strate LL, Naumann CR. (2010) The role of colonoscopy and radiological procedures in the management of acute lower intestinal bleeding. *Clinical Gastroenterology and Hepatology* 8 (4): 333–43.

Case history 4.15: Emergency: rectal prolapse

A 72-year-old woman presents to the emergency department with a 6-hour history of a soft-tissue swelling protruding from her anus. She became aware of this when she was attempting to open her bowels on the toilet that morning. She is alarmed but is otherwise well. There is no preceding history of this. She is chronically constipated for which she has taken lactulose and senna for several years. At times over the past few months she has noticed a prominent swelling on attempting to open her bowels, which she has managed to push back manually upon finishing on the toilet. She has also noticed some faecal staining and streaks of bright red blood on her pants. She had attributed all these features to haemorrhoids and not sought any medical treatment. She denies any alternating bowel habit or weight loss. She has a past medical history of hypertension for which she is on ramipril. On rectal examination, rectal mucosa is seen to protrude from the anus for about 5 cm. The mucosa is soft, painless, and of normal colour. Abdominal and other systems examinations are unremarkable.

Questions

1. What are the differential diagnoses?
2. What is rectal prolapse?
3. How is rectal prolapse classified?
4. What is the pathophysiology of rectal prolapse?
5. What are the predisposing factors for rectal prolapse?
6. How does rectal prolapse present?
7. How is rectal prolapse managed?

Answers

1. What are the differential diagnoses?

The history and presentation are consistent with rectal prolapse.

Possible differentials include a prolapsing rectal tumour and internal haemorrhoids, the latter more so in smaller prolapses where the anatomy is less distinct. Features suggestive of rectal prolapse are concentric rings of mucosa and visible delineation of anus and rectum at the pectinate line.

On the other hand, haemorrhoids are delineated by radial folds with intervening grooves. Rectal tumours rarely prolapse but this would appear firm and irregular on digital examination, and be irreducible.

2. What is rectal prolapse?

This occurs where rectal tissue protrudes from the anus. It is very uncommon, occurring in less than 1% of the adult population. It is much more common in women over 60 years of age. It is six times more prevalent in women than in men.

3. How is rectal prolapse classified?

There are three types of rectal prolapse:

1. Complete or full-thickness prolapse (known as rectal procidentia): this involves prolapse of the actual rectum, resulting in protrusion of two layers of rectal wall, which contain peritoneal sac between them. This may contain small bowel. Rectal tissue and any contained small bowel are at risk of strangulation.

2. Incomplete or mucosal prolapse: this consists of mucosal lining only.

3. Concealed or internal prolapse: this occurs where the upper rectum invaginates into the lower rectum. Prolapse is internal and not visualized at the anus.

4. What is the pathophysiology of rectal prolapse?

The pathogenesis of rectal prolapse is still not definitively agreed upon. There are a number of factors that are thought to be at play. A clear understanding of the pelvic floor is required to understand these factors.

The pelvic floor consists of a muscular plate formed by a number of muscles that together constitute the levator ani: the pubococcygeus, puborectalis, and iliococcygeus. The most medial muscle, the pubococcygeus, arises from the pubis and the obturator fasica, and passes back horizontally to insert into the coccyx and sacrum. Its medial border forms the border of the urogenital diaphragm. The rectum is supported by the puborectalis, a muscular sling arising on both sides from the pubis symphysis and the fascia of the urogenital diaphragm to fuse around the rectum. The iliococcygeus muscle is the most lateral muscular aspect of the levator ani, arising from the inner ischium and obturator fascia, and inserting into the coccyx. Fibres of both pubococcygeus and iliococcygeus fuse in the space between the coccyx and anus to form the fibrous anococcygeal body or raphe. The pelvic floor is supplied by S3 and S4 sacral spinal nerves, as well as the pudendal, perineal, and inferior rectal nerves. The urethra, vagina, and anorectum pass through the urogenital diaphragm and are supported by muscular attachments (collectively termed pubovisceralis, which includes the puborectalis). The pelvic organs are supported by the fibrous anococcygeal raphe. Good muscular tone of the levator ani results in a horizontal pelvic floor on standing, which supports the rectum and upper vagina.

One theory is that anatomical weakness of the pelvic floor predisposes to pelvic organ prolapse. Weakness or atony of the levator ani muscles results in laxity, widening the urogenital diaphragm, and predisposing to herniation and prolapse of the pelvic organs. This may happen where nerve supply is damaged.

Another theory is that prolapse arises as a circumferential internal intussusception of the rectum approximately 8 cm proximal to the anal verge, and can progress to full-thickness prolapse. This could theoretically occur in the presence of a distended anus and redundant sigmoid colon.

5. What are the predisposing factors for rectal prolapse?

The condition is most commonly associated with chronic constipation, of which there is a preceding history in between one-third to two-thirds of prolapses. Factors associated with pelvic floor trauma, such as multiple pregnancies and vaginal deliveries, and pelvic floor surgery, such as prostatectomy, may contribute. Anatomical anomalies that may contribute are a large pouch of Douglas and a dilated anus. Other factors include spinal cord injury and cauda equina syndrome, which have been attributed to neurological weakness of the pelvic floor. Functional disorders include chronic withholding of stool, which is particularly prevalent in patients with psychiatric and developmental disorders.

6. How does rectal prolapse present?

Patients may present acutely with an irreducible prolapse or in the elective setting with recurring prolapse. Incomplete or mucosal prolapse is characterized by radial folds of mucosa, whereas a full-thickness prolapse is characterized by concentric mucosal folds.

Onset is usually gradual and patients will often report preceding symptoms that in hindsight are consistent with the development of rectal prolapse. Patients can report preceding mucus discharge, and faecal streaking and incontinence, which can occur when the rectum prolapses past the anal sphincter, which can thereby not function to prevent this. Mucus discharge may also result in pruritus ani. Trauma to the prolapsing mucosa may result in occasional bleeding that is light and self-limiting in nature.

Concealed and full-thickness prolapse may also be preceded with a history of rectal fullness and the sensation of tenesmus (incomplete defaecation), or the sensation of a protruding mass on straining (at toilet, sneezing, or physical activity generating an increase in intra-abdominal pressure). It is common for patients to report detecting a protruding mass that they have to manually reduce.

Clinical features usually progress as the prolapse worsens. Patients may present late due to embarrassment. Advanced presentation can result in ulcerated mucosa, which typically results in more profuse rectal bleeding.

Patients may present to the acute surgical take with a complete mucosal prolapse or as an elective referral to colorectal clinic with a history suggestive of prolapse. This is usually dependent on how quickly the prolapse progresses or how late the patient leaves it before seeking medical attention.

In the presence of pelvic floor weakness, patients may also report features of urinary incontinence and a bulging sensation within the vagina, suggestive of prolapse of other urogenital organs. Urinary incontinence is reported in a third of patients and vaginal prolapse in approximately a fifth.

7. How is rectal prolapse managed?

The rectal prolapse should be manually reduced with gentle pressure, to slide the distal end of the prolapse in and back up past the anal sphinchter. If there is mucosal oedema, this can be reduced by applying sugar to the mucosa, which reduces oedema through osmosis. Once the oedema has reduced, reduction can be attempted.

Strangulation of full-thickness prolapse is very rare, but should be rapidly identified, as the patient will require emergency surgical intervention by an experienced colorectal surgeon. The prolapse cannot be digitally reduced and may be associated with severe pain. The Altemeier surgical approach may be used in this situation, with a temporary protective ileostomy.

In patients in whom prolapse has reduced, rigid sigmoidoscopy can assess the anorectal mucosa for signs of ulceration and any evidence of anorectal malignancy that may be associated with prolapse. In patients presenting in the elective setting with a history consistent of prolapse, this diagnosis should be first confirmed. This can be done at the bedside following initial clinical examination by asking the patient to strain to stool for a brief period, followed by repeated clinical examination for evidence of prolapse. A defaecating proctogram is diagnostic of all types of prolapse, particularly internal prolapse, which will not manifest externally on clinical examination. This is a radiological procedure that allows assessment of the mechanics of defaecation and assessment of important structures, such as the pelvic floor, in the process. The patient's rectum is filled with barium and the patient is positioned on a commode alongside a fluoroscope, which can visualize the rectal vault and lower pelvis during defaecation of the barium.

Treatment is both through lifestyle modifications and surgical repair.

Patients should avoid constipation, and stool softeners such as laxatives and bulking agents may be used.

Surgical approach is either through abdominal or perineal approach:

- Abdominal approach is invasive with a relatively higher risk of morbidity but a lower recurrence risk. These procedures are, therefore, undertaken in younger, fitter patients with longer life-expectancies and the promise of good quality of life. Complications include bowel injury, bleeding, anastomotic leak, and infection. Damage to the nerve supply to the pelvic floor is associated with a small risk of altered bladder function and retrograde ejaculation in men.

  In non-constipated patients, rectopexy can be carried out. This involves dissection down to the level of the coccyx posterior to the rectum and fixing the rectum to the presacral fascia. This may be with sutures (suture rectopexy) or a non-absorbable mesh (Marlex rectopexy or Ripstein procedure, laparoscopic ventral mesh rectopexy).

  In constipated patients, resection rectopexy (Frykman–Goldberg procedure) can be carried out. Sigmoid colectomy is performed to remove redundant sigmoid, and bowel anastomosed to the rectum, followed by suture rectopexy.

- Perineal approaches have higher recurrence rates but lower morbidity and are much less invasive than abdominal approaches, and are, therefore, safer for comorbid patients who are not surgically fit for major surgery. There is a potential risk for outlet obstruction. Perineal procedures include:

- Delorme mucosal sleeve resection. The anal mucosa is resected circumferentially near the dentate line, stripped down from the rectum to the apex and excised. The underlying muscle is pleated with a suture to draw it back up.

- Perineal proctosigmoidectomy (Altemeier procedure). A circumferential full-thickness incision is made 1 cm above the dentate line, redundant rectum is resected along with its mesorectum, and colo-anal anastomosis is performed. There is a potential risk for anastomotic leak.

After a brief period of postoperative surveillance to ensure the patient has recovered from surgery, long-term follow-up is not indicated and patients should be referred back should they develop recurrence.

Further reading

Varma M, Rafferty J, Buie WD (2011) Practice parameters for the management of rectal prolapse. *Diseases of the Colon and Rectum* 54 (11): 1,339–46.

Williams JG (2012) Rectal prolapse, pp. 421–38 *in* Brown SR, Hartley JE, Hill J, Scott N, Williams JG (eds) *Contemporary Coloproctology*, first edition. Springer Publishers, London.

Chapter 5

Breast surgery

Jenna Morgan and Lynda Wyld

Case history 5.1: Elective: breast lump

A 32-year-old woman was referred by her GP with a 1-week history of a discrete breast lump in the upper-outer quadrant. She reports associated tenderness over the area and denies any history of trauma to the breast. She is nulliparous and takes only the oral contraceptive pill, with no other medical or surgical history. Of note in her family history, both her mother and maternal aunt were diagnosed with breast cancer at the ages of 36 and 40, respectively.

On examination the lump is firm and smooth, and measures approximately 1 cm in diameter. It is not tethered to either the skin or underlying muscle and is fairly mobile. There are no overlying skin changes, and examination of the contralateral breast and both axillae are normal.

Questions

1. What are the key differential diagnoses and which is most likely?
2. How should the lump be assessed?
3. What is a fibroadenoma and how should it be managed?
4. What are breast cysts and how should they be managed?
5. How significant is this woman's family history and what methods are available to calculate her risk?
6. How would you manage a woman of 32 if she was at a high familial risk of breast cancer?
7. What hereditary gene mutations may cause breast cancer to run in the family?

Answers

1. What are the key differential diagnoses and which is most likely?

The top differential diagnoses are fibroadenoma, a focal area of benign breast change, a breast cyst, and a breast abscess. In a pregnant or lactating woman, pregnancy-associated glandular changes and galactocoele should be considered. Breast cancer is much less common in this age group but must be excluded with triple assessment in the usual way, especially in the presence of a strong family history. In view of the age of the patient and the features of the lump, the most likely diagnosis would be a fibroadenoma.

2. How should the lump be assessed?

All new presentations of breast lumps should be assessed in a specialist fast-track breast clinic by triple assessment. A full history should be taken, including details of any recent trauma to the area, risk factors, family history, cycle variation, possible pregnancy/lactation, and current medication. On examination, particular attention should be paid to the size, contour, and consistency of the lump, as well as to whether there is any tethering to the skin or underlying structures. Cancerous lumps tend to be hard and irregular, whereas benign lumps tend to have a distinct, smooth outline, and be more mobile, although this is not always the case: a rapidly growing/high-grade cancer may have a pushing margin and feel like a fibroadenoma. Overlying skin changes should be noted, including any subtle distortions on raising the arms or contracting the pectoralis major muscle that can be caused by an invasive cancer. Both breasts should be examined to assess for further lumps in other quadrants or on the contralateral side. Both axillae should also be examined for palpable lymphadenopathy. Following clinical assessment the lumps should be given a score according to the level of suspicion:

- P_1 normal.
- P_2 benign.
- P_3 indeterminate.

- P_4 suspicious for malignancy.
- P_5 malignant.

The patient should then undergo imaging with mammography (in patients aged 40 years or more) and ultrasound, regardless of age. Women under the age of 40 years are initially assessed with only ultrasound due to the high tissue density of the breast at that age, which reduces the value of X-ray mammography. An imaging score is also given:

- M_1/U_1 no abnormal features.
- M_2/U_2 benign abnormality, e.g. cyst, fibrocystic change.
- M_3/U_3 indeterminate features.
- M_4/U_4 suspicious of malignancy.
- M_5/U_5 overtly malignant.

Solid lesions are then biopsied to confirm a histological diagnosis and given a score:

- B_1 insufficient/acellular.
- B_2 benign.
- B_3 atypical, probably benign.
- B_4 atypical, probably malignant.
- B_{5A} malignant *in situ*.
- B_{5B} malignant invasive.

Each of these scores is compared at the MDT meeting to ensure concordance. Concordance between assessments is a failsafe to ensure a correct diagnosis and discordance should prompt re-assessment or further tests. For example, an M_5 mammogram with a P_5 clinical assessment but a B1 biopsy would be discordant and probably suggest the lesion had been missed at biopsy; a repeat biopsy would be indicated.

3. What is a fibroadenoma and how should it be managed?

Fibroadenomas are benign breast tumours of hyperplastic fibrous and glandular tissue that account for around 13% of all breast lumps. They are commonest in women of child-bearing age (aged 15–40 years) and are sometimes referred to as a 'breast mouse' due to their small size and mobility. Clinically, they present as a firm, mobile, painless lump with a clearly defined border. They may be lobulated and multiple or bilateral. They are oestrogen-responsive and so may be associated with cyclical pain. Diagnosis should be by triple assessment, including core biopsy, as they may be difficult to distinguish from phyllodes tumours on imaging alone. Pathologically they have a well-defined capsule, encasing glandular/cystic tissue surrounded by fibroblastic stroma. Treatment is reassurance where the fibroadenoma is <3 cm in diameter and not symptomatic. Surgical excision should be considered in those larger than 3 cm, if they are prominent, painful, or where the histological diagnosis is not certain. If left *in situ*, 10% will increase in size and will require reassessment, 30% will decrease in size and may disappear, and 60% will remain the same.

4. What are breast cysts and how should they be managed?

Breast cysts are fluid-filled distended breast lobules. They are commonest in peri-menopausal women (aged 40–55 years). Clinically, they present as smooth, round, discrete breast lumps that may exhibit fluctuance. They usually appear rapidly and may diminish after menstruation. Diagnosis should be by triple assessment, with mammography and targeted ultrasound in women aged 40 years and over (ultrasound only in those <40 years), and needle aspiration to dryness under image-guidance. Aspirate may be clear, green, or brownish. The following features should prompt further assessment, as approximately 1% of breast cysts may be associated with a cancer:

- Blood-stained aspirate.
- Persistence of a cyst following aspiration or repeated refilling.
- Irregular or thickened cyst wall on imaging.

5. How significant is this woman's family history and what methods are available to calculate her risk?

An individual's risk of developing breast cancer depends on:

- The number of relatives diagnosed with breast, ovarian, or a related cancer.

- The age at which those relatives were diagnosed.

- The age of the individual.

- Previous diagnosis of high-risk breast pathologies, such as lobular carcinoma *in situ* (LCIS) and atypical duct hyperplasia (ADH).

- Other risk factors related to lifestyle and personal characteristics, such as post-menopausal obesity, menstrual age range, pregnancy and lactation, and use of oestrogen-containing preparations, such as HRT or the pill.

For the purposes of enhanced surveillance of women at raised breast cancer risk and treatment, the National Institute of Clinical Excellence categorizes individuals above 20 years of age according to their lifetime risk of developing breast cancer into near population, moderate and high risk.

In addition, there are several online risk calculators, such as the IBIS II or BOADICEA, which will calculate the patient's lifetime risk (from age 20), as well as their likelihood of being a gene carrier.

Using online risk calculators, this patient falls into the 'high-risk' category and has a greater than a 10% chance of being a gene carrier. She should have a full and thorough family history taken and be offered referral for genetic testing.

Near population -risk patients have less than 17% lifetime risk and are reassured. Moderate-risk patients have between 17 and 30% lifetime risk. This group are usually offered annual breast screening from age 40 to 60 and may be offered 5 years of prophylactic tamoxifen, or an aromatase inhibitor or raloxifene if post menopausal. High-risk patients have over 30% lifetime risk of developing breast cancer. If they also have greater than a 10% chance of being a gene carrier, they may be offered genetic testing. High risk women are offered additional screening (which may be with mammograms and with MRI from the age of 30 if gene carriers), prophylactic tamoxifen, aromatase inhibitor or raloxifene, or prophylactic mastectomy/oophorectomy may be offered. There is good evidence that prophylactic aromatase inhibitors (AIs) are even more effective than selective oestrogen-receptor modulators (SERMS) in high-risk post-menopausal women.

6. How would you manage a woman of 32 if she was at a high familial risk of breast cancer?

This patient would be offered genetic counselling to discuss the implications of an affected family member having a gene test if willing and still living (diagnostic testing). If a gene is identified the unaffected family members are tested for this mutation (predictive testing). If no such relative is available, the woman herself may be tested. There are several options available to women at high familial risk of breast cancer (summarized in Figure 5.1.1) and it is an individual choice.

Regular screening to attempt to identify any cancers at an early stage is an option. Mammographic screening of younger women is generally less effective than of older women due to increased breast density. There are also concerns regarding exposing young women to regular doses of ionizing radiation. Magnetic resonance imaging has a much higher sensitivity that mammography in younger women but is far less specific, leading to additional imaging and biopsies. In

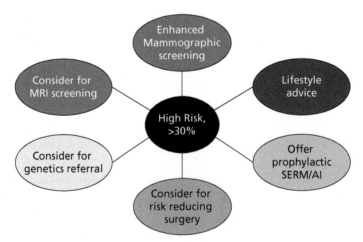

Figure 5.1.1 Potential management options for patients at high risk of familial breast cancer.

Reproduced courtesy of Jenna Morgan.

high-risk women, such as this patient, annual surveillance with both MRI and mammography is considered better than either test alone.

Some women with high familial risk of breast cancer, particularly those known to have a BRCA 1/2 mutation, may decide to undergo surgery in the form of bilateral risk-reducing mastectomies to remove most of the breast tissue, which reduces their risk of breast cancer by around 90-95%. This is, however, a major undertaking and patients should be adequately counselled pre-operatively. It is associated with a greater than 90% breast cancer risk reduction and improved survival rates in these women.

Women known to have a BRCA mutation may also consider risk-reducing bilateral salpingo-oophorectomy to reduce their risk of ovarian and breast cancer. The exact age at which this should be performed is still uncertain, although many centres advocate performing this procedure in patients' early 40s, after they have completed their family. This reduces the ovarian cancer risk by over 99% and the breast cancer risk by 50% (if performed pre-menopausally).

Chemoprevention (with tamoxifen, an aromatase inhibitor or raloxifene) is also an option for women at high risk of developing breast cancer, although they are less effective than risk-reducing surgery and have the potential for serious adverse events. Additionally, they may be less effective in BRCA 1 gene carriers, where ER negative cancers predominate. The uptake of chemoprevention is relatively low, despite favourable national guidance by NICE.

7. What hereditary gene mutations may cause breast cancer to run in the family?

Most cases of breast cancer (75%) are sporadic, with no genetic predisposition. The term familial breast cancer is used to describe a family with an unusually high number of members affected by breast, ovarian, or related cancers, which may be a sign of a genetic mutation. Around 20% of breast cancers may have some genetic contribution from weaker genes (70 single nucleotide polymorphisms have been identified that increase risk and a number of moderate penetrance mutations, such as ATM, PALB2, BRIP, and CHEK2, to name but a few), which only increase the woman's risk to a small or moderate degree and are not presently tested for. However, 5–8% of women with breast cancer carry highly penetrant, usually autosomal dominant, gene mutations, which give the individual up to an 80% lifetime risk of developing breast cancer (i.e. BRCA1, BRCA2, Li Fraumeni syndrome/TP53, TPEN, CDH1, STKII (Peutz–Jegher's), mutations, etc.) (Table 5.1.2).

Table 5.1.2 High-risk genes

Syndrome	Gene	Cancers	Lifetime risk of breast cancer
Breast–ovarian	BRCA1	Female breast, ovarian	40–80%
Breast–ovarian	BRCA2	Female and male breast, ovarian, prostate, pancreatic	20–80%
Li-Fraumeni	TP53	Breast, sarcoma, leukaemia, brain, adrenocortical, lung	56-90%
Cowden's	PTEN	Breast, thyroid, endometrial	25–50%
Peutz–Jegher's	STK11	Breast, ovarian, pancreatic, uterine, testicular, colon	32–54%
Hereditary diffuse gastric cancer	CDH1	Early onset diffuse gastric cancer, lobular breast cancer	60%

Adapted from Apostolou P and Fostira F (2013) 'Hereditary breast cancer: The era of new susceptibility genes', *Biomed Research International*, Copyright © 2013 Paraskevi Apostolou and Florentia Fostira, DOI: 10.1155/2013/747318, under the Creative Commons Attribution License 3.0 Unported (CC by 3.0).

Further reading

Apostolou P, Fostira F (2013) Hereditary breast cancer: the era of new susceptibility genes. *Biomedical Research International*, vol 2013, *Article ID* 747318, 11 pages, 2013. Doi: 10.1155/2013/747318.

Cuzick J, Sestak I, Bonanni B, Costantino JP, Cummings S, DeCensi A et al. (2013) Selective oestrogen receptor modulators in prevention of breast cancer: an updated meta-analysis of individual participant data. *Lancet* 381: 1,827–34.

Cuzick J, Sestak I, Forbes JF, Dowsett M, Knox J, Cawthorn S et al. (2014) Anastrozole for prevention of breast cancer in high-risk postmenopausal women (IBIS-II): an international, double-blind, randomised placebo-controlled trial. *Lancet* 383: 1,041–8.

Mavaddat N, Peock S, Frost D, Ellis S, Platte R, Fineberg E et al. (2013) Cancer risks for BRCA1 and BRCA2 mutation carriers: results from prospective analysis of EMBRACE. *Journal of the National Cancer Institute* 105: 812–22.

NICE (2013) Familial breast cancer: classification and care of people at risk of familial breast cancer and management of breast cancer and related risks in people with a family history of breast cancer. NICE Clinical Guideline 164. Available at: www.guidance.nice.org.uk/cg164

Case history 5.2: Elective: nipple discharge

A 54-year-old woman was referred by her GP with a 2-month history of left-sided nipple discharge. The discharge is clear and spontaneous, occurring two or three times per week, and is unilateral. She is otherwise fit and well with no past medical, surgical, or family history.

On examination there are no palpable abnormalities in either breast or axilla. There are no distortions or changes to the overlying skin. When expressed, the discharge is clear and appears to originate from a single duct.

Questions

1. What are the key features in determining surgically significant nipple discharge?

2. What are the differential diagnoses for nipple discharge and which is most likely?

3. Triple assessment picks up no visible abnormality on imaging. What would you do?

4. The patient returns 12 months later following her routine screening mammogram, which has identified a 2-cm area of fine, linear calcification centrally behind the nipple on the ipsilateral breast. How would you assess her?

5. What do you know about breast screening?

6. She undergoes triple assessment and her pathology results confirm DCIS. What are her treatment options?

7. What is 'overtreatment' and how is this important to breast screening?

Answers

1. What are the key features in determining surgically significant nipple discharge?

It is important to ascertain potentially malignant nipple discharge from benign nipple discharge. Key features of surgically significant nipple discharge (i.e. with a potentially malignant aetiology) include:

- Persistent.
- Unilateral.
- Uniductal (from a single duct).
- Spontaneous.
- Bloody or clear.

2. What are the key differential diagnoses for nipple discharge and which is most likely?

Key differential diagnoses for nipple discharge, with the typical colour of the discharge, are seen in Table 5.2.1. In this case, the most likely diagnosis would be a ductal papilloma but a breast cancer needs to be excluded.

Table 5.2.1 Aetiology of nipple discharge

Colour of nipple discharge	Aetiology
Clear, watery	Physiological
	Papilloma
	Breast cancer
Red, blood-stained	Papilloma
	Breast cancer
Yellow, purulent	Abscess
	Peri-ductal mastitis
Green/greenish brown	Duct ectasia
White, milky	Lactation, post-partum
	Drugs
	Prolactinoma

Reproduced courtesy of Judith Ritchie.

3. **Triple assessment picks up no visible abnormality on imaging. What would you do?**

The patient needs further assessment as the discharge is clear, unilateral, and uniductal so potentially pathological. A microdochectomy can be performed to excise part of the affected duct for pathological assessment. This procedure is performed under general anaesthetic and the breast is examined to identify the discharging duct prior to incision. A fine probe is placed into the affected duct and approximately 2–3 cm of the duct is removed with a cuff of surrounding breast tissue. Alternatively, a total duct excision may be performed. This involves identifying the central ducts immediately behind the nipple, ligating and dividing them, and excising approximately 2 cm of ductal tissue for assessment.

4. **The patient returns 12 months later following her routine screening mammogram, which has identified a 2-cm area of fine, linear calcification centrally behind the nipple on the ipsilateral breast. How would you assess her?**

She should undergo triple assessment of the new area, including a clinical examination, targeted ultrasound, and a core biopsy, in the same way as any new patient with a screening abnormality. This is covered in the Case 5.1 in Question 2.

5. **What do you know about breast screening?**

A screening programme needs to fulfil the criteria set out by the World Health Organization in 1966:

- The condition should be an important health problem.
- The natural history of the disease is well understood.
- There should be a treatment for the condition.
- Treatment is better at an earlier stage.
- There is a latent and recognizable early stage of the disease.
- A suitable test exists to detect the disease at an early stage.
- The test should be acceptable.
- Adequate facilities for both diagnosis and treatment should be available.

- Screening should be a continuous process, performed at regular intervals.

- It should be cost-effective.

In addition, screening tests themselves should also be simple and cost-effective, both sensitive (few false-negatives) and specific (few false-positives), safe and easy to perform and analyse.

The NHS BSP started in 1987 with the aim of reducing breast cancer deaths by identification and treatment of pre-clinical early disease. Women are invited to attend for mammographic screening every 3 years between the ages of 50 and 70 years. This age range is being extended to 47–73 over the next few years as part of a national randomized clinical trial. Women over this age can still self-refer every 3 years. Two radiological views are taken: cranio-caudal, which allows visualization of the medial breast; and medio-lateral oblique, which visualizes the lateral breast and axilla. All images are double-reported to improve sensitivity and specificity.

Patients are recalled if an abnormality is detected for further imaging (e.g. mammographic compression views, targeted ultrasound), and/or clinical examination and core biopsy of the area. Around 5% of women are recalled (this rate decreases with age and decreasing breast density), and of these, approximately two-thirds will have no worrying features on additional investigation. Between 6 and 8 women per 1,000 screened will be diagnosed with breast cancer.

The NHS BSP tends to identify smaller, lower grade, node-negative cancers and more non-invasive disease compared to symptomatic presentations. The result is that patients are more likely to be offered breast-conserving surgery, as opposed to mastectomy, and also less likely to require adjuvant chemotherapy.

However, breast screening is not without its disadvantages, which include:

- Recall for benign disease causing anxiety and unnecessary investigation.

- False-negative screening (missed cancers).

- 'Radiation exposure' (negligible).

- Over-diagnosis (and hence potential overtreatment) of breast cancer. This is where a very low-risk cancer or area of ductal carcinoma *in situ* (DCIS) is identified and treated, which would never have become symptomatic during the woman's lifetime. It is estimated that up to 29% of all cancers may fall into this category, resulting in psychological distress and treatments conferring harm but no benefit (see The Marmot Review in Further reading).

- Discomfort and anxiety.

- Interval cancers (i.e. those cancers that are diagnosed between screening visits).

6. She undergoes triple assessment and her pathology results confirm the presence of DCIS. What are her treatment options?

Ductal carcinoma *in situ* (DCIS) is a pre-malignant condition where the proliferation of malignant cells has not breached the ductal basement membrane and hence it is not able to metastasize. Around 40% of large areas of high-risk DCIS will progress to become invasive breast cancers. However, for small areas of low-grade DCIS, it is thought that probably only around 5% will progress to invasive disease after 20 years. At present we cannot predict which lesions will progress and hence all lesions are treated, but this is almost certainly a cause of unnecessary treatment morbidity.

Treatment is the surgical removal of the affected area, either by mastectomy or wide local excision (WLE), depending on the relative size of the area compared to breast volume (up to 50% breast volume removal may be compatible with WLE). Up to 10–15% may be resected with simple wide excision, 15–25% volume loss will benefit from level 1 oncoplastic techniques and larger volumes, up to 50%, may be excised with level 2 oncoplastic techniques in certain cases. More than 50% would mandate a mastectomy, plus or minus reconstruction (see Clough in Further reading). As the disease is close to the nipple in this patient, this would most likely be a central WLE, which would also involve excision of the nipple. Nipple conservation may be appropriate if the disease is 2.5 cm or more away from the nipple. Axillary surgery is not usually performed in patients with DCIS unless a mastectomy is undertaken, when sentinel lymph node biopsy (SLNB) is usually performed at the time, as the surgeon is already operating in the low axilla anyway. Axillary surgery is not performed when wide excision is planned for DCIS.

Patients who have had breast conservation are usually offered adjuvant radiotherapy, unless they have only a very small area of low-grade DCIS.

The IBIS II trial showed a reduction in the number of high-risk women (including those who had had excision of previous DCIS) developing breast cancer at 5 years with anastrazole. However, the use of anti-oestrogen therapy in patients with DCIS is still contentious and is not currently used routinely in all centres the UK.

The LORIS trial is looking at whether women who have small areas of low-grade DCIS may be able to avoid treatment altogether. LORIS aims to compare the long-term outcome (over 10 years) of women who undergo surgery for DCIS with those who have yearly surveillance of the area with mammography.

7. What is 'overtreatment' and how is this important to breast screening?

Overtreatment refers to the treatment of disease that is not clinically relevant. In terms of breast screening, it is likely that a subset of patients with DCIS will never progress to invasive breast cancer in their lifetimes and so traditional management may represent overtreatment. DCIS was rarely diagnosed before the introduction of the NHS BSP but it now accounts for around 20% of screen-detected cancers in the UK. Since DCIS alone poses no threat to life, the aim of treatment is to prevent progression to invasive cancer. It was thought that the introduction of the NHS BSP would eventually see a reduction in the number of cases of invasive disease, however this has not happened and, consequently, the issue of overtreatment of low-risk DCIS has been raised.

Further reading

Barnes NLP, Ooi JL, Yarnold JR, Bundred NJ (2012) Ductal carcinoma *in situ* of the breast. *British Medical Journal* 344: e797.

Clough KB, Kaufman GJ, Nos C, Buccimazza I, Sarfati IM (2010) Improving breast cancer surgery: a classification and quadrant per quadrant atlas for oncoplastic surgery. *Annals of Surgical Oncology* 17: 1375–91.

Marmot M et al. (2012) The benefits and harms of breast cancer screening: an independent review. Independent UK Panel on Breast Cancer Screening. *Lancet* 380: 1778–86.

Case history 5.3: Elective: breast cancer

A 72-year-old woman attends outpatients following a 2-week wait referral from her GP with a 10-day history of a lump in the upper-outer quadrant of the right breast. She has a history of hypertension that is well-controlled on medication, she is a smoker and is overweight with a BMI of 36. She has moderate-sized (DD cup), moderately ptotic (grade 2) breasts.

On examination there is a 3-cm irregular, firm lump in the upper-outer quadrant of the right breast (P_5). Examination of the contralateral breast is normal, as are the axillae. The patient undergoes triple assessment, which reveals a 32-mm spiculated M_5 mass on mammography (Figure 5.3.1), which coincides with an ill-defined 35-mm hyper-echoic U_5 lesion on ultrasound. Imaging assessment of the axilla shows a single pathologically enlarged node, which biopsy confirms as containing metastatic breast cancer. An ultrasound-guided core biopsy of the mass is taken and pathology comes back as a B_{5b} grade 2, invasive lobular carcinoma, oestrogen receptor score positive, HER2 receptor negative.

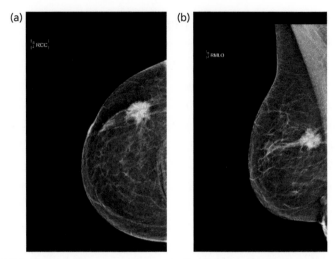

Figure 5.3.1 Mammogram images demonstrating the spiculated breast tumour (white mass) in the breast tissue. RCC = right craniocaudal view; RMLO = right medio-lateral view.

Reproduced courtesy of Judith Ritchie.

Questions

1. What are the aetiological factors in the development of breast cancer?

2. Breast cancer is classified in a number of ways: histopathological morphology-based but also more complex systems based on receptor expression patterns. Describe these systems and identify which subtype this patient has.

3. Describe the surgical management options for this patient.

4. The patient requests a mastectomy. What are her potential reconstructive options?

5. Following surgery her histology shows she had a 35-mm grade 3 pleomorphic lobular cancer with 5 out of 12 nodes positive, ER score 8/8, Her 2 score negative, and Ki67 proliferation index of 32%. What methods of estimating her prognosis are available and what is her 10 year survival likely to be without adjuvant therapy?

6. What adjuvant therapies would you offer this woman?

Answers

1. What are the aetiological factors in the development of breast cancer?

There is an increased risk of breast cancer with increased exposure to oestrogens, so that the following are all risk factors for its development:

- Increasing age.
- Early menarche (<12 years).
- Late menopause (risk is double for women who go through the menopause at 55 compared to 45 years).
- Nulliparous (or first child born after the age of 30 years).
- Hormone replacement therapy (HRT) for 5 years, doubles the risk.
- Oral contraceptive pill (OCP) increases the risk by 1.2-fold.
- A positive family history of breast or ovarian cancer.
- Past medical history of either breast cancer, DCIS, LCIS, or benign proliferative changes with atypia. Also a past history of mantle radiotherapy for lymphoma.
- Post-menopausal obesity.
- Excessive alcohol intake.

2. Breast cancer is classified in a number of ways: histopathological morphology-based but also more complex systems based on receptor expression patterns. Describe these systems and identify which subtype this patient has.

The most common staging system used for breast cancer in the UK is the TNM (tumour, nodes, metastases) system.

75% of invasive breast cancers are invasive ductal carcinomas of no special type. However, other pathological types include:

- Invasive lobular carcinoma (10%).
- Mucinous carcinoma.
- Medullary carcinoma.
- Papillary carcinoma.

◆ Tubular carcinoma.

◆ Cribriform carcinoma.

Invasive carcinomas are graded according to the degree of glandular formation, the degree of nuclear pleomorphism, and the frequency of mitoses, known as the Bloom and Richardson grading system:

◆ Grade I: well differentiated.

◆ Grade II: moderately differentiated.

◆ Grade III: poorly differentiated.

Four biologically distinct subtypes of breast cancer have been described, according to their immunohistochemical profiles: Luminal A, Luminal B, HER2-enriched, and Triple Negative. In general, adjuvant systemic therapy is guided by the subtype of invasive breast cancer (see Table 5.3.1).

Table 5.3.1 Four main biological sub-types of breast cancer

	ER/PR	HER2	Proliferative markers (e.g. Ki67)	Adjuvant systemic therapy recommendation
Luminal A	ER & PR positive	Negative	Low	Endocrine therapy
Luminal B	ER positive PR positive/ negative	Negative	High	Endocrine therapy + chemotherapy
HER2-enriched	Negative	Over-expressed or amplified		Trastuzumab + chemotherapy
Triple negative	Negative	Negative		Chemotherapy

Reproduced courtesy of Judith Ritchie.

3. Describe the surgical management options for this patient.

Management for this patient would include the choice between wide local excision (WLE) or mastectomy for the surgical treatment of the primary breast cancer.

WLE involves excision of the lesion with a margin of normal tissue and can usually be performed in tumours smaller than 5 cm in diameter or where <20% of the breast tissue would be removed. Patients undergoing WLE are required to have post-operative adjuvant radiotherapy.

Mastectomy involves removal of the breast tissue on that side and is usually required for large or multi-centric tumours. Radiotherapy is not always required following mastectomy but is advocated in patients with a high risk of local recurrence, e.g. high-grade disease plus nodal involvement, T3 disease (primary greater than 5 cm), T4 disease, or involved margins where further surgery is not possible or not desired.

She will also require axillary surgery, and in the case of this patient, where a pre-operative ultrasound-guided biopsy has confirmed the presence of cancer in a lymph node, this will take the form of an axillary node clearance. Women without known nodal disease have an axillary staging procedure called a sentinel node biopsy and only proceed to a later axillary node clearance, usually as a second operation, if this is positive. However, some centres perform intra-operative SLNB analysis using a number of techniques, including frozen section, touch imprint cytology, and one-step nucleic acid amplification to detect a specific breast cancer cytokeratin in the nodal tissue (OSNA), so that patients can proceed to axillary clearance under the same anaesthetic if lymph node metastases are identified.

4. The patient requests a mastectomy. What are her reconstructive options?

The simplest type of 'reconstruction' is to wear an external prosthesis inside a special bra, using a prosthesis that is designed to match the contralateral breast for size and shape.

Surgical reconstruction may be categorized as immediate/primary (at the time of mastectomy) or delayed (months or even years after the original surgery). Immediate reconstruction is usually combined with a skin-sparing mastectomy to preserve the skin envelope and, in some instances, the nipple may also be spared, providing a much better cosmetic outcome. Reconstruction of the breast mound may be achieved either with saline or silicone implants, or by use of the patient's own tissues, so called autologous reconstructions. These latter techniques may move tissue from the back, abdomen, thighs, or buttocks to recreate breast volume. These are also known as myocutaneous flaps, which may be 'pedicled', as in the latissimus dorsi (LD) or the thoracodorsal perforator flap (TDAP), or 'free' as in the transverse rectus abdominis myocutaneous flap (TRAM), or deep inferior epigastric perforator flap (DIEP), superior or inferior gluteal artery perforator flap (S and I-GAP), and the transverse upper gracillis (TUG) flap. These techniques may also be combined with implants to increase the size of the reconstruction in women with larger breasts.

Implants may be simply placed under the pectoralis major and the anterior and lateral chest wall muscles (submuscular implant reconstruction), which provides extra coverage and helps to prevent distortion or erosion. This technique is good for creating small, non-ptotic breasts. For slightly larger breasts, expander implants may be use to stretch the overlying muscle and allow the use of larger sized implants. More recently, better implant pocket sizes and a more natural breast shape have been achieved by supplementing the chest wall musculature with either the de-epithelialized inferior mastectomy flap (dermal sling technique) or use of a range of acellular dermal matrices derived from bovine or porcine dermis/pericardium to support the inferior pole of the implant.

Complications of reconstructions depend on their type, but include:

- Flap or skin necrosis, occasionally resulting in loss of the reconstruction.
- Infection.
- Donor site problems in flap reconstructions, e.g. abdominal wall hernias in TRAM flaps.
- Fibrous capsule formation with associated pain and deformation.
- Implant rupture.
- Implant malposition and asymmetry.

For most patients where the nipple has been excised, nipple reconstruction techniques can be used in combination with tattooing to improve appearance. This is usually performed as a secondary procedure and patients may consider adhesive artificial nipples in the interim.

Other available techniques include reduction mammoplasty for women with larger breasts (+/– contralateral breast reduction or mastopexy for symmetrization) or contralateral augmentation mammoplasty for symmetrization for women with smaller breasts.

This patient would be a good candidate for a therapeutic mammoplasty since she has a relatively large lateral tumour and cosmesis with standard breast conservation is likely to be poor. She has relatively large ptotic breasts, which facilitates this type of surgery. However, she may be at a higher risk of surgical complications as she is a smoker and hypertensive. She would be considered unsuitable for a TRAM/DIEP flap as she would have a high risk of flap failure with a BMI of over 35 and she is a smoker.

5. **Following surgery her histology shows she had a 35-mm grade 3 pleomorphic lobular cancer with 5 out of 12 nodes positive, ER score 8/8, Her 2 score negative, and Ki67 proliferation index of 32%. What methods of estimating her prognosis are available and what is her 10 year survival likely to be without adjuvant therapy?**

Several methods of assessing prognosis are available. They may also aid patient understanding of their disease and clinical decision-making regarding additional adjuvant treatment requirements.

The Nottingham prognostic index is a simple calculation based on tumour grade, size, and lymph node stage, using the formula:

$$NPI = [0.2 \times S] + N, +G$$

where S is the size of the tumour in centimentres, N is the number of lymph nodes involved (no nodes = 1, 1–3 nodes = 2, >3 nodes = 3), and G is the tumour grade (grade I = 1, grade II = 2, grade III = 3). So, for example, for this patient:

$$NPI = [0.2 \times 3.5] + 3 + 3 = 6.7.$$

The NPI score can give a projected 5-year survival for the patient (Table 5.3.2).

Table 5.3.2 Correlation of Nottingham prognostic index with 5-year survival

NPI Score	5-year survival
2–2.4	93%
>2.4–3.4	85%
>3.5–5.4	70%
>5.4	50%

Adapted from *British Journal of Cancer,* Volume 56, Issue 4, pp. 489–92, Todd JH, Dowle C, Williams MR, et al., 'Confirmation of a prognostic index in primary breast cancer', Copyright © 1987, by permission of Macmillan Publishers Ltd on behalf of Cancer Research UK.

More recently, online prognostic calculators have become available that take into account more clinical information. Examples include Predict (see Figure 5.3.2) and Adjuvant! Online.

Adjuvant! Online considers the patients age, level of comorbidity, ER status, tumour grade and size, and number of positive lymph nodes. Using this method, the patient's 10-year survival without any adjuvant treatment is estimated to be 27.7%. Predict considers the patient's age, mode of cancer detection, tumour size and grade, ER,

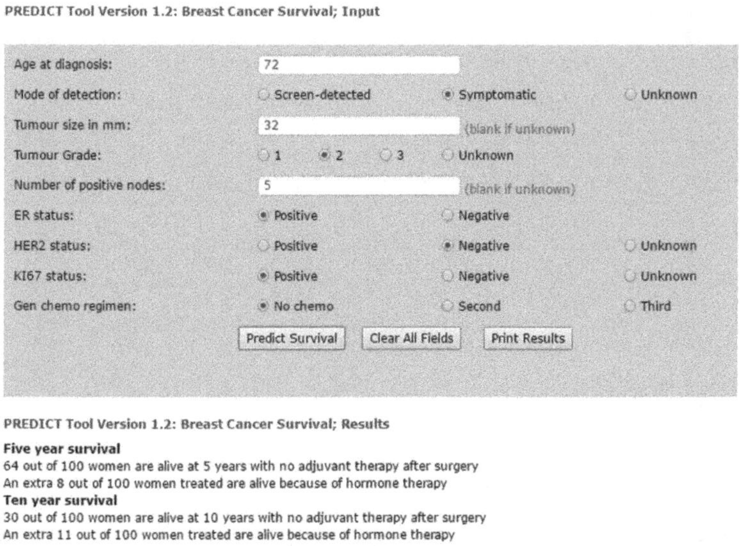

PREDICT Tool Version 1.2: Breast Cancer Survival; Input

PREDICT Tool Version 1.2: Breast Cancer Survival; Results

Five year survival
64 out of 100 women are alive at 5 years with no adjuvant therapy after surgery
An extra 8 out of 100 women treated are alive because of hormone therapy
Ten year survival
30 out of 100 women are alive at 10 years with no adjuvant therapy after surgery
An extra 11 out of 100 women treated are alive because of hormone therapy

Figure 5.3.2 Output from Adjuvant! Online showing calculation of risk of mortality and benefit of adjuvant therapy for this patient.

credit line: Adjuvant! Online

HER2 and Ki67 status, and number of positive lymph nodes. Using this method, the patient's 10-year survival without any adjuvant treatment is estimated to be 13.6%.

6. What adjuvant therapies would you offer this woman?

She will also receive adjuvant endocrine therapy as she has ER positive disease. This will usually be in the form of an aromatase inhibitor (AI) for 5 years, since she is post-menopausal. However, in patients with significant osteopenia or those who don't tolerate the side-effects of AIs, tamoxifen may be used as an alternative.

This patient has a very high-risk cancer and would normally be offered chemotherapy, although the evidence for chemotherapy benefit in the over 70s is weak. The MDT will review her case and her fitness level and decide whether, on balance, she will gain more benefit than risk from chemotherapy. Adjuvant chemotherapy is usually considered only for patients at high risk of recurrence, including:

+ Young, pre-menopausal patients.
+ Lymph-node positive.
+ ER negative.
+ HER2 positive.
+ Grade III.
+ Large tumour size.
+ Lymphovascular invasion.

  In certain specific situations a multigene array test, Oncotype DX may also be performed to assess the risk of recurrence.

The Adjuvant! Online and Predict programs give useful information about how much benefit a patient will gain with chemotherapy, which is useful both for clinician and patient decision-making.

Further reading

Goldhirsch A, Wood WC, Coates AS, Gelber RD, Thürlimann B, Senn H-J, Panel members (2011) Strategies for subtypes—dealing with the diversity of breast cancer: highlights of the St Gallen International Expert Consensus on the Primary Therapy of Early Breast Cancer 2011. *Annals of Oncology* 22: 1,736–47.

NICE (2009) Early and locally advanced breast cancer: diagnosis and treatment. NICE Clinical Guideline 80. Available at: www.guidance.nice.org.uk/cg80

Case history 5.4: Emergency: breast abscess

A 34-year-old woman attends the emergency department with a painful lump in her left breast for the last week. She feels unwell with a fever and malaise. She is 4 weeks post-partum and has been breast-feeding. She has no relevant past medical history and takes no regular medication.

On examination the left breast is red, swollen, and tender to palpation. She has a pyrexia of 37.9°C.

Questions

1. What are the differential diagnoses?
2. What are the likely causative organisms?
3. How would you manage this patient?
4. What advice would you give regarding breast-feeding?
5. How does the management change for non-lactational breast abscesses?
6. What is the main underlying cause of non-lactational abscesses?
7. What are the hormonal regulatory mechanisms for lactation?

Answers

1. What are the differential diagnoses?

Differential diagnoses include lactational mastitis and lactational abscess. Inflammatory cancer is very rare in this age group but may need to be considered if the symptoms fail to resolve as expected after a few weeks. In view of her young age, the fact that she has a discrete lump and is lactating—an abscess is the most likely diagnosis. Acute mastitis occurs in around 2–3% of women who are breast-feeding, with less than 10% of these developing an abscess. Infection usually occurs within the first 6 weeks of breast-feeding and in severe cases may result in septicaemia. There is usually a history of cracked nipple or skin abrasion, and drainage of milk for the affected segment is often reduced.

2. What are the likely causative organisms?

Lactational breast abscesses arise when cracks in the nipple act as an entry point for bacteria. As such, the most common causative bacteria is *Staphylococcus aureus*. However, other skin commensals, such as *Staphylococcus epidermidis* and streptococci are occasionally isolated.

3. How would you manage this patient?

The first-line antibiotic of choice is usually flucloxacillin, with erythromycin used in penicillin allergies. Tetracyclines and ciprofloxacin should be avoided in breast-feeding patients.

Patients should undergo ultrasound to identify any purulent collection within the breast.

Ultrasound-guided needle aspiration is usually performed in patients with fluctuance or significant collections seen on imaging. This may need to be repeated several times to achieve resolution. If a solid lesion is identified on ultrasound, there is no collection, or the patient fails to respond to treatment, full triple assessment with imaging (ultrasound is used in this age group, as mammography has very low sensitivity in women in this age group, especially when lactating) and core biopsy should be performed to rule out an inflammatory breast cancer.

Additionally, patients should be advised to use simple analgesia (paracetamol should be used first line, with ibuprofen as an alternative) to relieve the pain. The use of warm compresses can also help to relieve discomfort and encourage the milk to flow. Many women find that not wearing a bra also helps with the discomfort due to swelling.

In severe cases, if there is overlying skin necrosis or no resolution with repeated aspirations, incision and drainage may rarely be required but carries the risk of creating a lactational fistula. This is a communication between the skin and a lactating milk duct. This may necessitate discontinuance of breast-feeding before it will close and may be quite a high-volume fistula and very unpleasant. For this reason, surgical drainage should be avoided if possible in lactating women unless there is no alternative.

4. What advice would you give regarding breast-feeding?

Breast-feeding can continue from both breasts and is safe for the infant, although it may be necessary to express milk from the affected side (by hand or pump), as the infant often refuses to feed if there is ongoing infection and it may cause excessive pain on that side. Patients can then resume breast-feeding from the affected side as soon as it is pain-free.

5. How does the management change for non-lactational breast abscesses?

Non-lactating breast abscesses are usually seen in smokers and the causative organisms are most commonly *Staphylococcus aureus*, followed by anaerobes.

All patients should undergo triple assessment. Antibiotics of choice should include anaerobic cover, so either co-amoxiclav or flucloxacillin in combination with metronidazole should be prescribed. Erythromycin plus metronidazole can be used in patients with penicillin allergy.

Patients should be advised to stop smoking otherwise relapse commonly occurs. Pus should be aspirated under ultrasound guidance with a needle in the first instance, the same approach as for lactational abscesses, with incision and drainage reserved for non-responders, progressive disease, if there is multi-loculation or overlying skin necrosis. Chronic disease may result in fistula formation, which always requires surgical fistulectomy to resolve.

6. What is the main underlying cause of non-lactational breast abscesses?

Non-lactational abscesses can be separated into those that occur centrally in the peri-areolar region and those that occur peripherally. Peri-areolar abscesses are most common and are often associated with duct ectasia and periductal mastitis, which is why they are usually located centrally. Current evidence suggests that cigarette smoking is a significant causative factor in the development of peri-areolar non-lactational breast abscesses and it is thought substances within the cigarette smoke either directly or indirectly damage the wall of the subareolar breast ducts making them more prone to infection.

Peripheral non-lactational breast abscesses are less common and can be associated with underlying conditions, such as diabetes mellitus, rheumatoid arthritis, steroid use, granulomatous lobular mastitis, and trauma.

Very rarely, non-lactating infections can occur due to infection of an area of comedo necrosis associated with DCIS. After treatment, the palpable abnormality can resolve completely, and for this reason, all patients aged over 35 years should have a mammogram following resolution of an infective episode.

7. What are the hormonal regulatory mechanisms for lactation?

Prior to birth, from the 24th week of pregnancy, hormones are produced to stimulate the growth of the milk duct system within the breasts. The hormones involved at this stage include:

- Progesterone—this has an influence on the growth of the ducts and lobules. High levels of progesterone at this stage inhibit milk production during pregnancy.
- Oestrogen—this stimulates the growth and differentiation the ducts and lobules. Again, high levels at this stage inhibit milk production before birth.
- Prolactin—this contributes to the growth and differentiation of the milk duct system. The high levels at this stage and during lactation increase insulin resistance, increase growth factor levels, and modify lipid metabolism in preparation for breast-feeding.
- Growth hormone and thyroid stimulating hormone—both are galactopoietic hormones.
- Human placental lactogen (HPL)—this is thought to be important in breast, nipple, and areola growth during pregnancy.

At birth, delivery of the placenta results in a sudden drop in progesterone, oestrogen, and HPL levels, triggering the onset of copious milk production. Serum prolactin levels increase when the breast is stimulated, which in turn triggers production of milk by the alveoli. Oxytocin is responsible for the milk-ejection reflex, it causes contraction of the smooth muscle layer surrounding the alveoli, causing milk to move into the ducts. Milk production is driven by the endocrine system for the first few days post-partum, but once feeding is more established, the autocrine system takes over. At this stage, the more milk that is expressed from the breasts, the more milk will be produced.

Further reading

Dixon M (ed.) (2015) *ABC of Breast Diseases (ABC Series)*, third edition. Wiley–Blackwell, London.

Chapter 6

Endocrine surgery

Jenna Morgan and Saba Balasubramanian

Case history 6.1: Elective: goitre and thyroid cancer

A 65-year-old man is referred to surgical outpatients with a large goitre. This has been present for a few years, but seems to have grown in size more recently. He has no other neck symptoms. He is clinically and biochemically euthyroid, and has no significant past medical or family history. There is no past history of exposure to radiation.

An ultrasound of his neck shows multiple nodules in both thyroid lobes with a 4-cm dominant nodule in the right thyroid lobe. This was aspirated under ultrasound guidance. Cytology was indeterminate (Thy3f as per UK Royal College of Pathologists classification or Bethesda type IV as per the American classification), suggesting a follicular neoplasm.

Questions

1. What are the causes of goitre and when should it be investigated further?

2. What is a fine-needle aspiration and when is it performed?

3. What are the implications of a Thy3f cytology result?

4. What risks would you explain to a patient undergoing thyroid surgery?

5. The patient eventually recovers from surgery and sees you in the follow-up clinic. Histology shows papillary thyroid cancer. Describe the different types of thyroid cancer and how this will impact on the prognosis.

6. What are the commonly used treatment modalities in the management of differentiated thyroid cancer?

7. What features are unique to differentiated thyroid cancer in comparison to other solid-organ malignancies?

Answers

1. What are the causes of goitre and when should it be investigated further?

The term goitre describes an enlarged thyroid gland. Physiologic causes of a goitre include puberty and pregnancy. The most common cause of pathological goitre worldwide is iodine deficiency. In the UK, thyroid epithelial hyperplasia and/or varying amounts of colloid accumulation can result in the formation of diffuse or multinodular goitre. Other benign causes of goitre include follicular hyperplasia, adenoma, cysts, and rarely, abscesses. Less common causes of multinodular goitre include long-term lithium and amiodarone treatment. There are many types of thyroid cancer causing goitre, these will be discussed later (Section 6.1, Question 5).

Goitre can be detected on assessment of patients with symptoms or may be an incidental finding on clinical examination or radiology performed for other reasons. Enlarged glands can occasionally extend retrosternally or compress adjacent structures such as the trachea, oesophagus, or recurrent laryngeal nerves (Figure 6.1.1). Symptomatic patients include those with symptoms of hypo- or hyperthyroidism, or patients presenting with compression of adjacent structures such as the oesophagus (dysphagia), trachea (shortness of breath on lying flat), or the recurrent laryngeal nerve (stridor, hoarse voice).

Not all goitres need to be investigated and treated. Asymptomatic multinodular goitres that are mild to moderate in size, longstanding, and confined to the neck do not require intervention.

Patients with a solitary or dominant nodule, goitre with compressive symptoms, and goitre with associated hyperthyroidism need further investigations. This usually includes an ultrasound scan and often a fine-needle aspiration cytology, in addition to thyroid function tests, to determine the presence and severity of thyroid dysfunction.

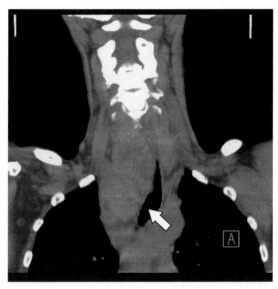

Figure 6.1.1 A coronal image of a CT scan of the neck and chest demonstrating retrosternal extension of a goitre. The goitre is displacing and compressing the trachea (delineated by a white arrow).

Reproduced courtesy of Saba Balasubramanian.

2. What is a fine-needle aspiration and when is it performed?

The fine-needle aspiration (FNA) is a minimally invasive, safe procedure that allows the clinician to obtain an aspirate of the nodule for diagnostic cytological analysis in a relatively quick and painless manner. Indications for FNA are set out by the Society of Radiologists in Ultrasound and are useful in the following situations:

♦ Dominant or solitary nodules over 1 cm.

♦ Nodules with concerning features on ultrasound (such as hypoechogenicity, microcalcifications, and increasing size).

♦ Nodule in the presence of clinical risk factors, including childhood head and neck radiation, family or personal history of thyroid cancer, and MEN2 oncogene.

FNA can be performed on palpable nodules in the outpatient clinic or by ultrasound guidance.

The patient should be consented for the procedure after explanation of the need for the procedure and pertinent risks, including infection, bleeding into the nodule, pain, and the risk of not obtaining a diagnostic sample (10% of cases).

3. What are the implications of a Thy3f cytology result?

The results of thyroid cytology in the UK are reported in accordance to the guidance from the Royal College of Pathologists and classified into five categories: 'Thy1' to 'Thy5'. The likelihood of malignancy increases with increasing Thy category. The cytology report should be correlated with clinical and ultrasound findings but, in general, the implications of the various Thy categories are as follows:

- Thy1—this indicates a 'non-diagnostic' sample. This category includes samples with insufficient epithelial cells for diagnosis or those reflecting lesions such as cysts. Thy1c indicates cyst fluid with insufficient colloid and epithelial cells. Thy1 result usually requires further assessment with US and repeat cytology.

- Thy2—this indicates a non-neoplastic or benign result, such as can be obtained from a colloid nodule, thyroiditis, and normal thyroid tissue. Cyst samples with abundant colloid can be categorized as Thy2c. Surgery is not mandatory for these lesions. The risk of malignancy has been cited at 0–3%.

- Thy3—indicates an indeterminate lesion, possibly neoplastic. This is further subdivided into Thy3a and Thy3f. Thy3a lesions show atypical features that are not enough to warrant placement into any other category. Repeat cytology may allow reclassification into another category; an alternative option may be a diagnostic hemi-thyroidectomy. Thy3f lesions are those suspicious of follicular neoplasms; potential diagnoses include a hyperplastic nodule, follicular adenoma, follicular carcinoma, or follicular variant of papillary carcinoma. Definitive diagnosis requires surgical excision; usually in the form of a diagnostic hemi-thyroidectomy. However, a total thyroidectomy may be appropriate for patients with associated diseases, such as Graves' disease, and a multi-nodular goitre. Risk of malignancy is 5–15% for Thy3a lesions and 15–30% for Thy3f lesions.

- Thy4—indicates a lesion suspicious (but not definite) of malignancy. These lesions are associated with malignant histology in about 60–75% of cases. Patients in this category should usually undergo at least a diagnostic hemi-thyroidectomy.

- Thy5—indicates thyroid cancer. The type of malignancy should be stated in the report. Treatment should be tailored according to tumour type but surgery is almost always required. Exceptions include thyroid lymphoma and unresectable anaplastic cancer.

For this patient with a Thy3f lesion, malignancy cannot be excluded using FNA cytology (FNAC) alone. He should be advised to undergo a diagnostic hemi-thyroidectomy.

4. What risks would you explain to a patient undergoing thyroid surgery?

Risks of thyroid surgery include those common to any procedure occurring under a general anaesthetic. These include infection and, rarely, cardio-respiratory complications and venous thrombo-embolism. Those risks specific to thyroid surgery should also be discussed, these include:

- *Haemorrhage with neck haematoma*. This may result in airway oedema and obstruction—this requires an urgent assessment by a senior member of the surgical and/or anaesthetic team and, occasionally, emergency re-exploration of the neck.

- *Laryngeal nerve damage*. The recurrent laryngeal nerve (RLN) is at risk of injury in thyroid surgery. Injuries may be unilateral or bilateral, complete or incomplete, transient or permanent. Transient damage occurs in around 5–10% and long-term/permanent rates should be approximately 1%.

  - Unilateral incomplete injury may go unnoticed or may result in a weak or hoarse voice and often requires no treatment. Unilateral complete injury may result in a weak, hoarse voice, a bovine cough, difficulty in swallowing liquids, and/or aspiration. In the short term, conservative management, including dietary advice and/or speech therapy, is the standard treatment. Long term, persistent palsy may need surgical treatment in the form of cord medialization.

♦ A bilateral incomplete injury results in inspiratory stridor and partial airway obstruction, often requiring a tracheostomy in the immediate post-operative period. The voice can be surprisingly good. A bilateral complete injury results in complete loss of voice. However, respiration is still possible, but patients may become dyspnoeic on exertion. Treatment is usually with tracheostomy with a speaking valve.

♦ *The external laryngeal nerve (ELN)* is at risk when the superior pedicle is ligated and may result in a weak voice, particularly on singing or shouting. Speech therapy may be of use.

♦ *Hypocalcaemia.* This may be temporary or permanent. This is most commonly due to hypoparathyroidism, where there is damage/bruising from handling the gland during thyroidectomy, devascularization, or inadvertent removal of the parathyroid glands. It may also occur as a result of 'hungry bone disease' in patients with thyrotoxicosis (this is discussed in more detail in the Parathyroid case (6.2) in this chapter). Signs and symptoms of hypocalcaemia include perioral tingling, paraesthesia in the fingertips, cramps, tetany, and (in severe cases) convulsions. Treatment is with administration of calcium and active vitamin D (alfacalcidol or calcitriol), usually by the oral route. Occasionally, intravenous administration is required in the severely symptomatic patient.

♦ *Tracheomalacia.* This is a very rare complication and occurs following the excision of very large and longstanding goitres that have been compressing the trachea. Removal of the goitre results in the collapse of the tracheal wall and subsequent airway obstruction, necessitating ventilation and sometimes tracheostomy.

- *Thyroid crisis.* In patients requiring thyroidectomy for thyro-toxicosis, thyrotoxic crisis (also known as thyrotoxic storm) is a rare but potentially life-threatening complication that may occur when patients are not rendered euthyroid pre-operatively and manipulation of the gland causes excess hormone release. It may also be precipitated by stress, infection, or iodine administration. Patients develop hyperpyrexia, tachycardia, dyspnoea, diarrhoea, jaundice, and neurological symptoms, which range from agitation to delirium or coma. Heart failure or myocardial infarction may also occur. Patients should be treated in an intensive care setting with inorganic iodine (e.g. Lugol's iodine) and anti-thyroid drugs (e.g. carbimazole or propylthiouracil) are administered with beta-blockers, oxygen, temperature control, and careful fluid balance. Digoxin, mechanical ventilation, and corticosteroids may also be required.

- For those undergoing total thyroidectomy, patients should be informed that they will be rendered hypothyroid and will need thyroxine supplements for life.

- Patient should be counselled about the possibility of hyper-trophic scarring and keloid formation which may be prominent on the neck.

5. **The patient eventually recovers from surgery and sees you in the follow-up clinic. Histology shows papillary thyroid cancer. Describe the different types of thyroid cancer and how this will impact on the prognosis.**

The types and subtypes of thyroid cancer are as follows:

- Differentiated thyroid cancer (commonest type with the best prognosis):
  - Papillary (commonest subtype with the best prognosis).
  - Follicular.
  - Hurthle cell cancer.
  - Poorly differentiated thyroid cancer.
  - Anaplastic thyroid cancer.

- Medullary thyroid cancer.

- Lymphoma.

- Metastatic (secondary) deposits in thyroid (very rare).

Differentiated thyroid cancer These account for around 95% of all thyroid malignancies. They may occur at any age but the peak incidence is between the 3rd and 5th decades. They arise from the follicular epithelial cells of the thyroid gland, are slow-growing, often multifocal, and sometimes encapsulated. The commonest subtype (papillary) tends to metastasize to lymph nodes, while the follicular subtype has the propensity to spread via the bloodstream. They can be successfully treated with surgery with/without radio-iodine ablation and lifelong high-dose thyroxine therapy for TSH suppression, as these tumours are TSH-dependent. Overall, prognosis is good, with a 90% 10-year survival rate.

Medullary thyroid carcinoma This type accounts for up to 5% of all thyroid malignancies and may occur at any age. They are associated with familial syndromes in around 25% of cases. Pathologically, these tumours arise from parafollicular C-cells and secrete calcitonin. The tumour grows locally, may be multifocal, and readily spreads to the regional lymph nodes and via the bloodstream to the liver, lungs, and bone. Treatment is with total thyroidectomy and central +/– lateral neck dissection. Prognosis is dependent on lymph node involvement and distant metastases at presentation. Excellent 10-year survival figures of 90% have been reported, but this drops to 70% if cervical lymph node metastases are present, and to 20% in the presence of distal metastases.

Anaplastic thyroid cancer This type accounts for less than 2% of thyroid malignancies and occurs in elderly patients, with peak incidence in the 7th decade. These are undifferentiated, rapidly growing tumours that are locally invasive and metastasize via lymphatics and bloodstream to lymph nodes, lungs, bone, and brain. Surgical resection is rarely possible due to the local extent of the disease and treatment options usually include debulking surgery and palliative radiotherapy. Tracheal stents may be required in some patients. Prognosis is poor with an average survival of between 3 and 6 months after diagnosis; 90% of patients die within 1 year.

Poorly differentiated thyroid cancers lie in a spectrum between the differentiated and anaplastic varieties and have an intermediate prognosis. Thyroid lymphomas and metastases from other sites are rare but can occasionally occur. The prognosis for primary thyroid lymphomas is reasonably good as they respond well to chemotherapy. The prognosis for metastases to the thyroid is dependent on the primary cancer.

6. What are the commonly used treatment modalities in the management of differentiated thyroid cancer?

- *Surgery.* Surgery is the mainstay of treatment of differentiated thyroid cancer. Hemi-thyroidectomy (also called total thyroid lobectomy) is the minimum operation for suspected thyroid malignancy and may be sufficient for small papillary and follicular cancers. Total or near-total thyroidectomy is the usual operation for most other types of thyroid cancers. Near-total thyroidectomy involves leaving a small remnant of thyroid tissue/capsule on one or both sides, and is done to preserve the blood supply to the parathyroid glands or to avoid damage to the laryngeal nerves. Central and lateral neck dissections are performed in patients with lymph node disease. In patients without clinical or radiological evidence of lymph node disease, a prophylactic central neck dissection may be performed in the presence of certain high-risk factors that indicate an increased risk of recurrence.

- *TSH suppressive doses of thyroxine.* TSH is thought to be a growth factor for thyroid cancer and suppression of TSH with high doses of thyroxine is thought to reduce the risk of recurrence.

- *Radioactive iodine ablation.* Iodine is selectively taken up by thyroid tissue and, therefore, radioactive iodine can be used as ablative treatment to ensure destruction of any residual thyroid tissue or metastases. Radioactive iodine ablation is performed after surgery; in some high-risk patients, a further dose may be administered 6 months later.

- *External beam radiotherapy*. Differentiated thyroid cancer is relatively resistant to external beam radiotherapy. However, in some patients, external beam radiotherapy may have a role. These include patients where the primary tumour has been incompletely resected and where at least part of the tumour is poorly differentiated or undifferentiated. This may help control locally aggressive tumours and reduce the risk of local recurrence.

7. What features are unique to differentiated thyroid cancer in comparison to other solid-organ malignancies?

Differentiated thyroid cancers have some unique features differentiating them from other types of solid-organ cancers:

- They are slow growing and hence have the best prognosis amongst all solid cancers, with a survival rate of over 90% at 10 years.

- They have a specific affinity to an element (i.e. iodine), which is unique. Iodine is an essential component of thyroid hormones. This affinity for iodine can be used for therapeutic benefit in the treatment of these cancers with radio-active iodine.

- They are relatively radio- and chemo-resistant, unlike other solid cancers.

- In most solid-organ cancers, lymph node metastasis is a sign of systemic spread of disease and carries a poor prognosis. However, in papillary thyroid cancer (the commonest subtype of thyroid cancer), lymph node metastases do not have a significant bearing on prognosis and does not feature in the American Joint Committee on Cancer (AJCC) tumour node metastases TNM classification.

Further reading

British Association of Endocrine Surgeons (2003) *Guidelines for the Surgical Management of Endocrine Disease and Training Requirements for Endocrine Surgery*. Available at http://www.baets.org.uk/

Frates MC, Benson CB, Charboneau JW, Cibas ES, Clark OH, Coleman BG et al. (2005) Society of Radiologists in Ultrasound. Management of thyroid nodules detected at US: Society of Radiologists in Ultrasound consensus conference statement. *Radiology* 237: 794–800.

Perros P, Colley S, Boelaert K, Evans C, Evans RM, Gerrard GE et al. on behalf of the British Thyroid Association (2014) British Thyroid Association Guidelines for the Management of Thyroid Cancer, third edition. *Clinical Endocrinology* 81 (Suppl. 1): 1–136.

Case history 6.2: Elective: parathyroid disease

A 34-year-old man presented to A&E 2 days ago with severe, left-sided loin pain radiating into his groin. This pain was associated with nausea but no vomiting, and lasted for approximately 4 hours. He describes a recent history of constipation and low mood but is otherwise well. He does not take any regular prescription medication and denies any family history of stone disease.

Physical examination and an abdominal X-ray were unremarkable. Urinalysis demonstrated microscopic haematuria and a non-contrast CT scan confirmed the presence of a left-sided, 5-mm, ureteric calculi. His blood results on admission are shown in Table 6.2.1.

The urologists query a diagnosis of primary hyperparathyroidism (PHPT) and refer him to you to consider a parathyroidectomy.

Table 6.2.1 Blood results

Hb	165
WCC	8.0
Platelets	220
Sodium	135
Potassium	3.5
Urea	6.5
Creatinine	83
Adjusted calcium	3.5
Phosphate	1.0
ALP	140

Questions

1. How can hyperparathyroidism be classified?

2. How would you confirm the diagnosis of primary hyperparathyroidism?

3. Following the diagnosis, would you request any imaging tests? If so, explain the role of imaging in these patients.

4. The patient is diagnosed with primary HPT. How will you decide if he requires an operation?

5. On the day after the operation, you are called to review him on account of his symptoms (tingling and numbness in fingers and toes, and feeling unwell) and an adjusted calcium of 1.9 mmol/l. What further information do you need to formulate a management plan? Discuss the possible mechanisms of hypocalcaemia in this scenario and the principles of management.

6. At his post-operative follow-up visit, he reports that his father, who died of a brain tumour, apparently had a 'high calcium' problem. What does this mean and how would you take this further?

Answers

1. How can hyperparathyroidism be classified?

Hyperparathyroidism (HPT) is characterized by the over-production of parathyroid hormone. There are three types of hyperparathyroidism:

- *Primary HPT (PHPT)*. This refers to autonomous parathyroid activity with partial or complete loss of negative-feedback mechanisms. High levels of parathyroid hormone (PTH) result in hypercalcaemia and a normal or raised urinary calcium excretion. The effects are depicted in Table 6.2.2. The pathology is usually single gland disease (parathyroid adenoma) and, uncommonly, due to multi-gland disease (multiple adenoma or hyperplasia).

- *Secondary HPT*. High levels of PTH is a physiological response to metabolic pathology, commonly vitamin D deficiency or renal failure. In chronic renal failure, parathyroid growth and

Table 6.2.2 Clinical features of hypercalcaemia

Site	Features
Central nervous system	Lethargy
	Weakness
	Confusion
	Coma
Gastrointestinal	Nausea
	Constipation
	Anorexia
	Pancreatitis
	Gastric ulcer
Genitourinary	Polyuria
	Nocturia
	Nephrolithiasis
	Ureteric calculi
Musculoskeletal	Bone pain

Reproduced courtesy of Jenna Morgan.

proliferation is stimulated by hypocalcaemia, hyperphosphatemia, and impaired renal activation of vitamin D. In these patients, the calcium is low to normal and the PTH is high. Treatment should focus on the underlying pathology, but occasionally surgery is required in renal disease.

- *Tertiary HPT.* This is autonomous overproduction of PTH arising as a consequence of chronic secondary HPT after the causative pathology has been treated. An example would be following renal transplantation for chronic kidney disease. Usually, both calcium and PTH levels are elevated. Surgical treatment is often required.

2. How would you confirm the diagnosis of primary hyperparathyroidism?

Diagnostic workup requires:

- Serum adjusted calcium.
- Serum PTH level.
- Urinary calcium measurement.

The biochemical diagnosis of primary HPT requires the demonstration of elevated levels of corrected serum calcium in the presence of a raised or normal PTH level.

Hypercalcaemia due to other causes would result in suppression of PTH. It is important to note that normocalcaemia does not exclude hyperparathyroidism. In addition, urinary calcium excretion should be normal or elevated. This can be demonstrated in a 24-hour urine calcium collection or a calculation of fractional excretion of calcium based on concurrent urine and blood samples. A low urine calcium in the presence of elevated serum calcium and PTH should lead to the consideration of familial hypocalciuric (or benign) hypercalcaemia (FHH or FBH); a condition where parathyroid surgery is contraindicated.

3. Following the diagnosis, would you request any imaging tests? If so, explain the role of imaging in these patients.

Parathyroid imaging is not required to confirm the diagnosis of primary hyperparathyroidism. Failure to localize an abnormal parathyroid gland on imaging doesn't negate the diagnosis. Primary hyperparathyroidism is caused by a solitary benign adenoma in 80–85% cases but may be due to multiple adenomata or diffuse or nodular hyperplasia in the remainder. Bilateral neck exploration to examine all four glands has traditionally been considered the gold standard for patients undergoing surgery for primary hyperparathyroidism. The glands can often be identified on the basis of their anatomical location, soft consistency, and characteristic reddish-brown colour. Figure 6.2.1 shows an example of an enlarged gland.

However, targeted or minimally invasive parathyroidectomy is equally effective in patients with single gland disease and this can be facilitated by the pre-operative identification of the enlarged gland on imaging. Parathyroid imaging is, therefore, useful to identify those suitable for this type of approach by identifying a solitary abnormality and establishing the location of the single enlarged gland. Although the type of imaging used varies, most centres perform 99Tc Sestamibi scanning and high-resolution ultrasonography.

A bone mineral density assessment with a dual X-ray absorptiometry (DEXA) scan is essential to diagnose osteoporosis, the

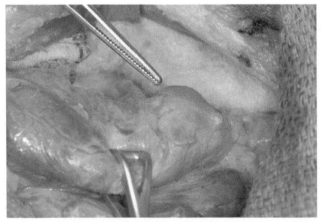

Figure 6.2.1 Intra-operative image of the retracted thyroid and parathyroid gland. The forceps are pointing at a parathyroid gland.

Reproduced courtesy of Saba Balasubramanian.

presence of which is an indication for surgery, even if hypercalcaemia is mild and the patient is asymptomatic.

Ultrasound of the kidneys help to determine the presence of renal stones or nephrocalcinosis, which are also indications for parathyroid surgery in an asymptomatic patient with mild hypercalcaemia. However, ureteric calculi may very well lead to clinical presentation of the parathyroid disease, such as with this patient.

4. This patient is confirmed to have primary HPT. How will you decide if he requires an operation?

Surgery is clearly indicated in this patient as he presented with symptomatic renal stone disease. Surgical excision is the mainstay of treatment of PHPT and should be considered for all patients, as it is not possible to predict deterioration in calcium levels or the occurrence of end-organ damage, such as osteoporosis or renal disease. Clear indications for surgery include symptoms and the presence of end-organ damage. Asymptomatic patients over the age of 50 with mild hypercalcaemia without osteoporosis, renal stone disease, renal impairment or hypercalciuria may be managed conservatively.

5. On the day after the operation, you are called to review him on account of his symptoms (tingling and numbness in fingers and toes, and feeling unwell). He has an adjusted calcium of 1.9 mmol/l. What further information do you need to formulate a management plan? Discuss the possible mechanisms of hypocalcaemia in this scenario and the principles of management.

The management of post-operative hypocalcaemia depends on the severity of hypocalcaemia and PTH level. Information on the extent of parathyroidectomy would also be useful in formulating a management plan.

There are two main mechanisms underlying post-operative hypocalcaemia following parathyroid surgery. The first is hypoparathyroidism (either from a subtotal parathyroidectomy or inadvertent devascularization or damage of normal parathyroid glands). This condition requires treatment with calcium and active vitamin D (alfacalcidol or calcitriol). The second mechanism is 'hungry bone syndrome', referring to the increased bone turnover and remineralization of the skeleton that follows the surgical treatment of primary hyperparathyroidism. In this latter scenario, PTH levels are secondarily elevated and treatment is primarily with calcium supplements. Active vitamin D is often not required, but any co-existing vitamin D deficiency needs to be treated with inactive vitamin D (cholecalciferol). This can last for weeks, during which time patients should be closely monitored and may be treated on an outpatient basis, where possible.

6. At his post-operative follow-up visit, he reports that his father, who died of a brain tumour, apparently had a 'high calcium' problem. What does this mean and how would you take this further?

It is likely that the cause of this patient's primary hyperparathyroidism is due to multiple endocrine neoplasia type I (MEN I or Werner) syndrome. MEN syndromes consist of clusters of endocrine tumours and have an autosomal dominant mode of inheritance. Primary hyperparathyroidism is often sporadic; however, 95% of patients with MEN I syndrome will present with primary hyperparathyroidism due to four gland hyperplasia. Parathyroid neoplasia is also a feature of MEN IIa (or Sipple) syndrome. In patients suspected of having a MEN syndrome, referral for counselling and genetic testing should be done. Patients shown to have a mutation for MEN1 or MEN2 should undergo initial (biochemical and radiological) screening for the presence of specific endocrinopathies, followed by regular surveillance, details of which are beyond the scope of this book. Other familial syndromes include HPT–JT (hyperparathyroidism–jaw tumour) syndrome and familial hyperparathyroidism.

Table 6.2.3 Common and uncommon endocrine tumours seen in patients with MEN1, MEN IIa, and MEN IIb syndromes

	Tumours in MEN I	Tumours in MEN IIa	Tumours in MEN IIb
Common	◆ Parathyroid hyperplasia	◆ Medullary carcinoma of the thyroid	◆ Medullary carcinoma of the thyroid
	◆ Pancreatic and duodenal endocrine tumours:	◆ Phaeochromocytoma	◆ Mucosal and ganglioneuromas
	◆ Zollinger-Ellison		◆ Marfanoid appearance
	◆ Insulinoma		◆ Phaeochromocytoma
	◆ PP-oma (pancreatic polypeptide)		
	◆ Pituitary adenoma:		
	◆ Prolactinoma		
	◆ ACTH-oma		
Uncommon	◆ Thyroid tumours	◆ Parathyroid tumours	
	◆ Adrenal adenoma or carcinoma		
	◆ Foregut or midgut carcinoid		
	◆ Lipoma		

Reproduced courtesy of Jenna Morgan.

Table 6.2.3 shows the common and uncommon endocrine tumours seen in patients with MEN1, MEN IIa, and MEN IIb syndromes.

Further reading

Mihai R (2014) Surgical management of hyperparathyroidism. *Surgery* (Oxford) **32** (10): 548–51.

Case history 6.3: Elective: adrenal lesion

A 60-year-old man with severe hypertension is referred to the surgical clinic for abdominal pain. He has no past medical history apart from an appendicectomy as a child. He takes no medication, has no known drug allergies, and is a non-smoker. Physical examination reveals a soft, non-tender abdomen with no palpable masses or organomegaly. His observations in clinic are as follows: pulse rate is 85, BP is 135/80, and respiratory rate of 12 breaths a minute.

Ultrasound followed by a CT scan show a retroperitoneal lesion superior to the left kidney. An ultrasound guided biopsy is arranged. During the procedure, he develops chest pain and is diagnosed to have had a myocardial infarction.

A further detailed history reveals episodes of 'panic attacks' over a 2-year period associated with a feeling of anxiety, headaches, and nausea.

Questions

1. What diagnosis should be suspected at this stage? What is the take-home message for clinicians investigating abdominal masses of uncertain aetiology?

2. What is a phaeochromocytoma?

3. What tests will help confirm the suspected diagnosis?

4. Following confirmation of the diagnosis, what further investigations should be performed in such a patient before treatment?

5. Describe the pre-operative management of such pathology.

6. What are the peri-operative risks in this patient?

Answers

1. What diagnosis should be suspected at this stage? What is the take-home message for clinicians investigating abdominal masses of uncertain aetiology?

A phaeochromocytoma should be suspected. Most patients with phaeochromocytoma do not have the classic triad of headaches, palpitations, and hyperhidrosis with hypertension. Some present with one or more symptoms, while others may be asymptomatic and found on routine scanning for an unrelated condition.

Adrenal lesions are often an incidental finding in asymptomatic patients on cross-sectional imaging for other indications. As well as phaeochromocytoma, other potential differential diagnoses include an adrenal adenoma, adrenocortical cancer, adrenal metastasis from a distal primary (e.g. colon tumour), and adrenal myelolipoma.

A phaeochromocytoma or paraganglioma (also called extra-adrenal phaeochromocytoma) should be considered in the differential diagnosis of all retroperitoneal lesions. Biopsy is seldom required in the diagnosis and management of adrenal lesions; diagnosis relies more on imaging and biochemical screening. Even if a biopsy is considered in the investigation of an adrenal lesion, it must only be performed after biochemical screening has ruled out a phaeochromocytoma.

2. What is a phaeochromocytoma?

Phaeochromocytoma is a catecholamine-secreting paraganglioma derived from chromaffin cells that are found predominantly in the adrenal medulla but can be located in extra-adrenal tissue. These patients present with features that arise from the high levels of catecholamines and their effects on the sympathetic nervous system: headache, sweating, palpitations, tremor, anxiety, abdominal pain, nausea, weakness, constipation, and weight loss.

Between 10 and 20% of tumours are malignant, with a higher risk of malignancy in extra-adrenal phaeochromocytomas. Familial conditions should be suspected in patients presenting below 40 years of age.

3. What tests will help confirm the suspected diagnosis?

The chromaffin cells of the adrenal medulla metabolize tumour-derived catecholamines to normetanephrine and metanephrine, and these can be reliably assayed in the diagnostic workup. Therefore, if phaeochromocytoma is suspected, the levels of catecholamines and their metabolites in the blood and/or urine should be measured. In many centres, one or two 24-hour urine collections are performed to measure both catecholamines and their metabolites. More recently, plasma-free metanephrines have been considered as the gold standard test for the diagnosis of phaeochromocytoma; sensitivity and specificity are thought to be better than urine estimations with the added advantage of increased convenience for the patient.

It is important to note that the results of these tests may be affected by the concurrent use of drugs, such as calcium-channel blockers, monoamine oxidase inhibitors, tricyclic antidepressants, alpha-blockers, and beta-blockers. Patients on such medications should be tested for a phaeochromocytoma in a specialist endocrine unit and appropriate modifications to medications made before biochemical testing.

4. Following confirmation of the diagnosis, what further investigations should be performed in such a patient before treatment?

Following biochemical confirmation of the diagnosis, the lesion should be localized on cross-sectional imaging, if this has not already been done. This further tests may need to be considered before planning surgical treatment:

- Further cross-sectional imaging, such as MR scanning, may help in cases where findings on CT is equivocal.
- Functional imaging, such as an iodine-131-labelled meta-iodobenzylguanide (MIBG) scan, is useful in patients where there is a suggestion of familial disease or malignancy. This will help in ruling out other extra-adrenal foci of disease, which occurs in 15–20% of cases.
- Some phaeochromocytomas are associated with cortisol hypersecretion. Failure to identify this problem may result in adrenal

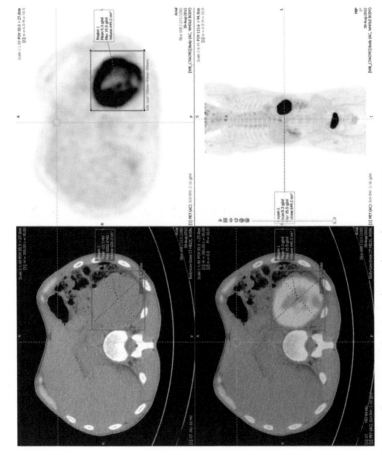

Figure 6.3.1 A transverse image from PET-CT showing a large phaeochromocytoma.

Reproduced courtesy of Judith Ritchie.

insufficiency in the post-operative period due to contralateral adrenal suppression. A biochemical assessment for hypercortisolism should, therefore, be done in all such patients.

5. Describe the pre-operative management of such pathology.

Adrenal surgery for phaeochromocytoma is a major undertaking, even when performed laparoscopically. All patients should undergo a detailed pre-operative assessment prior to surgery. Liaison with the anaesthetic and medical teams is crucial. A detailed cardiology assessment (including an electrocardiogram and echocardiogram) will help identify co-existing cardiac illness and may help optimize the patient before surgery. Any anaemia or electrolyte imbalances should be fully corrected. A hypertensive crisis resulting in a myocardial infarction or stroke is a real risk during or after surgery for phaeochromocytoma. To reduce this risk, patients should be on maximally tolerated doses of alpha-adrenergic blockers (such as phenoxybenzamine). To counteract the effects of alpha-blockade and reduce the severity of hypotension immediately following excision of a phaeochromocytoma, patients should be adequately hydrated in the days leading to the operation. Beta-blockers are not required in most patients for pre-operative preparation, but may be needed in a minority of patients who develop symptomatic and severe tachycardia on alpha-blockers. Beta-blockers should not be administered to patients with a phaeochromocytoma without ensuring adequate alpha-blockade first. Other precautions similar to that required for patients undergoing any major surgery include thromboprophylaxis and the availability of appropriately cross-matched blood for transfusion.

6. What are the peri-operative risks in this patient?

The risks specific to surgery for phaeochromocytoma are hypertensive crisis (as explained above) and post-excision hypotension. Devascularization and excision of the gland results in a dramatic drop in circulating vasoactive catecholamines and their metabolites, resulting in hypotension. The risk of these complications is reduced by adequate pre-operative preparation (including alpha-blockade and hydration) and the appropriate intra-operative use of fluid resuscitation, vasodilators, and/or inotropes by an experienced anaesthetist. Close monitoring of blood pressure with an arterial line during and after surgery is mandatory. Intra-operative arrhythmias may occur and this may be related to gland manipulation and the release of catecholamines. The ECG should, therefore, be closely monitored intra-operatively for arrhythmias.

Other risks include bleeding (during mobilization of the gland as phaeochromocytomas are very vascular) and risk of damage to adjacent structures, such as the spleen, liver, and inferior vena cava.

Hypoglycaemia occasionally occurs in the first few hours following excision of a phaeochromocytoma and should be anticipated. If co-existing hypercortisolism is not detected and managed appropriately (as explained before), adrenal insufficiency may occur following surgery.

Generic risks that should be discussed with the patient include infection, abdominal wall herniae, and venous thromboembolism.

Further reading

Balasubramanian SP, Harrison BJ (2014) Investigation and management of adrenal disease. *Surgery* (Oxford) **32** (10): 552–57.

Case history 6.4: Emergency: peri-operative management of the thyroid patient

A 34-year-old woman with severe thyrotoxicosis is an inpatient in the endocrinology unit. She developed severe leukopenia following the initiation of anti-thyroid drugs, and the endocrinologist has requested that she be considered for an urgent thyroidectomy for definitive disease control.

The patient is clinically toxic, reporting palpitations, tremor, feelings of anxiousness, and increased sweating. She reported some weight loss over the last few months. She has no relevant past medical history and is currently on beta-blockers and cholestyramine.

On examination, she has a diffuse goitre. Her most recent bloods are shown in Table 6.4.1.

Table 6.4.1 Blood results

Hb	140
WCC	6.5
Platelets	280
Sodium	136
Potassium	3.8
Urea	5.5
Creatinine	93
TSH	<0.01
Free T4	42
Free T3	9.1

Reproduced courtesy of Jenna Morgan

Questions

1. What are the causes of thyrotoxicosis?

2. Describe various medications that can be used in the control of thyrotoxicosis and their mechanisms of action.

3. What are the definitive treatment options for thyrotoxic patients? What are the pros and cons of each approach?

4. How would you prepare this patient for a thyroidectomy?

5. Following pre-operative treatment to normalise her thyroid hormone levels, she undergoes a total thyroidectomy. On the evening of the operation, you are called by the nurse as she is concerned about some swelling around the wound and reports that the patient's breathing has become noisy. On examination the patient appears to be in respiratory distress. What are the mechanisms of respiratory distress following thyroid surgery?

6. Outline your initial approach to acute respiratory distress post thyroidectomy and the principles of management.

Answers

1. What are the causes of thyrotoxicosis?

Thyrotoxicosis is a syndrome of clinical features that result from excessively high levels of circulating thyroid hormones. The diagnosis of thyrotoxicosis is confirmed by measurement of serum levels of TSH, and T4 and T3 hormones: the T4 and T3 are raised, whereas the TSH is appropriately suppressed in the vast majority of cases.

There are a number of causes (Table 6.4.2). The most common cause is Graves' disease, characterized by features of thyrotoxicosis, goitre, and extra-thyroid signs such as eye signs. Circulating stimulating autoantibodies against TSH receptor stimulate thyroid hormone production and release.

Table 6.4.2 Causes of thyrotoxicosis

Group	Disease	Relative frequency
Thyrotoxicosis of thyroidal origin (overproduction)	Graves' disease	70%
	Toxic adenoma	5%
	Multinodular toxic goitre	20%
	Iodine-induced thyrotoxicosis	<1%
	TSH-secreting adenoma	<1%
	Neonatal thyrotoxicosis	<1%
Associated with thyroid destruction	Subacute thyroiditis	3%
	Silent thyroiditis	3%
	Amiodarone-induced thyrotoxicosis (type 2)	<1%
Thyrotoxicosis of non-thyroidal origin	Factitious thyrotoxicosis	Very rare
	Thyroid hormone poisoning	Very rare
	Struma ovarii	Very rare
	Metastatic thyroid cancer	Very rare

2. **Describe various medications that can be used in the control of thyrotoxicosis and their mechanisms of action.**

Anti-thyroid drugs are very effective drugs that are used for first-line management of hyperthyroidism. These include thionamides, such as carbimazole, methimazole, and propylthiouracil. The drugs interfere with several steps of the thyroid hormone synthesis pathway, including interfering with the incorporation of iodine into tyrosine residues on the thyroglobulin molecule and preventing the intra-thyroglobulin coupling of iodotyrosines. Propylthiouracil also blocks peripheral conversion of T4 to T3. They control hyperthyroidism within several weeks, so can be effective for short-term control ahead of surgery. There are rare but serious side-effects. In particular, these drugs can cause bone marrow suppression, and resulting neutropenia and agranulocytosis can result in serious life-threatening sepsis. In these instances, anti-thyroid drugs would have to be discontinued, as in this case. Beta-blockers are also effective in controlling the symptoms of thyrotoxicosis (anxiety and palpitations) and are commonly used. Some beta-blockers, such as propanalol, also help by reducing the peripheral conversion of T4 to T3.

Other treatment options that can be used in the rapid control of thyrotoxicosis include:

- Intravenous or oral iodine preparations (such as Lugol's iodine) in high doses paradoxically inhibits the synthesis and release of thyroid hormones (Wolf–Chaikoff effect) and help to render patients euthyroid in the short term. The effects are transient and thought to only last for a few weeks, during which time surgery should be performed.

- Steroids are occasionally used as an adjunct in the management of uncontrolled thyrotoxicosis. They help in reducing thyroid hormone synthesis and also reduce conversion of T4 to T3.

- Cholestyramine is a bile acid sequestrant and interferes with extra-hepatic circulation of thyroid hormone conjugates, helping to significantly and rapidly reduce blood levels of thyroid hormones. Cholestyramine can also interfere with the absorption and effectiveness of other drugs used in treating hyperthyroidism.

Care should, therefore, be taken to appropriately schedule administration of cholestyramine in such a way as to reduce its impact on the delivery of other medications when it is used.

3. What are the definitive treatment options to surgery for thyrotoxic patients? What are the pros and cons of each approach?

Treatment options include:

+ Radioactive iodine ablation of the thyroid.

+ Total thyroidectomy.

Radioactive iodine (I^{131}) is preferentially taken up by the thyroid tissue, which is then destroyed in the process. It is given as a single oral dose and causes damage to the follicular cells that produce thyroid hormone. Radioactive iodine will render more than 60% of patients euthyroid in 1 year, and the remaining patients may require additional doses to achieve a euthyroid state. It is easy and safe to administer, but is contraindicated in pregnancy and breast-feeding patients, as well as those who work with children. Patients should have limited social contact (particularly with children) in the initial short-term treatment period. However, as with surgery, adequate control of thyrotoxicosis is essential before radio-iodine is used. Oral iodine cannot be used in the treatment of the toxic patient, as it will render the use of radio-iodine ineffective. In addition, in patients with thyroid eye disease (which this patient probably has), radioiodine ablation is associated with an increased risk of worsening of eye disease compared to surgery. This risk may be reduced with the use of steroids.

Surgery in the form of total or near-total thyroidectomy in patients with hyperthyroidism is effective and immediate in rendering patients euthyroid. It is used in patients where radio-iodine is contraindicated and particularly suitable for patients with a large goitre, eye signs, or those planning a possible pregnancy. Thyroid function should be normalized as much as possible pre-operatively to avoid the risks of a thyrotoxic storm. Surgery requires a general anaesthetic and there is the potential for post-operative complications (see Case 6.1).

4. How would you prepare this patient for a thyroidectomy?

When a thyroidectomy is planned in a toxic patient, all attempts should be made to render the patient euthyroid before surgery to reduce the risk of a peri-operative thyrotoxic crisis (also referred to as thyroid storm). This is a life-threatening hypermetabolic state caused by release of excessive levels of thyroid hormone. Features include fever and sweating, nausea, vomiting and diarrhoea, respiratory distress, tachycardia, hypertension, congestive heart failure, and, rarely, seizures.

In a patient with complications such as the one presented, managing thyrotoxicosis may be exceptionally challenging. However, the judicious use of a combination of drugs (outlined above) with appropriate dose escalation in the days leading to surgery is often successful in achieving the objective.

Other measures in the preparation of this patient include a general anaesthetic assessment, a pre-operative laryngoscopy to confirm normal vocal cord function, and calcium and vitamin D levels. Patients with Graves' disease are at higher risk of post-thyroidectomy hypocalcaemia due to both parathyroid damage and hungry bone syndrome. This risk can be reduced by meticulous surgical attention to avoid damaging the parathyroid glands and their blood supply. Pre-operative detection and treatment of co-existing vitamin D deficiency has also been demonstrated to reduce the risk of post-operative hypocalcaemia.

A pre-operative ECG will help in the detection and management of arrhythmias secondary to thyrotoxicosis.

5. Following pre-operative treatment to normalise her thyroid hormone levels, she undergoes a total thyroidectomy. On the evening of the operation, you are called by the nurse as she is concerned about some swelling around the wound and reports that the patient's breathing has become noisy. On examination the patient appears to be in respiratory distress. What are the mechanisms of respiratory distress following thyroid surgery?

Respiratory distress is a potentially life-threatening complication following thyroid surgery and may be caused by one of several mechanisms:

- Haemorrhage with neck haematoma—small volumes of bleeding into the thyroid bed have potential to cause respiratory distress by increasing compartment pressures and impeding venous and lymphatic draining from the larynx. This results in laryngeal mucosal oedema and airway compromise. The routine use of drains is not common practice now as drains often become blocked.

- An incomplete, bilateral, recurrent laryngeal nerve injury and tracheomalacia are other rare but serious complications that have the potential to compromise the airways (see Case 6.1 for detailed discussion).

6. Outline your initial approach to acute respiratory distress post thyroidectomy and the principles of management.

Airway compromise following thyroid surgery is a medical emergency and should initially be managed using the CCrISP approach and ABC assessment. Early input from a senior thyroid surgeon and anaesthetist is mandatory.

The patient should be propped up, started on high flow oxygen, and IV access should be ensured. Although the definitive management plan will depend on the cause of respiratory distress, laryngeal oedema is an essential component of the pathogenesis of the complication. Intravenous hydrocortisone and the use of nebulized adrenaline may help reduce the oedema and are reasonable first steps that can be quickly administered.

For patients who have a neck haematoma and associated respiratory distress, which is progressive, early intubation is ideal. However, this is best performed by an experienced anaesthetist, as multiple attempts by the inexperienced will worsen airway oedema and make future attempts more difficult. In this situation, evacuation of the haematoma may need to be performed at the bedside, especially if respiratory distress is significant or worsening rapidly. This is usually achieved by opening the skin sutures; the open wound is covered by a moist swab until the patient is taken to the operating theatre for a formal exploration.

The measures outlined above often result in stabilization of the patient's airway until the arrival of expert help, and facilitate controlled airway access and exploration (to evacuate haematoma and control bleeding) in the operating theatre.

Patients with recurrent laryngeal nerve injury or tracheomalacia will often require tracheostomy for safe and secure access to the airway.

Further reading

Kane EG, Shore S (2014) Thyroidectomy. *Surgery* (Oxford) 32 (10): 543–47.

Truran P, Aspinall S (2014) Thyrotoxicosis and thyroiditis. *Surgery* (Oxford) 32 (10): 537–42.

Chapter 7

Emergency surgery

Jonathan Wild, Emma Nofal,
Imeshi Wijetunga, and Antonia Durham-Hall

Case history 7.1: Emergency: acute abdominal pain

A 72-year-old female presented with a 1-day history of sudden onset lower abdominal pain. On admission the pain had become more generalized and was worse on movement. She had vomited twice but with no haematemesis reported. Bowels had been opened 2 days ago and she was passing flatus. Past medical history included polymyalgia rheumatica, hypothyroidism, and osteoarthritis. Drug history included oral prednisolone, thyroxine, and paracetamol. She was an ex-smoker and occasional social drinker only.

She appeared flushed and to be in severe discomfort. Her GCS score was 15/15, blood pressure was 90/70, pulse was 110 beats per minute, temperature was 37.4°C. Her respiratory rate was 24 breaths per minute and oxygen saturations were 98% on 2 l of supplementary oxygen. There was no evidence of jaundice, anaemia, or cervical lymphadenopathy. Chest examination was normal. Her abdomen appeared distended. There were no scars from previous surgery. On abdominal examination she was generally tender across the lower abdomen, with no guarding or rebound tenderness evident. There was no palpable abdominal aortic aneurysm. Digital rectal examination revealed soft stool in the rectum only. The patient's blood results are show in Table 7.1.1.

An erect chest radiograph revealed free air under the right hemidiaphragm, indicating a visceral perforation (see Figure 7.1.1). Plain abdominal radiograph did not reveal any dilated bowel loops.

Table 7.1.1 Blood results

Blood results	
Hb	11.0
WCC	22.1
Platelets	240
Sodium	138
Potassium	4.9
Urea	5.6
Creatinine	130
Amylase	41
INR	1.3
Bilirubin	31
AST	62
ALP	42
CRP	108
Lactate	3.3

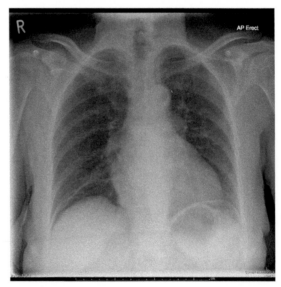

Figure 7.1.1 An erect plain chest radiograph revealing free air arising as a consequence of a colonic diverticular perforation seen under the left hemi-diaphragm.

Reproduced Courtesy of Mathew Kaduthodil.

Questions

1. What are the key differential diagnoses?

2. What are the important factors to consider in the initial assessment of a patient who presents with acute abdominal pain?

3. What are the key features that should be determined in assessing a patient who presents as a surgical emergency and how can these impact on management?

4. What are the key features that should be determined in assessing someone presenting with acute abdominal pain?

5. What are the key features to identify in the physical examination in a patient who presents with acute abdominal pain?

6. What investigations should you consider in the acute abdomen?

7. How should this patient be managed?

8. How is pre-operative mortality risk estimated? Why is this necessary?

Answers

1. What are the key differential diagnoses?

Acute abdominal pain can be defined as pain lasting less than 1 week in duration, requiring hospitalization, and that has not been previously treated or investigated. Acute abdominal pain remains a diagnostic challenge. The differential diagnosis is far-ranging, from benign to life-threatening, and encompasses medical, surgical, intra-abdominal, and extra-abdominal elements, with so-called atypical presentations a frequent occurrence. Undifferentiated or non-specific abdominal pain remains the diagnosis for around one in four patients who present to the emergency department with acute abdominal pain, with 80% of those patients improving or becoming pain free within 2 weeks of presentation.

Surgical causes of non-traumatic acute abdominal pain can be classed by the originating system:

Gastrointestinal

- Acute appendicitis.
- Gallstone disease.
- Acute cholecystitis.
- Acute pancreatitis.
- Gastritis.
- Gastroenteritis.
- Peptic ulcer disease.
- Peritonitis: from perforated viscus (duodenum, bowel, appendix); spontaneous bacterial peritonitis.
- Hepatitis.
- Small bowel obstruction.
- Mesenteric ischaemia.
- Mesenteric adenitis.
- Inflammatory bowel disease.
- Irritable bowel syndrome.
- Diverticular disease.

- Large bowel obstruction.
- Volvulus (sigmoid, caecal).
- Hernia (internal, inguinal, femoral, obturator, Richter's).
- Ruptured or expanding thoraco-abdominal aortic aneurysm.
- Haematoma: retroperitoneal; rectus sheath.

Genitourinary

- Ectopic pregnancy.
- Pelvic inflammatory disease.
- Ovarian torsion.
- Ovarian cyst disease.
- Endometriosis.
- Urosepsis.
- Ureteric stone disease.
- Testicular torsion.

Medical causes resulting in referred pain should also be taken into account. These include:

- Lower lobe pneumonia.
- Pulmonary embolus.
- Diabetic ketoacidosis.
- Sickle cell crisis.
- Hypercalcaemia.
- Infectious mononucleosis.
- Henoch–Schonlein purpura.

2. What are the important factors to consider in the initial assessment of a patient who presents with acute abdominal pain?

The surgeon's aim in the initial clinical assessment of a patient who presents with acute abdominal pain is to determine:

- The patient's current clinical status, including the need for resuscitation and optimization.

- A list of differential diagnoses and likely diagnosis.
- If sepsis is present, to administer early antibiotics in addition to supportive care, as well as considering source control.
- Whether early surgical or radiological intervention is required or not required.
- The patient's pre-operative risk of mortality, appropriateness of further investigation intervention, and to decide on any ceilings to care.
- If additional investigations are required, and the timing of such investigations.

3. **What are the key features that should be determined in assessing a patient who presents as a surgical emergency and how can these impact on management?**

From the patient's history it is important to elicit details of the characteristics of the abdominal pain.

In addition, the patient's age, gender, past medical and surgical history, and medications will be relevant.

- *Age.* The elderly are more likely to present with more severe disease and with atypical symptoms. Intra-abdominal malignancy, mesenteric ischaemia, ruptured abdominal aortic aneurysm (AAA), and atypical presentation of a myocardial infarction are more likely in patients over 50 years of age.
- *Gender.*
    - In women of childbearing age, it is vital that pregnancy status is determined promptly.
    - In the pregnant patient, the differential diagnosis expands to include ectopic pregnancy, pre-eclampsia, and placental abruption, which should be excluded as a matter of urgency.
- *Medications.* Patients may be taking drug therapies that may impact on the differential diagnoses and subsequent potential surgical management. A decision will need to be made whether certain drugs are to be stopped, replaced, or temporarily administered by another route. Some important examples include:

- *Diabetic medication.* This may need to be stopped if a patient is maintained nil by mouth for investigation and subsequent surgical management. Peri-operative glycaemic control has a significant impact on post-operative infective complications. Therefore, close monitoring of blood glucose levels is required, with a target range of 6–10 mmol/l. Given prolonged starvation periods encountered by patients undergoing assessment and operative intervention in the acute setting, anti-diabetic medication should be withheld and variable rate intravenous insulin infusion commenced once blood glucose levels exceed 10 mmol/l. Of note, metformin should ideally also be omitted, along with other nephrotoxic drugs, in patients undergoing urgent CT with intravenous contrast, in order to minimise the risk of contrast nephropathy.

- *Anti-platelet and anticoagulation therapy.* These need to be identified, especially when urgent surgical intervention is required, as the effect of these drugs may need to be reversed promptly. Patients on warfarin will need their clotting levels normalizing with IV vitamin K and fresh frozen plasma, and discussion with haematology, where they are actively bleeding, for consideration of prothrombin complex concentrate such as Beriplex P/N®.

- *Diuretics and ACE inhibitors.* These should ideally be withheld the day before surgery, in order to prevent volume depletion, potassium derangement, and refractory hypotension during anaesthesia; however, this may not be possible if urgent surgery is required.

- *Prednisolone and other immunosuppressants.* These may mask the classic symptoms and signs of intra-abdominal sepsis and peritonitis, and this must be taken into account in the assessment and decision-making process. Patients taking long-term steroids may also have iatrogenic adrenal insufficiency and may require intravenous glucocorticoid coverage during the peri-operative period in order to prevent adrenal crisis. Another consideration is that the use of steroids and non-steroidal anti-inflammatory drugs predisposes to peptic ulceration and gastrointestinal bleeding.

- *Past medical history.*

  - Of note, a history of cardiovascular and peripheral arterial disease increases the risk of mesenteric ischaemia and abdominal aortic aneurysm.
  - Previous intra-abdominal surgery increases the risk of adhesional bowel obstruction.

The social history is also of importance. Excessive alcohol intake places patients at risk of pancreatitis, gastroduodenitis, hepatitis, cirrhosis, and spontaneous bacterial peritonitis. A good social history is also needed to gain an impression of the functional status and quality of life of the patient. Combined with knowledge gained on the severity of co-existing medical conditions, this information is useful to inform decisions regarding a patient's fitness for surgery or whether there should be a ceiling for investigation and care in, for example, frail patients with poor functional status and quality of life, and a poor prognosis.

4. **What are the key features that should be determined in assessing someone presenting with acute abdominal pain?**

   SOCRATES is a simple mnemonic for assessing and documenting features of abdominal pain. This includes:

   - Site.
   - Onset (time of onset, sudden or gradual, intermittent or constant).
   - Character (dull, ache, crushing, etc.).
   - Radiation.
   - Associated features (vomiting, fever, change in bowel habit, etc.).
   - Time course (pattern).
   - Exacerbating or relieving factors.
   - Severity.

   Site

   The location of the abdominal pain can narrow the differential diagnosis, although any diagnosis should not be based solely on the location of the pain, as the two often may not correspond.

The source of the abdominal pain can be divided into three categories: visceral, parietal (or somatic), and referred:

- Visceral pain originates from the walls of hollow organs and capsules of solid organs. It is often caused by inflammation, distension, or ischaemia. Such pain is dull and poorly localized in the midline and is perceived in the abdominal region corresponding to embryonic origin of the disease viscera in question. Visceral pain from foregut structures (distal oesophagus, stomach, proximal duodenum, pancreas, liver, and gallbladder) manifests in the epigastrium, visceral pain from the midgut (distal duodenum, small bowel, and proximal large bowel) to the periumbilical region, with visceral pain from the hindgut (from distal third of transverse colon to rectum) manifesting as suprapubic pain.

- Parietal pain, caused by noxious stimulation of the parietal peritoneum, is transmitted via the ipsilateral dorsal root ganglia at the same dermatomal level as the origin of the pain. Such pain is, therefore, more localized and distinct.

- Referred pain, which is pain perceived at a location distant from the diseased organ, is caused by a shared pathway for afferent neurones from different locations with the pain being located in the dermatome of the shared spinal segment. Classically, this occurs with pathologies such as cholecystitis (referred shoulder tip pain) and localized peritonitis from appendicitis (referred pain in the left iliac fossa on palpation or percussion, termed Rozving's sign).

Onset and character

Features relating to the onset and character of the pain are important. Sudden onset of significant pain can reflect organ perforation or ischaemia, aortic rupture or dissection, ovarian torsion or cystic rupture, or obstruction of tubular structures such as the biliary tract or ureters. More gradual onset of pain suggests an inflammatory or infective process.

Associated features

Associated symptoms can help narrow the diagnosis. An underlying surgical pathology is more likely if vomiting occurs after the onset of pain. Bilious vomiting occurs due to an obstruction distal to the duodenum. Distension and constipation are also features of bowel obstruction. Diarrhoea often indicates an infective or inflammatory cause, such as colitis or diverticulitis. Diarrhoea, often bloody in nature, may also occur in mesenteric ischaemia. One should always inquire about relevant extra-abdominal symptoms, such as cough, dyspnoea, chest pain, and back pain. These can be covered in a comprehensive systemic enquiry at the end of the history. Significant genitourinary symptoms should also be identified. In women presenting with lower abdominal pain, any abnormal vaginal bleeding and discharge, and changes in menstruation, should be determined. In men, penile discharge, scrotal pain, and swelling should also be inquired about.

Timing

Colicky abdominal pain is consistent with distension of hollow viscera, such as in bowel or ureteric obstruction.

Exacerbating and relieving factors

Exacerbating and relieving factors can also help determine the diagnosis. Movement or coughing can aggravate the pain in peritonitis, yet relieve the pain in renal colic. Sitting forward can relieve the pain in acute pancreatitis and the pain can increase when the patient reclines. Pain from a peptic ulcer can be relieved with a meal, yet biliary colic can be brought on by food.

5. **What are the key features to identify in the physical examination in a patient who presents with acute abdominal pain?**

The physical examination should begin by assessing the patient's vital signs (respiratory rate, oxygen saturations, blood pressure, pulse, and GCS), especially seeking evidence of hypovolaemia and sepsis. Of note, while a pyrexia with abdominal pain increases the suspicion of intra-abdominal sepsis, the elderly and immunosuppressed may not be capable of mounting a fever, with sepsis in the elderly often presenting with hypothermia. An elevated respiratory rate is a significant finding, and can be a sign of a metabolic acidosis or mounting systemic inflammatory response to intra-abdominal sepsis.

Important features of abdominal pain include:

+ The actual location of pain.
+ Presence of peritonism. Localized peritonism certainly warrants further investigation and a diagnostic laparoscopy may be considered, especially if appendicitis is suspected. Diffuse guarding and rigidity of generalized peritonitis often indicates that explorative surgery is urgently required. Early administration of opiate analgesia and re-examination will often facilitate better examination to determine whether a patient is truly peritonitic, as well as improve patient discomfort.

Physical examination should include:

+ Systemic palpation of all nine quadrants.
+ Examination of the femoral and inguinal hernia orifices for hernias, as these can be clinically occult and present as pain, as well as bowel obstruction.
+ Palpation of the abdominal aorta in all patients over 50 years to assess for an aneurysm.
+ Rectal examination is recommended for patients with lower abdominal pain, constipation, or lower GI bleeding in order to detect faecal impaction, palpable mass, or blood in the stool.
+ A pelvic examination should be carried out in suspected gynaecological conditions.

6. What investigations should you consider in the acute abdomen?

Basic investigations include:

+ Blood tests: full blood count, urea and electrolytes, liver function tests, coagulation screen, glucose, amylase, lactate and blood group, and save are required. A β-HCG should be performed in females of childbearing age. Such tests are required to assess for the presence of organ dysfunction, systemic inflammatory response, and to assess the severity of sepsis, if present. An arterial blood gas is useful in patients with oxygen saturations below 92%, signs of severe chest disease, or systemic dysfunction, as the parameters can indicate the degree of metabolic or respiratory disturbance.

- Blood cultures should be taken if the patient is febrile.

- Urinalysis should be carried out in all patients with acute abdominal pain.

- A plain erect chest radiograph is the initial test for suspected visceral perforation; however, it only has a sensitivity of approximately 75% and further investigations may be required if a plain erect chest radiograph does not reveal free air under the diaphragm, yet perforation is still clinically suspected. A chest radiograph is also useful at excluding lower lobe pneumonia.

- The use of abdominal radiography should be limited to cases of suspected bowel obstruction or exacerbation of colitis to assess for toxic megacolon.

- Ultrasonography is the first-line investigation in suspected acute biliary disease, with a high sensitivity for the diagnosis of acute cholecystitis. It is also useful for the investigation of right iliac fossa pain in female patients of childbearing age, to assess for gynaecological causes of acute abdominal pain. It may also visualize an inflamed appendix but it is not reliable for making this diagnosis. Ultrasonography is also useful in identifying and monitoring abdominal aortic aneurysms, urinary tract disease, and rectus sheath haematomas.

Further investigations are patient-specific and include:

- Computed tomography (CT) can play an important role in the assessment of acute abdominal pain. It is extremely useful in the detection of gastrointestinal perforation, obstruction, diverticulitis, colitis, and abdominal wall disorders. CT is also useful in the assessment of suspected acute appendicitis, which is described in more detail in Case 7.2 in this chapter. It may occasionally detect features of established mesenteric ischaemia, and CT angiogram can also detect bleeding. However, CT is expensive and exposes the patient to radiation. It should, therefore, be reserved for patients where there is uncertainty in the diagnosis or in the decision to operate after initial assessment.

- ♦ Laparoscopy significantly improves surgical decision-making when used as a diagnostic tool and is of particular use in investigation of suspected appendicitis, especially in females, and in the acute abdomen, where the need for a laparotomy remains uncertain after clinical, laboratory, and radiological assessment.

7. How should this patient be managed?

Clinical assessment and bloods indicated severe intra-abdominal sepsis with a differential diagnosis of complicated acute diverticulitis, mesenteric ischaemia, and intestinal obstruction. The patient was, therefore, resuscitated with oxygen, IV crystalloid fluids, and IV tazocin, and a urethral catheter inserted, in accordance with the *Surviving Sepsis* guidelines. Parenteral analgesia was administered and venous thrombo-prophylaxis prescribed.

On re-assessment, the patient's blood pressure had only transiently responded to 2 l of crystalloid fluid and she remained tachycardic. There remained no peritonism on abdominal examination, although diffuse tenderness was elicited. An arterial blood gas revealed a persistent raised lactate at 3.5 mmol/l. Potentially, given the lack of generalized peritonism on examination, a CT scan may have been of value if the perforation was due to localized diverticulitis, which may be amenable to a non-operative approach. However, given that the patient had severe sepsis with haemodynamic compromise, was on steroids that may mask any peritonism, had an elevated lactate that could indicate mesenteric ischaemia, and had an acute kidney injury that would contraindicate the use of intravenous contrast, a decision was made to carry out an urgent diagnostic laparoscopy and proceed.

At laparoscopy, there was four-quadrant faecal peritonitis from perforated sigmoid diverticulitis (Hinchey IV). Given the extent of contamination, the operation was converted to an open procedure with a midline incision and a Hartmann's procedure (excision of rectosigmoid colon with stapling off of rectal stump and end colostomy) was performed, along with extensive lavage of the peritoneal cavity. Abdominal and pelvic drains were left *in situ* to minimize the occurrence of post-operative collections.

The patient was sick following surgery. She remained intubated until the third post-operative day and required 7 days of critical care before being discharged back to the ward. The post-operative course was further complicated by pneumonia and a wound infection with superficial dehiscence, which required a negative pressure wound therapy (VAC®) dressing. Following stoma education, the patient was discharged on the 18th post-operative day to a rehabilitation unit. On review in surgical outpatients 8 weeks following discharge, the patient was making steady progress back towards her normal level of function. The wound was healing well, no longer required VAC® dressing, but still required regular dressing changes from the district nurses. The patient was coping well with her colostomy and a plan was to review again in 6 months to consider a reversal of Hartmann's, although at this stage the patient had expressed an opinion that she would prefer to live with her stoma rather than undergo a further high-risk operation.

8. How is peri-operative mortality risk estimated? Why is this necessary?

The average mortality of emergency laparotomy lies between 15 and 20%. This figure rises to 25–40% in those over 80 years of age. Approximately one-third of emergency laparotomy patients are admitted to intensive care post-operatively, compared with routine intensive care admission for elective cardiac surgery. Variation in outcome across the UK, and high mortality rates associated with emergency general surgery, have recently been highlighted. This has led to hospitals formalizing their peri-operative pathways for emergency general surgery in order to improve patient outcomes. Research in the UK has indicated that a higher risk sub-group accounts for over 80% of post-operative deaths and routine identification of patients most at risk following an emergency laparotomy can permit care and resources, such as critical care, to be allocated more effectively. Routine peri-operative mortality risk estimation also allows us to compare outcomes between all providers of emergency laparotomy in national audits, such as the National Emergency Laparotomy Audit (NELA).

Objective risk assessment should take place for all elective and emergency patients. Although at present this often involves simply using the American Society of Anaesthesiologists (ASA) score, this method is too subjective and the use of more robust risk assessment tools should become the routine. The Portsmouth Physiological and Operative Severity Score for the enumeration of Mortality and Mortality (P-POSSUM) is the best validated method. It encompasses 12 physiological and 6 operative parameters for its calculation and is readily available online (Table 7.1.2). The operative

Table 7.1.2 P-POSSUM parameters used for modelling and predicting risk of morbidity and mortality

Age	<61 years old	61–70 years old	>70 years old	
Physiological parameters				
Cardiac failure	No cardiac failure	Diuretic, digoxin, angina/ hypertension treatment	Peripheral oedema, warfarin, borderline cardiomyopathy	Raised JVP, cardiomyopathy
Respiratory	No dyspnoea	Dyspnoea on exertion, mild COAD	Limiting dyspnoea, moderate COAD	Dyspnoea at rest, pulmonary fibrosis/ consolidation on X-ray
ECG	ECG normal	AF, rate 60–90	Any abnormal rhythm, >4 ectopics/minute, Q waves, ST/T changes	
Systolic BP (mmHg)	110–130	100–109 or 131–170	>170 or 90–99	<90

(continued)

Table 7.1.2 Continued

Age	<61 years old	61–70 years old	>70 years old	
Physiological parameters				
Pulse rate (bpm)	50–80	40–49 or 81–100	101–120	<40 or >120
Hb (g/dl)	13–16	11.5-12.9 or 16.1-17	10-11.4 or 17.1-18	<10 or >18
WBC	4–10	10.1–20 or 3.1–4	>20 or <3	
Urea	<7.6	7.6–10	10.1–15	>15
Sodium (mmol/l)	>135	131–135	126-130	<126
Potassium (mmol/l)	3.5–5	3.2-3.4 or 5.1–5.3	2.9–3.1 or 5.4–5.9	<2.9 or >5.9
GCS	15	12–14	9–11	<11
Operative parameters				
Operation type	Minor operation	Moderate operation	Major operation	Complex major operation
Number of procedures	One	Two	More than two	
Operative blood loss (ml)	<100	101–500	501–999	>1,000
Peritoneal contamination	No soiling	Minor soiling	Local pus	Free bowel content, pus or blood
Malignancy status	Not malignant	Primary malignancy only	Malignancy and nodal metastases	Malignancy and distant metastases
CEPOD	Elective	Urgent/ emergency	Emergency (within 2 hours)	

Reproduced Courtesy of Jonathan Wild.

detail can be estimated pre-operatively and then updated after surgery. This lady had a predicted mortality risk of over 10% using the P-POSSUM tool.

P-POSSUM risk has been used by the Royal College of Surgeons of England to produce guidance on patient care, as well as to inform discussion with patients and their families. Patients with a predicted mortality of over 5% should be managed as 'high risk.' There should be active input from a consultant surgeon and consultant anaesthetist, and the patient should arrive in theatre within 1 hour of the decision to operate. Operations on very high-risk patients (predicted mortality of over 10%) should be conducted under the direct supervision of a consultant surgeon and consultant anaesthetist, unless the responsible consultants are satisfied that the surgical and anaesthetic trainees are sufficiently competent to perform the procedure unsupervised. All high-risk patients should be considered for a critical care bed post-operatively and all patients with over a 10% risk of death should be admitted onto the critical care unit.

Further reading

Dellinger RP, Levy MM, Rhodes A, Annane D, Gerlach H Opal SM et al. (2012) Surviving sepsis campaign: international guidelines for management of severe sepsis and septic shock. *Critical Care Medicine* Feb; **41**(2): 580–637.

Manterola C, Vial M, Moraga J, Astudillo P. (2011) Analgesia in patients with acute abdominal pain. *Cochrane Database Systematic Reviews* (1): CD005660; PMID 21249672.

Paterson-Brown S. (2014) *Core Topics in General and Emergency Surgery*, fifth edition. Elsevier.

RCSEng (2011) *The Higher Risk General Surgical Patient: Towards Improved Care for a Forgotten Group*. Royal College of Surgeons and Department of Health. London See: https://www.rcseng.ac.uk/library-and-publications/college-publications/docs/the-higher-risk-general-surgical-patient/.

Smith JJ, Tekkis PP. *Risk Prediction in Surgery*. See: http://www.riskprediction.org.uk/ Last accessed 25/10/2015.

The National Emergency Laparotomy Audit (NELA). See: www.nela.org.uk Last accessed 25/10/2015.

Rhodes A, Evans LE, Alhazzani W, Levy MM, Antonelli M, Ferrer R et al. (2017) Surviving sepsis campaign: international guidelines for management of sepsis and septic shock: 2016. *Intensive Care Medicine* Mar;**43**(3): 304–77.

Case history 7.2: Emergency: acute appendicitis

A 62-year-old otherwise fit and well male presented with a 24-hour history of central abdominal pain that subsequently moved to the right iliac fossa. The pain persisted despite paracetamol and was made worse by moving and coughing. This was associated with an episode of loose stool and nausea but no vomiting. The patient denied recent weight loss, change in bowel habit, or any urinary symptoms. There was no significant past medical, drug, or family history reported.

On examination the patient's pulse was slightly elevated at 96 bpm, but otherwise cardiovascular and respiratory examinations were normal. There was no evidence of jaundice or anaemia; however, he appeared flushed with a temperature of 37.4°C. On palpation there was localized tenderness in the right iliac fossa with guarding. The abdomen was otherwise soft and non-tender. Rosving sign was positive. Digital rectal examination was normal and examination of the hernial orifices and external genitalia also revealed no abnormalities. The patient's blood and ward urine analysis results are shown in Table 7.2.1.

Table 7.2.1 Blood and ward urine results

Blood results	
Hb	14.5
WCC	15.2
Platelets	295
Sodium	140
Potassium	4.2
Urea	4.5
Creatinine	75
INR	1.1
Amylase	35
CRP	43
Urine dipstick	
RBC	+
WCC	++
Nitrites	–
Ketones	++
Glucose	–

Reproduced Courtesy of Jonathan Wild.

Questions

1. What are the key differential diagnoses?
2. What is the pathophysiology of appendicitis?
3. How do patients with acute appendicitis present?
4. What investigations should you consider when suspecting acute appendicitis?
5. How should this patient be managed?
6. What operative strategy and techniques should be considered?
7. How is suspected acute appendicitis in pregnancy diagnosed and managed?

Answers

1. What are the key differential diagnoses?

Acute appendicitis is a common consideration in right iliac fossa pain. There are many conditions that can cause right iliac fossa pain and may, therefore, mimic appendicitis, thereby making the early diagnosis of acute appendicitis a challenge. Viral or bacterial gastroenteritis, ileocaecal Crohn's disease, and Meckel's diverticulitis should be considered. Mesenteric adenitis is a common cause of right iliac fossa pain in children and young adults, and is associated with a viral upper respiratory tract infection. Intussusception is another consideration in the paediatric patient, whereas caecal malignancy and colonic diverticulitis should be suspected in the older patient. Pathologies originating from the upper gastrointestinal tract, which may mimick acute appendicitis, include acute cholecystitis, perforated peptic ulceration, and acute pancreatitis. Urinary tract pathologies to consider include a right-sided ureteric calculus, ascending urinary tract infection, right-sided pyelonephritis, and cystitis. Pain originating from right-sided inguinal or femoral hernias may also cause right iliac fossa pain.

Differential diagnoses specific to male patients include epididymoorchitis, testicular torsion, or torsion of hydatid of Morgagni.

In women the differential diagnoses are wider and should also include ectopic pregnancy, ovarian cystic disease, pelvic inflammatory disease, tubo-ovarian abscess, endometriosis, and ovarian malignancy. Physiological mid-cycle ovulation pain, or *Mittelschmerz,* may also mimick appendicitis.

Despite serial assessments and baseline investigations, in approximately two-thirds of all patients who present to the emergency general surgeon with acute right iliac fossa pain, no firm diagnosis is made, so the diagnosis of non-specific abdominal pain is common.

2. What is the pathophysiology of appendicitis?

Appendicitis results from inflammation of the vermiform appendix and is the most common abdominal condition requiring emergency surgery. Appendicitis is caused by the obstruction of the appendiceal lumen. Commonly this is caused by an appendiceal faecolith or hyperplasia of surrounding lymphoid tissue. Less common causes of appendiceal obstruction include caecal or appendiceal tumours and parasitic infections.

Luminal obstruction causes an increase in intraluminal pressure with a subsequent build-up of mucus and inflammatory cells, eventually producing pus. Aerobic organisms predominate early in the course, while mixed infection is more common in late appendicitis. The prolonged build-up of pus and on-going obstruction produces a high pressure that exceeds the venous pressure and occludes the outflow of blood. This subsequently causes arterial ischaemia of the appendix wall that eventually leads to necrosis, perforation, and localized abscess formation, or suppuration of pus into the peritoneum resulting in peritonitis. Common organisms involved in gangrenous and perforated appendicitis include *Escherichia coli*, *Streptococcus*, *Bacteroides fragilis*, and *Pseudomonas* spp.

3. How do patients with acute appendicitis present?

The clinical presentation of acute appendicitis is notoriously inconsistent. Typically, acute appendicitis presents with a 24-hour history of vague central abdominal pain that migrates to the right iliac fossa. This is often accompanied by anorexia, nausea, and sometimes vomiting, and either constipation or loose stools. A tachycardia and low-grade pyrexia are common but may be absent. Abdominal examination may reveal localized tenderness in the right iliac fossa with guarding, rigidity, and percussion or rebound tenderness, depending on the degree of inflammation involving the overlying peritoneal lining. A swelling may be palpable if an appendiceal mass or collection has formed. Often the site of maximum tenderness is located at McBurney's point, which lies two-thirds along a line from the umbilicus to the anterior superior iliac spine. Pain may be exacerbated by movement and by asking the patient to cough, which will often localize the pain to the right iliac fossa (Dunphy sign). Palpation of the left iliac fossa may cause pain in the right iliac fossa, suggesting peritoneal irritation (Rosving sign), which was elicited in this patient.

The variation in presentation of appendicitis can be caused by the different anatomical positions of the appendix. An inflamed retrocaecal appendix can cause right loin tenderness rather than right iliac fossa tenderness due to its more posterior position with the caecum lying in between it and the anterior abdominal wall. A retrocaecal appendix may also cause irritation of the right psoas muscle and the patient may lie with their hip flexed to alleviate pain. On examination, extension of the right hip causes right-lower quadrant pain (psoas sign).

An inflamed appendix lying in the pelvis is more likely to cause urinary frequency and loose stools due to the tip of the appendix lying in contact with the bladder or rectum causing irritation. Localized tenderness of the pouch of Douglas or rectovesical pouch on rectal examination indicates pelvic suppuration. Right iliac fossa pain reported with internal and external flexion of the right hip suggests that an inflamed appendix is located in the right hemipelvis (obturator sign).

Inflamed appendix making contact with the ileum can result in vomiting and diarrhoea due to irritation of the ileum.

4. What investigations should you consider when suspecting acute appendicitis?

* Routine blood tests: full blood count, urea and electrolytes, liver function test, amylase, and C-reactive protein. The white cell count and C-reactive protein are often elevated in acute appendicitis. The positive predictive value is increased by having both a raised white cell count and C-reactive protein, although if the duration of symptoms is less than 12 hours, then a rise in C-reactive protein may not be seen. In patients with normal inflammatory markers and a low clinical suspicion of appendicitis, a watch and wait policy or imaging is advocated.

* Routine urinalysis should always be performed in patients presenting with right iliac fossa pain. This can aid the diagnosis of urinary tract infection or calculi. A pelvic or retrocaecal appendix may lead to a false-positive urinalysis with red blood cells and leucocytes often present in the absence of nitrites. A urinary

pregnancy test should be performed in females in order to exclude ectopic pregnancy.

♦ Plain erect chest (CXR) and abdominal (AXR) radiograph are of limited value in the diagnosis of appendicitis, however a CXR may be required as part of pre-operative workup.

♦ Ultrasound (USS) can be used to exclude alternative pathology relating to the liver, gallbladder, pancreas, kidney, or pelvic organs and assess for the presence of free peritoneal fluid. Transvaginal approach can give superior imaging of the female reproductive tract over the transabdominal approach. The main advantages of USS over other imaging modalities is that it is non-invasive, quick, and cheap to perform with a lack of ionizing radiation, making it safer for patients and operators. USS is operator-dependent and as a result the reported sensitivity and specificity can vary between 76–90% and 83–100%, respectively. Given its advantages, USS is, therefore, commonly used in female, paediatric, and pregnant patient populations in whom appendicitis is suspected.

♦ Computed tomography (CT) scan is often the next imaging modality of choice where ultrasound is equivocal. Although CT has been shown to have a high diagnostic accuracy, with a sensitivity of 90–100% and specificity of 90–100%, the major limitation of CT is the use of ionizing radiation. It is for this reason that CT should be reserved for those cases of possible appendicitis with equivocal presentations or for cases of right iliac fossa pain in patients over 50 years of age, as in this case, in order to help rule out caecal malignancy or colonic diverticulitis. The patient in this case underwent a CT scan, which identified features consistent with acute appendicitis (see Figure 7.2.1).

♦ Diagnostic laparoscopy is often used instead of CT, especially in young female patients, in order to prevent unnecessary radiation exposure with the added benefit of giving appropriate access to deliver definitive treatment at the same setting as

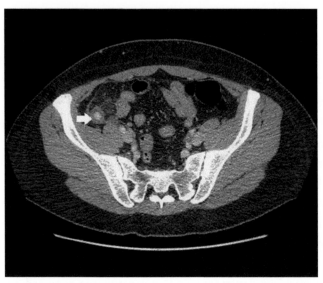

Figure 7.2.1 CT abdomen and pelvis with contrast demonstrating acute appendicitis. An appendiceal faecolith is clearly viable with thickened appendiceal wall (white arrow). There is no free fluid or collections seen.

Reproduced Courtesy of Mathew Kaduthodil.

the investigation. Laparoscopy is, however, also associated with increased morbidity and is more expensive.

Scoring systems have been developed to aid diagnosis by estimating the probability of appendicitis occurring in the individual patient. The best known is the Alvarado scale (Figure 7.2.2). Patients with an intermediate score require serial reassessment of physical findings and often complementary diagnostic imaging. Meta-analysis has demonstrated that an Alvarado score of <5 performs well as a test to 'rule out' appendicitis, with a sensitivity of 99%. However, a score >7, recommended for 'ruling in' appendicitis and proceeding to surgery, performs poorly in comparison, with a specificity of 83%, and therefore overpredicts the probability of appendicitis, especially in children and women of childbearing age, resulting in an increased negative appendicectomy rate. Imaging modalities are, therefore, often required to aid the accurate diagnosis of appendicitis, especially in women. These scoring systems are not in mainstream clinical use.

Fetaure	Score
Migratory right iliac fossa pain	1
Anorexia (or ketones in urine)	1
Nausea or vomiting	1
Tenderness in right iliac fossa	2
Rebound tenderness	1
Elevated temperature (>37.3°C)	1
Leucocytosis (WBC >10^9/L)	2
Shift of neutrophils to the left	1
Total	**10**

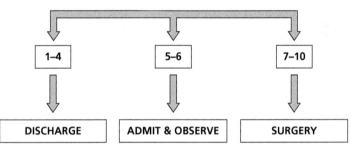

1–4	5–6	7–10
DISCHARGE	ADMIT & OBSERVE	SURGERY

Figure 7.2.2 The Alvarado scoring system and suggested clinical management strategy. The Alvarado scoring system comprises of eight weighted clinical indicators—three symptoms, three signs, and two laboratory findings. The pneumonic MANTRELS can be used to remember each feature.

Source: data from Alvarado A, 'A practical score for the early diagnosis of acute appendicitis', *Annals of Emergency Medicine*, Volume 15, Issue 5, pp. 557–64, Copyright © 1986, Published by Mosby, Inc., http://www.sciencedirect.com/science/article/pii/S0196064486809933

5. How should this patient be managed?

Appendicectomy remains the standard of care for most patients with acute appendicitis. A non-operative strategy, including antibiotics, supportive care, and close observation, has been proposed, reserving appendicectomy for those who fail to respond to this conservative approach; however, this is still under debate and research studies are looking at the feasibility and safety of this management approach. Early data suggest that 50% of patients treated with antibiotics only as their first approach will have treatment failure and undergo appendicectomy, with 15–25% of those initially successfully treated non-operatively subsequently developing recurrent appendicitis. Therefore, non-operative management should be reserved for the subset of patients least likely to fail this approach, high-risk surgical candidates, and patients who refuse surgery. Conservative treatment followed by interval appendicectomy should be considered in patients who present with an appendiceal mass. Antibiotics and percutaneous drainage should be considered in patients who present with an appendicular collection.

Once the CT diagnosis was obtained for this patient, broad-spectrum intravenous antibiotics were delivered according to local microbiology protocol and the patient was then prepared for an appendicectomy.

6. What operative strategy and techniques should be considered?

While laparoscopic appendicectomy has gained widespread acceptance, there are both benefits and limitations of the laparoscopic approach. Compared with the open approach, laparoscopic appendicectomy is associated with reduced analgesic requirements, reduced length of stay, reduced wound complications, and quicker return to work. However, the laparoscopic approach is associated with increased operative time and use of more expensive equipment than the open procedure.

The choice of laparoscopic or open appendicectomy depends on surgeon experience, institutional capabilities, severity of disease, body habitus, or previous history of lower abdominal or pelvic surgery. The principles of consent for the two procedures are similar: patients should be consented to the risk of bleeding, injury to surrounding viscera and structures, post-operative pain, infection (including wound and intra-abdominal collections that may require further surgery or intervention to treat), thromboembolism, wound-healing complications, scarring, and incisional hernia, either at the port site or within the incision of an open appendicectomy. Laparoscopic appendicectomy should also be consented for the risk of conversion to an open procedure. Previous open

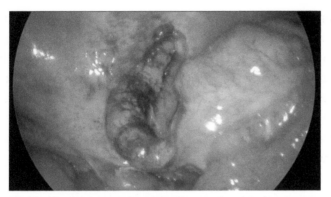

Figure 7.2.3 Intra-operative image showing a non-perforated necrotic retrocaecal appendix, viewed through a laparoscope.

Reproduced Courtesy of Jonathan Wild.

abdominal surgery increases the risk of adhesions within the abdominal cavity, which can make establishment of pneumoperitoneum and a safe field of view difficult, if not impossible, so patients with this history should be warned that their risk of conversion to an open procedure is likely to be higher. Laparoscopic is the preferred approach when the diagnosis is uncertain, especially in female patients, and also preferable in obese patients and in the elderly patient population.

An open appendicectomy is best performed via a Lanz incision; however, in the patient with four-quadrant peritonitis, a lower midline incision is sometimes preferred in order to adequately drain the pus and perform an effective washout of the peritoneal cavity.

In this case the patient underwent a laparoscopic appendicetomy and was found to have a necrotic retrocaecal appendix that had not perforated (Figure 7.2.3).

7. How is suspected acute appendicitis in pregnancy diagnosed and managed?

Diagnosing appendicitis in pregnancy remains a challenge. The classical abdominal findings can be distorted by the upward displacement of the appendix by the gravid uterus. Delayed intervention can result in perforated appendicitis, whereas unnecessary intervention with negative appendicectomy in pregnancy is associated with a high risk of miscarriage or preterm labour.

In suspected appendicitis in pregnancy, an urgent MRI scan should be performed when a USS is negative or indeterminate in order to improve diagnostic accuracy. However, if there is any clinical suspicion of acute appendicitis then urgent exploratory surgery is indicated in order to avoid serious maternal and foetal complications of a perforated appendicitis.

There is no evidence as to the preferred modality of surgery when comparing open and laparoscopic appendicectomy in pregnancy. Certainly, minimizing anaesthetic time is an important consideration and the surgical approach is often dependent on the surgeon's experience. It is advisable to mark the point of maximal tenderness, in addition to the gravid uterus in the third trimester, prior to anaesthesia. Laparoscopy in the third trimester may be more challenging due to limited working space. Port positions should be adapted for fundal height and a lower threshold for conversion to an open operation should be adopted. For open appendicectomy, some advocate making an incision over the site of maximal tenderness. However, MRI-based studies have demonstrated minimal displacement of the appendix during pregnancy with a standard transverse incision over McBurney's point, therefore providing adequate access.

Further reading

de Moya MA, Sideris AC, Choy G, Chang Y, Landman WB, Cropano CM et al. (2015) Appendectomy and pregnancy: gestational age does not affect the position of the incision. *American Surgeon* Mar; **81**(3): 282–8.

Ohle R, O'Reilly F, O'Brien KK, Fahey T, Dimitrov BD (2011) The Alvarado score for predicting acute appendicitis: a systematic review. *BMC Medicine* Dec; **9**: 139.

Sauerland S, Jaschinski T, Neugebauer EA (2010) Laparoscopic versus open surgery for suspected appendicitis. *Cochrane Database of Systematic Reviews* Art. No.: CD001546.

Walker HG, Al Samaraee A, Mills SJ, Kalbassi MR (2014) Laparoscopic appendicectomy in pregnancy: a systematic review of the published evidence. *International Journal of Surgery* **12**(11): 1235–41.

Case history 7.3: Emergency: sigmoid volvulus

An 82-year-old female nursing-home resident presented out of hours with a 2-day history of constant lower abdominal pain and distension. Her carers stated that she had last opened her bowels 3 days ago. The patient was unable to report the last time she had passed flatus. A phosphate enema had been prescribed by her GP 12 hours ago without any effect. Past medical history included Alzheimer's dementia, hypertension, chronic constipation, hypothyroidism and osteoporosis. Drug history included aspirin, bendroflumethiazide, magrocol sachets, thyroxine, alendronic acid, calcium and vitamin D supplements. At presentation her blood pressure was 160/90 and pulse was 90 and regular. Respiratory rate was 18 breaths per minute, oxygen saturations of 92% on air, and her temperature was 37.2°C. She had a long-term urinary catheter and urine output was adequate. She was mildly agitated with a GCS of 14, which was unchanged from her usual GCS. She had dry mucous membranes and reduced skin turgor. There was reduced basal air entry bilaterally without additional breath sounds and her abdomen was markedly distended, tympanic with generalized tenderness, but with no evidence of peritonism. Digital rectal examination (DRE) revealed an empty rectum. The patient's blood results are show in Table 7.3.1.

An erect chest X-ray revealed a raised right hemi-diaphragm due to distended abdominal viscus with clear lung fields and no evidence of pneumoperitoneum. A plain abdominal film demonstrated the characteristic 'coffee bean' sign of sigmoid volvulus (see Figure 7.3.1).

Table 7.3.1 Blood results

Blood results	
Hb	12.5
WCC	5.2
Platelets	190
Sodium	130
Potassium	3.1
Magnesium	2.0
Urea	8.7 (longstanding, stable)
Creatinine	165 (longstanding, stable)
INR	1.0
Amylase	23
CRP	19
Lactate (venous)	1.9

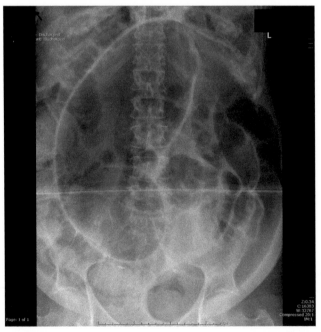

Figure 7.3.1 Plain supine abdominal radiograph reveals the classic 'coffee bean' sign of a sigmoid volvulus.

Reproduced courtesy of Mathew Kaduthodil.

Questions

1. What are the key differential diagnoses?
2. What is sigmoid volvulus?
3. What is the pathophysiology of sigmoid volvulus?
4. What is the epidemiology of sigmoid volvulus?
5. How do patients with sigmoid volvulus present?
6. What investigations should you consider when suspecting sigmoid volvulus?
7. How should this patient be managed?
8. How can recurrent sigmoid volvulus be prevented?

Answers

1. What are the key differential diagnoses?

The differential diagnoses include other causes of large bowel obstruction, both mechanical and functional, and is distinguished from other aetiologies based on clinical features and abdominal imaging. Colonic pseudo-obstruction and mega-rectum are causes of functional colonic obstruction that are also commonly encountered in elderly patients requiring nursing-home care with neuro-psychiatric conditions.

Pseudo-obstruction is a syndrome characterized by a flaccid dilatation of the colon with a clinical picture suggestive of mechanical large bowel obstruction in the absence of any demonstrable evidence of a mechanical cause of the obstruction. The exact pathophysiology of colonic pseudo-obstruction is unknown, however it is thought to be due to an imbalance in the autonomic nervous system. Pseudo-obstruction can be an acute presentation (known as Olgivie syndrome) or it can be chronic. This is discussed more in Case 4.14 in Chapter 4.

Mega-rectum is defined on contrast enema as rectal dilatation with a diameter of greater than 6.5 cm at the pelvic brim. This condition is characterized by faecal impaction, increased rectal compliance, hypomotility, and sensory dysfunction resulting in impaired rectal evacuatory function, delay in colorectal transit, and faecal impaction.

An additional differential diagnosis to consider is an ileosigmoid knot, also known as a compound volvulus. This is a rare condition where the ileum wraps round the base of the sigmoid colon and forms a knot causing a closed-loop obstruction that requires urgent surgical intervention.

2. What is sigmoid volvulus?

The term volvulus is derived from the Latin word *volvere* ('to twist') and refers to torsion of a segment of the alimentary tract. The commonest site for gastrointestinal volvulus is the sigmoid colon and caecum. Sigmoid volvulus occurs when the sigmoid colon twists on the sigmoid mesocolon, which can result in acute, subacute, or chronic colonic obstruction. It accounts for 6% of intestinal obstructions.

3. What is the pathophysiology of sigmoid volvulus?

Chronic constipation in Western societies and a high-fibre diet in developing nations leads to an overloaded sigmoid colonic loop and elongated mesentery with the weight of the loaded sigmoid making it susceptible to torsion along the axis of the mesocolon. Volvulus occurs when an air-filled loop of the sigmoid colon twists along its mesentery with luminal obstruction occurring when the degree of torsion exceeds 180°. Vascular perfusion is compromised with a 360° twist leading to ischaemic gangrene and perforation of the colonic wall, if left untreated.

4. What is the epidemiology of sigmoid volvulus?

Globally there appears to be a dual pattern of disease. In the Western world, sigmoid volvulus occurs in the elderly with a mean age of 70 years at first presentation. Patients are often institutionalized, and have neuro-psychiatric disease with a long history of consti-pation and laxative use. Higher frequencies of sigmoid volvulus are reported in Africa and the Middle East where 50% of large bowel obstruction is caused by sigmoid volvulus. These patients tend to be 15–20 years younger than in the West and are predominantly male. In these regions the inhabitants consume a high-fibre diet, which is thought to be the predisposing factor for the development of sig-moid volvulus. Hirschsprung disease in children may present with sigmoid volvulus with an aganglionic segment of colorectum distally thought to predispose to volvulus of the sigmoid. Additionally, in South America, approximately 10% of patients with megacolon as a result of Chagas' disease develop sigmoid volvulus.

5. How do patients with sigmoid volvulus present?

Often the patients presenting with sigmoid volvulus are elderly and bedridden with neuropsychiatric impairment and, therefore, only a limited history from carers is available. Around 50% of patients present with classic symptoms of 24–48-hour history of acute abdominal pain, distention, and absolute constipation. Vomiting tends to be a late feature. A previous history of chronic constipation is common and the patient may also describe similar previous episodes of abdominal pain, distension, and constipation, suggesting recurrent subclinical episodes of volvulus in the past. The older institutionalized patients often present insidiously 3–4 days after the onset of symptoms, which are often milder. Rarely, patients present with peritonitis and sepsis secondary to a gangrenous sigmoid colon.

On physical examination the abdomen is distended, tympanic, and generally tender on palpation. Sometimes there may be emptiness in the left iliac fossa with a mass palpable on the right side of the abdomen. Guarding and rigidity indicate peritoneal irritation from colonic ischaemia or perforation, indicating urgent surgical intervention, if appropriate. Digital rectal examination reveals an empty rectal ampulla, which can be a distinguishing feature from colonic pseudo-obstruction or megarectum, where rectal examination may reveal a distended rectum with liquid stool or impacted faeces, respectively.

6. What investigations should you consider when suspecting sigmoid volvulus?

* Routine blood tests: full blood count, urea and electrolytes, liver function tests, serum amylase, serum lactate, and clotting screen should be performed. A leucocytosis and hyperlactacaemia may indicate colonic ischaemia. Electrolyte disturbance may occur as a result of third-space sequestration of fluid into the obstructed colonic lumen.

* A plain abdominal radiograph is the initial radiological investigation of choice as it is useful, readily available, and cheap. Sigmoid volvulus can be diagnosed in approximately two-thirds of patients on plain radiograph with the classic 'coffee bean' sign of a U-shaped sigmoid colon lacking haustra extending from the pelvis towards the right-upper quadrant and diaphragm (see Figure 7.3.1). Frimann Dahl's sign of three dense lines converging towards the site of the obstruction and absent rectal gas are

also radiographic features of sigmoid volvulus. The diagnosis on plain radiography may not be clear in one-third of patients and, therefore, a CT scan of the abdomen and pelvis, ideally with intravenous and rectal contrast, is the gold standard radiological investigation, with the 'whirl sign' of the twisted sigmoid meso-colon diagnostic of volvulus. CT imaging can also help exclude other causes of large bowel obstruction, including obstructing neoplasms and pseudo-obstruction, but importantly can also assess for evidence of colonic ischaemia and perforation.

◆ A water-soluble contrast enema may be useful in situations where plain film radiography or CT are inconclusive for sigmoid vol-vulus, or where CT is not available. In addition to providing a diagnosis, the osmotic properties of gastrograffin may also offer a therapeutic effect by reducing the volvulus. This procedure should be performed under fluoroscopic control in patients deemed to be at low suspicion of perforation.

7. How should this patient's obstruction be managed?

The initial management of sigmoid volvulus is aimed at reliev-ing the obstruction and preventing bowel ischaemia. A treatment algorithm is provided in Figure 7.3.2. The patient in this case was initially treated with 2 l/min of supplemental oxygen and IV 0.9% saline with potassium chloride to rehydrate and correct her elec-trolyte abnormalities. Parenteral analgesia was also administered. As the diagnosis was confirmed with plain abdominal radiograph, and there was no clinical suspicion of colonic ischaemia or perfor-ation, a CT scan was not required in this case. Antibiotics were not indicated. Decompression of the sigmoid volvulus was performed at the bedside by inserting a rigid sigmoidoscope up to the point of torsion at the rectosigmoid junction, approximately 15 cm from the anal verge, with immediate effect and symptomatic relief. A rectal tube was also then inserted into the proximal sigmoid and was left in place for 3 days to help prevent immediate recurrence.

Successful decompression with rigid sigmoidoscopy is achiev-able in approximately 80% of patients with sigmoid volvulus. If this

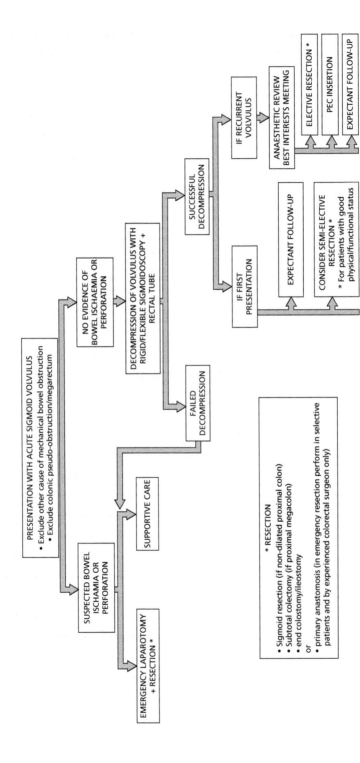

Figure 7.3.2 Treatment algorithm for sigmoid volvulus.

Reproduced Courtesy of Jonathan Wild.

approach is not achievable, e.g. if the site of torsion is out of reach of the rigid sigmoidoscope, then flexible sigmoidoscopy is advised to achieve non-operative reduction of the sigmoid loop. Success rates for decompression of sigmoid volvulus are higher with flexible sigmoidoscopy as opposed to rigid sigmoidoscopy, with endoscopic decompression also having the advantage of providing optimal views of the colonic mucosa to assess for ischaemia. Rigid sigmoidoscopy remains a valuable option as it is readily available, especially out of hours when access to flexible endoscopy is often limited.

Emergency operative intervention is reserved for failed endoscopic decompression or when there clinical or radiological features of colonic ischaemia, perforation, or peritonitis. A laparotomy, sigmoid resection with an end colostomy, and closure of the distal rectal stump is the procedure most commonly performed, although resection with primary anastomosis can be considered in selected haemodynamically stable patients with minimal peritoneal contamination when performed by experienced colorectal surgeons. Mortality rates for emergency resection for sigmoid volvulus are high, ranging from 10 to 60% in published case series.

8. How can recurrent sigmoid volvulus be prevented?

Approximately 60% of patients represent with recurrent sigmoid volvulus. The 'gold standard' treatment of surgical resection is often not the ideal treatment option for frail, elderly patients who typically develop sigmoid volvulus, given the mortality and morbidity associated with a major colonic resection. Alternative operative techniques that avoid a resection include sigmoidopexy and mesenteric plication procedures, but these have fallen out of favour due to high recurrence rates. Semi-elective resection, with either a sigmoid colectomy, if the proximal colon is normal, or sub-total colectomy with proximal mega-colon, should therefore be offered for patients with good physical and functional status after the first presentation of volvulus. Elective resection should be considered in higher risk patients only if they represent with recurrent volvulus.

Percutaneous endoscopic colostomy (PEC) does offer an option for high-risk patients unsuitable for colonic resection. PEC is a minimally invasive technique in which the sigmoid colon is fixed to the anterior abdominal wall with endoscopically placed venting tubes that are passed through the colon and anterior abdominal wall before being secured in place. PEC is, however, also associated with significant morbidity, especially infective stoma site complications often requiring tube removal, and mortality associated with faecal leakage and peritonitis. PEC should, therefore, only be considered in carefully selected cases.

In the case discussed already, non-operative management was successful, and as it was the first time this lady presented with sigmoid volvulus, she was discharged back to her nursing home with expectant management. If she was to present again with recurrent sigmoid volvulus, given her dementia and lack of capacity to consent for medical treatment, then a meeting between family, carers, and her consultant surgeon would be required in order to decide what management strategy is in the patient's best interests.

Further reading

Cowlam S, Watson C, Elltringham M, Bain I, Barrett P, Green S et al. (2007) Percutaneous endoscopic colostomy of the left side of the colon. *Gastrointestinal Endoscopy* 65(7): 1,007–14.

Hunt LM (2012) Colonic volvulus, *in* Brown SR (ed.) *Contemporary Coloproctology*. Springer–Verlag: London, pp. 449–64.

Oren D, Atamanalp SS, Aydinli B, Yildirgan MI, Basoglu M, Polat KY (2007) An algorithm for the management of sigmoid colon volvulus and the safety of primary resection: experience with 827 cases. *Diseases of the Colon and Rectum* 50(4): 489–97.

Safioleas M, Chatziconstantinou C, Felefouras E, Stamatakos M, Papaconstantinou I, Smirnis A et al. (2007) Clinical considerations and therapeutic strategy for sigmoid volvulus in the elderly: a study of 33 cases. *World Journal of Gastroenterology* 13(6): 921–4.

Tan KK, Chong CS, Sim R (2010) Management of acute sigmoid volvulus: an institution's experience over 9 years. *World Journal of Surgery* 34(8): 1,943–8.

Case history 7.4: Emergency: small bowel obstruction

An 85-year-old male presented with a 3-day history of central colicky abdominal pain and 36 hours of vomiting. He had not opened his bowels for 2 days and cannot remember passing flatus over this period. The patient reported three similar, but less severe, episodes over the last 4 months, associated with diarrhoea, which had resolved spontaneously, so he had not sought medical advice. Past medical history included non-insulin dependent type 2 diabetes, COPD, hypertension, and osteoarthritis. His exercise tolerance was 50 yards (45 m) on the flat. He had also undergone an open right hemicolectomy for a Duke's A caecal adenocarcinoma 7 years previously. Drug history included metformin, amlodipine, simvastatin, bendroflumethiazide, and apixaban. He lived alone with help from carers once a day. On physical examination, his blood pressure was 98/53, pulse 110 and irregularly irregular, respiratory rate of 16 breaths per minute, oxygen saturations of 92% on room air, and a temperature of 37.4°C. Dry mucous membranes were evident. Abdominal examination revealed a mildly distended abdomen with a transverse incision in the right iliac fossa noted. The abdomen was soft, mildly tender centrally, with no incisional or groin hernias palpable. High-pitched tinkling bowel sounds were also noted. The rectum was empty on rectal examination. The patient's blood results are shown in Table 7.4.1.

A plain supine abdominal radiograph revealed evidence of a proximal small bowel obstruction with dilated jejunal loops and stomach (see Figure 7.4.1). No free air was seen on erect chest radiograph. Given the previous history of abdominal surgery, a provisional diagnosis of adhesive small bowel obstruction (SBO) was made.

Table 7.4.1 Blood results

Blood results	
Hb	13.8
WCC	11.2
Platelets	210
Sodium	128
Potassium	2.9
Urea	7.8
Creatinine	178
Albumin	23
Bilirubin	18
ALP	78
AST	18
INR	1.1
Amylase	23
CRP	38
Lactate (venous)	1.9

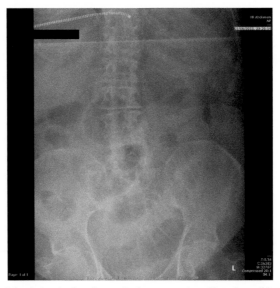

Figure 7.4.1 Plain abdominal radiograph demonstrating dilated small bowel loops lying in the pelvis and gas in the stomach. Prominent valvulae coniventes on the small bowel loops (white arrow) indicate these to be jejunal in keeping with a fairly proximal small bowel obstruction. Minimal gas seen in the colorectum is also a feature of small bowel obstruction.

Reproduced Courtesy of Mathew Kaduthodil.

Questions

1. How can small bowel obstruction be classified?
2. What is the pathophysiology of small bowel obstruction?
3. What is the aetiology of small bowel obstruction?
4. What clinical features may small bowel obstruction present with?
5. What investigations should be carried out?
6. How should this patient be managed?
7. What operative strategies and techniques for small bowel obstruction should be considered?

Answers

1. How can small bowel obstruction be classified?

Small bowel obstruction (SBO) can be classified by its aetiology, nature, level, and severity.

SBO can be *mechanical* (caused by a physical blockage arising from a structural abnormality) or *functional* (caused by absent or dysfunctional peristalsis of the small bowel). Functional small bowel obstruction is also called adynamic or paralytic ileus, which is characterized by similar manifestations as mechanical bowel obstruction in the absence of an obstructive lesion.

SBO can be classified as complete or, alternatively, as partial obstruction when gas or liquid stool can pass through the point of obstruction. These can be further characterized as *low-grade* or *high-grade*, depending on the severity of the narrowing.

SBO can also be acute, sub-acute, or chronic in nature, and can be classified by the level of obstruction—either *proximal* (high) or *distal* (low).

SBO can be *open-ended*, with a one-point obstruction interfering with the prograde propulsion of bowel content, or *closed-loop*, where the bowel lumen is occluded at two points, thereby preventing prograde and retrograde movement of bowel content. Finally, SBO can also be classified as *simple* or *complicated*. Complicated obstruction indicates that the blood supply to the bowel is compromised, resulting in ischaemia, infarction, and perforation.

2. What is the pathophysiology of small bowel obstruction?

SBO is the impendence of the normal passage of bowel content through the small bowel. Obstruction leads to progressive proximal dilatation of the intestine due to the accumulation of gastrointestinal secretions, swallowed air, and gas from bacterial fermentation. Bowel distal to the blockage will decompress. Bowel dilatation stimulates intestinal secretory cell activity resulting in further fluid accumulation and increased peristalsis above the level of the obstruction. As the process continues, the intraluminal pressure rises causing compression of the mucosal lymphatics and venous drainage. The bowel wall becomes oedematous as a result, with normal absorptive function lost. This results in the sequestration of fluid in the bowel lumen and subsequent massive third space losses of fluid, electrolytes, and protein into the intestinal lumen. Ongoing vomiting results in additional loss of fluid, resulting in severe dehydration with electrolyte disturbance. Bacterial overgrowth can occur in the normally sterile proximal small bowel, resulting in faeculent vomiting. Translocation of gut bacteria, facilitated by microvascular changes in the bowel wall, can also occur typically resulting in an *E. coli* bacteraemia.

Excessive bowel dilatation can result in compression of the intramural vessels that supply the bowel wall, resulting in the perfusion of the bowel wall being compromised. Subsequent ischaemia, necrosis, and perforation may ensue if the disease process is allowed to progress. Ischaemia and necrosis can also be caused by twisting of the bowel or its mesentery around a band adhesion, for example, or strangulation of the bowel mesentery by an internal hernial defect.

3. What is the aetiology of small bowel obstruction?

The leading cause of mechanical SBO in industrialized nations is post-operative adhesions (60%), followed by malignancy (20%), incarcerated hernias (10%), IBD (5%), and volvulus (3%). The causes of mechanical SBO can be categorized into three groups: luminal, intramural, and extramural (see Table 7.4.2). SBO due to mechanical obstruction must be differentiated from paralytic ileus by the clinical history and imaging. Paralytic ileus occurs to some degree after almost all open abdominal operations but is also caused by metabolic and electrolyte disturbance, especially hypokalaemia and also spinal trauma, retroperitoneal pathology, or it can be secondary to other causes of intra-abdominal sepsis.

Table 7.4.2 Causes of mechanical SBO

Luminal	◆ Foreign body
	◆ Gallstone (gallstone ileus)
	◆ Bezoar
Intramural	◆ Tumours—adenocarcinoma, lymphoma, GIST, melanoma, metastases
	◆ Inflammatory—Crohn's stricture, TB, eosinophilic gastroenteritis
	◆ Ischaemia
	◆ Radiation enteritis
Extramural	◆ Adhesions
	◆ Hernia—external and internal
	◆ Endometrioma
	◆ Abscess
	◆ Haematoma
	◆ External compression from mass

Reproduced Courtesy of Jonathan Wild.

4. What clinical features may small bowel obstruction present with?

Patients with SBO may present with sudden onset of abdominal pain associated with nausea, vomiting, and distension, or may report more intermittent symptoms that resolve and recur in recurrent or partial obstruction. Diarrhoea can be an early symptom, with constipation a later feature. Patients with recurrent, intermittent obstruction may report post-obstructive diarrhoea when the obstructive symptoms resolve.

The character and severity of abdominal pain is key in order to determine the level and nature of the SBO. Pain may sometimes be absent in cases of partial, more proximal obstruction, with vomiting decompressing the bowel and causing less distension and pain. Usually, proximal SBO presents with colicky pain that occurs over a shorter duration accompanied by bilious vomiting. Distension is often less of a feature in proximal SBO compared with more distal obstruction. More progressive pain lasting several days, accompanied by distension and faeculent vomiting, may be more typical of distal obstruction. Changes in the character of the abdominal pain may indicate the development of strangulation or ischaemia.

Features of the history that may point towards the underlying aetiology of the SBO should also be sought, particularly:

+ Previous abdominal surgery.
+ Weight loss.
+ Change in bowel habit.
+ History of malignancy (particularly colonic and ovarian).
+ Previous radiation therapy.

On physical examination, patients with SBO are often dehydrated with dry mucous membranes, and may be tachycardic and hypotensive with a reduced urine output. Abdominal inspection should examine for surgical scars. Abdominal distension may be present, with more marked distension in more distal obstruction, and the abdomen is often tympanic on percussion due to gas-filled bowel loops. A mass on palpation may indicate malignant obstruction and, importantly, abdominal and groin hernias should be excluded. A characteristic feature of acute mechanical SBO is high-pitched 'tinkling' bowel sounds. Bowel sounds are often absent or 'sluggish' in paralytic ileus. However, bowel sounds may also become 'muffled' as a later sign in mechanical SBO, when the bowel becomes progressively distended and the bowel sounds hypoactive. Blood on digital rectal examination may indicate an underlying malignancy or gut ischaemia.

During the clinical assessment it is essential to differentiate simple from complicated SBO. The presence of fever, persistent tachycardia, and peritoneal signs on examination indicate bowel strangulation and ischaemia irritating the peritoneum. Reassessment with serial examinations are important in order to detect early changes.

5. What investigations should be carried out?

- Routine blood tests: full blood count, urea and electrolytes, liver function tests, amylase, lactate, C-reactive protein, clotting, and group and save. These may denote the presence and severity of hypovolaemia, end-organ hypoperfusion, and electrolyte disturbance. A leucocytosis and elevated CRP may point to the presence of complicated SBO, with anaemia indicating specific underlying aetiologies such as malignancy or Crohn's disease. Clotting screen should be requested in view of potential surgical intervention.

- In patients who are systemically unwell or clinically concerning, investigations should include arterial blood gas, serum lactate, and blood cultures. A metabolic acidosis that persists after adequate fluid resuscitation can indicate bowel ischaemia, with a metabolic alkalosis resulting from severe vomiting.

- Plain radiography, with erect chest and supine abdominal films, should be performed quickly to help confirm the diagnosis. A typical finding on plain abdominal film is centrally placed dilated loops of bowel with air-fluid levels. Plain films can suggest perforation through pneumoperitoneum on erect chest films. Air visualized on both sides of the bowel wall is suggestive of bowel perforation (termed Rigler's sign) on abdominal films. However, plain abdominal radiographs have a sensitivity of around 80% and specificity of approximately 70%; they are less useful at differentiating the level of the bowel obstruction and mechanical obstruction from ileus. CT is, therefore, needed in order to identify the nature, severity, and aetiology of the SBO. CT, ideally with intravenous contrast, can locate the level of SBO (termed the transition point), identify hernias, volvulus, or mass lesions as a cause of obstruction, whilst also identifying any features of complicated SBO, including closed-loop obstruction, and features of ischaemia, venous thrombosis, and perforation.

In terms of other imaging modalities, ultrasonography is not appropriate for determining the level and cause of SBO. Magnetic resonance (MR) enterography is not a practical alternative to CT in the acute setting. It does, however, have a role in the assessment of small bowel Crohn's disease where patients may present with symptoms suggestive of low-grade chronic SBO. MR has the advantage over CT in reducing the exposure of ionizing radiation in younger patients. Barium studies, including small bowel enteroclysis and small bowel follow through, are now becoming obsolete in practice.

The administration of water-soluble contrast agent (WSCA), such as Gastrograffin®, can play a role in predicting which patients with simple adhesive small bowel obstruction can safely undergo non-operative management. The appearance of contrast in the colon within 4–24 hours after application has a sensitivity and specificity approaching 100% in predicting resolution of SBO. WSCA may also have a therapeutic effect due to its hyperosmolar properties and may reduce the need for surgical intervention.

6. How should this patient be managed?

The patient was treated as presumed simple adhesive SBO. Initial management included adequate intravenous fluid therapy via two large-bore peripheral lines with replacement of sodium and potassium. Parenteral opioid analgesia was administered and a nasogastric (NG) tube was inserted to decompress the distended stomach and proximal small bowel in order to relieve discomfort, and prevent vomiting and aspiration. A urinary catheter was also inserted and strict hourly fluid-balance monitoring was started. The patient was kept nil by mouth to limit bowel distention. With an acute kidney injury, metformin and bendroflumethiazide were omitted. With the potential of surgical intervention, the patient's apixapan, a direct factor Xa inhibitor, was also omitted, as this ideally should be stopped 48 hours prior to high-risk surgery.

As there was no evidence of strangulation or perforation, a trial of non-operative management was instituted. Other causes of mechanical SBO will often require an operation; however, the non-operative approach to adhesive SBO is successful in 65–80% of patients. During non-operative management, close monitoring with serial abdominal examination and laboratory investigations are required to ensure early recognition of complicated SBO.

A CT scan with intravenous contrast was requested once the serum creatinine returned towards normal following 24 hours of rehydration. The CT confirmed the diagnosis of adhesive SBO with a transition point at mid-jejunum. There were no clinical or radiological features of ischaemia or perforation. There was also no evidence on CT of other potential causes of mechanical SBO in this patient, specifically an incisional hernia or recurrent colorectal cancer.

At this stage the nasogastric output remained high and the patient had not opened his bowels. As the patient had not received nutritional intake for 5 days, total parenteral nutrition (TPN) was commenced. A 'Gastrograffin® challenge' was requested, with 100 ml of Gastrograffin® administered via the NG tube, followed by a plain abdominal radiograph 6 hours later. The plain film revealed contrast present in the colon (see Figure 7.4.2). The patient also opened

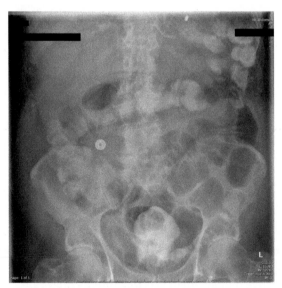

Figure 7.4.2 Plain abdominal radiograph performed 6 hours following nasogastric administration of gastrograffin. The gastrograffin is visible in the right colon along as far as the splenic flexure and also present in the upper rectum.

Reproduced Courtesy of Mathew Kaduthodil.

his bowels after administration of the Gastrograffin® and within 48 hours NG output had reduced, distension and pain resolved, bowels had opened further, and gradual enteral feeding had been introduced. Following this successful non-operative management of adhesive SBO, the patient was discharged with no routine follow-up required.

7. What operative strategies and techniques for adhesive small bowel obstruction should be considered?

Surgery is indicated for complicated SBO (closed-loop obstruction, ischaemia, perforation) and for failure of non-operative management. If the obstruction fails to resolve after 48 hours of conservative management, then surgical exploration is warranted, although in certain high-risk patients, a longer, non-operative approach may be required.

At present, laparotomy is the preferred approach for adhesive SBO. Common practice is to divide all adhesions so as to mobilize the small bowel fully from the ligament of Treitz down to the ileo-caecal junction. The viability and integrity of the small bowel should be assessed throughout and non-viable bowel resected. Selected patients may benefit from a laparoscopic approach with open access (Hasson technique) to establish pneumoperitoneum. Often this is used in patients with the first presentation of adhesive SBO, with proximal obstruction, and/or anticipated single-band adhesion.

With advances in laparoscopic techniques and growing expertise, laparoscopic treatment of adhesive SBO is on the increase. Several cohort studies have demonstrated several potential advantages of laparoscopic adhesiolysis for SBO, including reduced post-operative pain, earlier return to intestinal function, shorter hospital stay, earlier return to full activity, reduced wound complications, and decreased post-operative adhesion formation. At present, there has not been a randomized clinical trial (RCT) comparing laparoscopic with open adhesiolysis for SBO. However, a multi-centre prospective RCT from Finland is currently recruiting with results expected in 2018.

Further reading

Branco BC, Barmparas G, Schnuriger B, Inabal K, Chan LS, Demetriades D (2010) Systematic review and meta-analysis of the diagnostic and therapeutic role of water-soluble contrast agent in adhesive small bowel obstruction. *British Journal of Surgery* **91**: 470–8.

Di Saverio S, Coccolini F, Galati M, Smerieri N, Biffl WL, Ansaloni L et al. (2013) Bologna guidelines for diagnosis and management of adhesive small bowel obstruction (ASBO): 2013 update of the evidence-based guidelines form the world society of emergency surgery ASBO working group. *World Journal of Emergency Surgery* **8**: 42.

Kulaylat MN, Doerr RJ (2001) Small bowel obstruction, *in* Holzheimer RG, Mannick JA (eds) *Surgical Treatment: Evidence-Based and Problem-Orientated.* Munich: Zuckschwerdt, pp.1–15. Available from: http://www.ncbi.nlm.nih.gov/books/NBK6873/ Last accessed 02/09/2015.

NICE (2006) Nutrition support in adults: oral nutrition support, enteral tube feeding and parenteral nutrition. *NICE guidelines* [CG32] Feb. See https://www.nice.org.uk/guidance/cg32 Last accessed 02/09/2015.

Case history 7.5: Emergency: obstructed groin hernia

An 82-year-old female was admitted under the emergency medicine team 2 days ago with a 3-day history of being generally unwell with intermittent vomiting and diarrhoea. She had complained of lower left-sided abdominal pain and left hip pain. Past medical history included hypertension, osteoporosis, and osteoarthritis. She had had a right fractured neck of femur repaired 6 months earlier and a previous left hip arthroplasty. A diagnosis of gastroenteritis was made, along with pain secondary to osteoarthritis. Antibiotics, intravenous fluids, and analgesia were prescribed. Over the subsequent 24 hours the vomiting became more persistent with increasing abdominal distension. The medical team organized a plain abdominal radiograph, which revealed dilated, small bowel loops (see Figure 7.5.1) and an urgent surgical review was requested. The patient's blood results are show in Table 7.5.1.

The on-call surgical registrar reviewed the patient. Her blood pressure was 110/80, pulse was 100 beats per minute and regular, oxygen saturations of 96% on air, respiratory rate 20 breaths per minute, and temperature was 37.6°C. She was clinically dry with a kidney dish containing feculent vomit. Abdominal examination revealed a moderately distended soft abdomen. There was a 4 cm tender irreducible swelling in the left groin. An obstructed left femoral hernia was diagnosed.

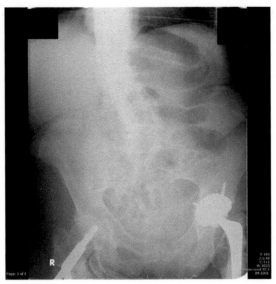

Figure 7.5.1 Plain supine abdominal radiograph revealed fairly featureless dilated small bowel which is secondary to an obstructed left femoral hernia. Lumbar scoliosis, right dynamic hip screw and left hemiarthroplasty noted.

Reproduced Courtesy of Mathew Kaduthodil.

Table 7.5.1 Blood results

Blood results	
Hb	13.8
WCC	16.2
Platelets	225
Sodium	138
Potassium	2.9
Urea	5.2
Creatinine	220
INR	1.2
Amylase	43
CRP	182

Questions

1. What are the key differential diagnoses?
2. What is a femoral hernia?
3. How do femoral hernias present?
4. How should this patient be managed?
5. What operative strategy and techniques should be considered for femoral hernia repair?

Answers

1. What are the key differential diagnoses?

The differential diagnoses of a groin swelling include other causes of groin swelling:

- Subcutaneous lesions: lipoma, sebaceous cyst, abscess.
- Hernia: direct or indirect inguinal; femoral.
- Inguinal lymphadenopathy: reactive or malignant.
- Femoral artery aneurysm/pseudo-aneurysm.
- Psoas abscess.
- Saphena varix.
- Undescended testes.
- Rupture of adductor longus with haematoma.

Ultrasound is the imaging modality of choice if a diagnosis of inguinal hernia cannot be made clinically. CT can also be used for further evaluation if ultrasound is indeterminate or further information is required, such as in a suspected psoas abscess, to assess the extent of the abscess and bony involvement.

2. What is a femoral hernia?

A femoral hernia is a protrusion of the peritoneal sac caused by a breakdown in the integrity of the transversalis fascia covering the femoral canal. The peritoneal sac and its contents emerge through the femoral ring into the femoral canal. Femoral hernias are:

- Not congenital.
- Rare in children.
- Twice as common on the right side than the left.
- Twice as common in females than males.
- Accountable for 1% of groin hernias in males, whereas the likelihood in females is 20%.
- Twice as common in women who have had children than in non-parous women.

3. How do femoral hernias present?

Femoral hernias typically present as mildly painful, non-reducible groin lumps, located inferiorly and lateral to the pubic tubercle. Femoral hernias tend to move superiorly to a position above the inguinal ligament, where they can be mistaken for an inguinal hernia. Clinical examination alone is inaccurate in distinguishing between inguinal and femoral hernias. Owing to the greater prevalence of femoral hernias in females, all groin hernias in women should be considered femoral until proven otherwise.

The cumulative probability of strangulation of femoral hernias is 22% at 3 months from diagnosis. This rises to 45% at 21 months, compared with the probability of strangulation of an inguinal hernia being 3 and 4.5%, respectively, over the same time periods. Elective femoral hernia repair is a safe procedure; however, given the high risk of strangulation, they should be referred urgently for elective repair.

In an emergency, patients with obstructed femoral hernias present with symptoms of bowel obstruction, including colicky abdominal pain, distension, and vomiting. Diarrhoea can also feature if there is intermittent obstruction.

As in this case, femoral hernias can be easily missed if not suspected. Around one-third of patients who present as an emergency with a femoral hernia complain of symptoms not directly attributable to the hernia. Femoral hernias are also typically small and can be easily missed on examination especially in obese patients. However, studies have demonstrated that 40% of hernias causing bowel obstruction are missed due to a lack of groin examination.

4. How should this patient be managed?

This patient requires emergency reduction and repair of the obstructed femoral hernia. Prompt resuscitation with intravenous fluids to correct electrolyte abnormalities is required. An NG tube should be placed in order to decompress the stomach and prevent future vomiting, and a urethral catheter placed to monitor the response to fluid therapy.

In a patient with acute SBO from a clinically obstructed and potentially strangulated hernia, a CT scan will not change the decision of a need to operate and, therefore, is not required. A CT may also cause unnecessary delay in getting the patient to theatre and, in this case, would have to be without IV contrast due to the acute kidney injury and would, therefore, provide inadequate images.

5. What operative strategy and techniques should be considered for femoral hernia repair?

The decision on the operative approach to repair a femoral hernia depends on the suspicion of bowel strangulation and, therefore, the need to perform a bowel resection. Classically, three approaches are described for open femoral hernia repair:

- Lockwood's infra-inguinal approach.
- Lotheissen's trans-inguinal approach.
- McEvedy's high approach.

The low infra-inguinal approach is preferred for elective repair or emergency femoral hernia repairs, where there is a low suspicion of strangulation. It can be performed easily under general anaesthetic. The femoral canal is approached via an oblique incision 1 cm below and parallel to the inguinal ligament. The hernia sac is defined and the lacunar ligament may need to be divided to enable reduction. Care should be taken when dividing the lacunar ligament as an abberant obturator artery (corona mortis) is present in approximately 25% of patients in whom it runs along the posterior part of the lacunar ligament. Suture closure of the femoral canal to prevent recurrence is then performed by approximating the medial inguinal ligament to the pectineal ligament with interrupted non-absorbable sutures, taking care to protect and avoid compression of the femoral vein laterally. Performing a repair of a right femoral canal, whilst standing on the left side of the patient, and vice versa, can aid visualization of the femoral vein during the repair. For wider defects, the use of a small piece of synthetic mesh to plug the femoral canal can be considered, although mesh should be avoided when necrotic bowel has been encountered within the hernia sac. A disadvantage of the low approach, however, is that it provides limited access if a resection of compromised bowel is required. If necrotic bowel is encountered via this approach, then a lower midline laparotomy is required in order to perform a small-bowel resection, thereby increasing post-operative pain and potential morbidity.

The trans-inguinal approach involves a skin incision 2 cm above the inguinal ligament and the external oblique divided to enter the inguinal canal, as for a standard open inguinal hernia repair. The transversalis fascia forming the posterior wall of the inguinal canal is divided from the pubic tubercle to the deep ring in order to access the pre-peritoneal space. The femoral hernia can be reduced from the inside and the sac divided to inspect its contents. The femoral canal is then obliterated with a suture repair from the inside. A benefit to this approach is that the peritoneal cavity can be accessed easily if a bowel resection is required and an inguinal hernia can be repaired if found. However, dissecting through the inguinal canal weakens it and can predispose to the formation of an incisional inguinal hernia. Although synthetic mesh can be used to reinforce the posterior wall of the inguinal canal, its use is contraindicated in the presence of necrotic bowel.

McEvedy's high approach utilizes a vertical incision over the lateral aspect of the lower rectus sheath, with the rectus muscle retracted medially to reveal the peritoneum. The femoral hernia can be reduced in the pre-peritoneal plane and the hernia repaired from the inside, or the peritoneal cavity can be entered in order to perform a bowel resection.

In practice, a single incision 1 cm over the medial half of the inguinal ligament permits all three approaches. The femoral hernia sac can be reached from below (Lockwood approach). If an uncomplicated femoral hernia is found, then this can be repaired in standard fashion. If an inguinal hernia is discovered, then the inguinal canal can be explored and an open inguinal hernia repair completed. If the femoral hernia contains compromised bowel requiring resection, then a modified high (McEvedy) approach can be achieved by developing a plane superficial to the external oblique aponeurosis. The rectus sheath is then divided 4 cm above the inguinal ligament along the semi-lunar line. This technique is often facilitated by lax skin in frail, elderly patients who often present with a complicated femoral hernia.

In addition, laparoscopy may also play a role for both elective and emergency repair of femoral hernias.

Further reading

Kingsnorth AN, Giorgobiani G, Bennet DH (2013) Abdominal wall, hernia and umbilicus, *in* Williams NS, Bulstrode CJK, O'Connell PR (eds) *Bailey & Love's Short Practice of Surgery*, twenty-sixth edition.CRC Press: FL, USA.

Sorelli PG, El-Masry Nabil, Garrett WV (2009) Open femoral hernia repair: one skin incision for all. *World Journal of Emergency Surgery* 4:44.

Whalen H, Kidd GA, O'Dwyer PJ (2011) Easily missed? Femoral hernias. *British Medical Journal* 343: d7668.

Case history 7.6: Emergency: blunt abdominal trauma

A 22-year-old male lost control of the car he was driving at 60 mph in wet conditions, with the car leaving the road and colliding head on with a tree. There was major damage to the vehicle, with intrusion into the passenger compartment. However, the patient had been wearing a seatbelt and front and side airbags had been deployed. There was no significant past medical or drug history.

On arrival in the emergency department a primary survey was carried out by the trauma team (see Table 7.6.1).

The patient remained haemodynamically stable, therefore an urgent whole-body CT scan was requested. CT head and C-spine was normal. CT chest revealed a non-displaced sternal fracture. CT abdomen demonstrated a grade II splenic injury with a 2-cm laceration without contrast extravasation. There was no free air or free fluid or any other evidence of solid- or hollow-organ damage seen. The patient's blood results are show in Table 7.6.2.

Table 7.6.1 Primary survey

Airway + C-spine:	Patent, C-spine immobilized with neck collar.
Breathing:	Trachea central, no distended neck veins.
	Good air entry both bases, no added breath sounds.
	No dullness or hyper-resonance on percussion but tender over sternum.
	Respiratory rate 22, oxygen saturations of 100% on 2 l O_2.
Circulation:	Blood pressure 110/70, pulse 120 regular, capillary refill time 3 s, normal heart sounds.
	Abdomen distended, tender across upper abdomen, no peritonism evident.
	No evidence of pelvic or long bone fractures.
	Two 16G intravenous cannulas inserted into ante-cubital fossae bilaterally.
	Full blood count, urea and electrolytes, amylase, liver function tests, clotting screen, group save/crossmatch requested.

(continued)

Table 7.6.1 Continued

	IV fluid therapy was initiated with 1-l bolus warmed Hartmann's solution.
	Urinary catheter was inserted.
Disability:	Glasgow coma score 15/15, mildly anxious.
	Pupils equal and reactive to light and accommodation, blood glucose 4.5.
Exposure:	No evidence of penetrating injuries, Temperature 37.6°C.
	Abrasions and bruising from seat-belt contact was noted across anterior chest and abdominal wall.

Table 7.6.2 Blood results

Blood results	
Hb	10.2
WCC	14.1
Platelets	240
Sodium	140
Potassium	4.2
Urea	4.5
Creatinine	75
INR	1.1
Amylase	35
CRP	43

Questions

1. How do you classify abdominal trauma?
2. What are the main principles in the management of penetrating abdominal trauma?
3. What are the main principles in the management of blunt abdominal trauma?
4. How are splenic injuries classified and managed?

Answers

1. How do you classify abdominal trauma?

Abdominal trauma is divided into blunt and penetrating types. Penetrating abdominal trauma is treated differently to blunt abdominal trauma with differences in the characteristics of injuries, relevant investigations, and methods and timing of intervention.

Road-traffic incidents are responsible for blunt abdominal trauma in 75% of cases. The organs most frequently injured in blunt abdominal trauma are the spleen (50%), liver (40%), and small bowel (10%). Penetrating abdominal trauma typically involves stab and gunshot wounds resulting from urban and domestic violence, and globally from military action and wars. Stab injuries traverse adjacent abdominal structures, commonly involving the liver (40%), small bowel (30%), diaphragm (20%), and colon (15%). Gunshot wounds transfer more kinetic energy to abdominal viscera, where additional intra-abdominal injuries can occur due to cavitation effect and bullet fragmentation.

2. What are the main principles in the management of penetrating abdominal trauma?

The initial assessment and management of patients with abdominal trauma should follow Advanced Trauma Life Support (ATLS®) principles with a systematic ABCDE primary survey to identify life-threatening injuries with simultaneous resuscitation. One must ensure that a secondary survey is also completed once all the life-threatening injuries from the primary survey have been identified and treated. The secondary survey involves a complete history and thorough head to toe examination in order to ensure all injuries sustained are identified.

Patients with penetrating abdominal trauma fall into three main categories:

- Pulseless.
- Haemodynamically unstable.
- Haemodynamically normal.

Patients who arrive in the emergency department with penetrating injury without palpable pulses but with witnessed recent or current signs of life (e.g. pulseless electrical activity) need an immediate laparotomy. In this group of patients there are very few survivors. For any chance of success there must be the ability to transfer the patient from the ambulance bay to operating table within 5 minutes. Another salvage option is to perform an emergency room thoracotomy in order to cross-clamp the descending thoracic aorta, if immediate access to an operating room is not available.

Patients with penetrating abdominal trauma who are unstable, i.e. non-responders or transient-responders to initial fluid bolus administration (100 ml/kg), require immediate laparotomy. There should be no delay in performing unnecessary investigations or attempting to resuscitate the patient prior to surgery.

Patients who are haemodynamically normal but have clinical signs of peritonitis or evisceration of bowel require an immediate laparotomy. There are several options for the assessment of patients with penetrating abdominal trauma who do not have signs of peritonitis:

- Serial physical examination supported by CT imaging can identify injuries that require surgical repair, whilst avoiding unnecessary surgery for those without significant intra-abdominal injury.

- Diagnostic laparoscopy can be useful in patients with suspected intra-abdominal injury with equivocal findings on CT, especially where there is documented or equivocal penetration of the abdominal wall fascia.

3. What are the main principles in the management of blunt abdominal trauma?

As above, a systematic approach following ATLS® principles should be followed. Identification of intra-abdominal injuries in blunt abdominal trauma is often challenging, as injuries may not manifest during the initial assessment. It is crucial to recognize that the *absence of abdominal pain or tenderness on physical examination does not rule out the presence of significant abdominal injury* and there should be a low threshold for obtaining diagnostic imaging. CT has a sensitivity and specificity of 97 and 98%, respectively, for identifying significant intra-abdominal injuries, especially liver and splenic injuries. CT can identify injuries that can be managed non-operatively, either by close observation and supportive care or with angiography and selective embolization. However, CT remains relatively insensitive for mesenteric, bowel, and pancreatic duct injuries. It is, therefore, important that a patient with suspected intra-abdominal injury, with a negative or indeterminate CT, undergoes a period of close observation with serial abdominal examination and repeat imaging to identify such injuries as early as possible.

Diagnostic laparoscopy can play a role in blunt abdominal trauma where intra-abdominal injury is suspected yet equivocal or negative findings are found on imaging. Diagnostic laparoscopy has been shown to decrease the rate of negative laparotomies and therefore minimizing the morbidity associated with a large incision. It also offers the best diagnostic accuracy for diaphragmatic injury when compared with imaging modalities.

Following blunt abdominal trauma, if the patient is haemodynamically stable for transfer to the scanner, then a CT scan should be requested. Whole-body CT scanning is commonly used in trauma centres as part of trauma assessment. If the patient is unstable and it is not safe to transfer to CT, then a focussed assessment with sonography for trauma (FAST) scan can play a role. FAST is a rapid bedside ultrasound that is performed in the emergency department that can be used to look for evidence of haemoperitoneum. If positive in the unstable patient, then an urgent laparotomy is required. However, even in experienced hands, FAST has a low sensitivity (82%), and in comparison to CT it cannot exclude intra-abdominal injury based on normal study. If the FAST scan is limited or negative in an unstable patient, then the surgeon needs to decide whether suspicion for intra-abdominal injury is sufficiently high enough to warrant an urgent laparotomy or to continue resuscitation and search for other sites of haemorrhage or causes of non-haemorrhagic shock. It should be borne in mind that mid-shaft fractures of the long bones can cause significant haemorrhage and subsequent hypovolaemia.

4. How are splenic injuries classified and managed?

The American Association for the Surgery of Trauma (AAST) has published a spleen injury grading scale based on CT findings (see Table 7.6.3). The grade of injury and degree of haemoperitoneum visualized on CT can correlate with the success of non-operative management. However, CT findings do not predict the need for initial operative intervention. This is a clinical decision.

The primary goal in the management of splenic trauma is identification and prompt management of potentially life-threatening haemorrhage. The initial management of splenic injury depends on the haemodynamic status of the patient, the grade of injury, and medical comorbidities. Preservation of functional splenic tissue by non-operative management or operative salvage techniques is a secondary aim. Techniques of splenic salvage described include suture

Table 7.6.3 The AAST CT classification of splenic trauma

Grade	Extent of splenic injury
I	Haematoma: subcapsular, <10% of surface area
	Laceration: capsular tear, 1 cm in depth into parenchyma
II	Haematoma: subcapsular, 10–50% of surface area
	Laceration: capsular tear, 1– 3cm in depth, but not involving a trabecular vessel
III	Haematoma: subcapsular, >50% of surface area or expanding, ruptured subcapsular or parenchymal haematoma >5 cm or expanding
	Laceration: >3 cm in depth or involving trabecular vessel
IV	Laceration: involving segmental or hilar vessels with major devascularization (i.e. >25% of spleen)
V	Haematoma: shattered spleen
	Laceration: hilar vascular injury which devascularizes spleen

Reproduced with permission from Moore EE, Cogbill TH, Jurkovich GJ, Shackford SR, Malangoni MA, Champion HR, 'Organ injury scaling: Spleen and liver (1994 revision)', *The Journal of Trauma and Acute Care Surgery*, Volume 38, Issue 3, pp. 323–4, Copyright © 1995 Wolters Kluwer.

repair (splenorrhapy), splenic wrapping, and partial splenectomy. Urgent laparotomy and splenectomy remains a life-saving measure in many patients.

Haemodynamically stable patients with low-grade (I–III) injuries, without active contrast extravasation on CT, may be initially observed safely without intervention. Non-operative management preserves functional splenic tissue whilst avoiding surgical morbidity. However, non-operative management is not appropriate in patients with generalized peritonitis or who require abdominal exploration for other injuries. Repeated CT imaging is indicated in patients whose clinical situation changes, such as falling haemoglobin, increasing abdominal pain, pyrexia, or if the clinical situation is unclear. The duration of inpatient observation depends on the grade of injury and the patient's clinical status, however a rule of thumb (that is not evidence-based) is that the number of days of observation is equal to the splenic injury grade plus one. Patients who fail observation require urgent embolization or surgery and abdominal exploration.

Splenic embolization is most beneficial in patients who are haemodynamically stable and have CT findings that include active contrast extravasation, splenic pseudoaneurysm, or large-volume haemoperitoneum. There is a higher failure rate with embolization with higher grade of injury, when there is contrast extravasation on CT and in older patients who have thinner, more friable splenic capsules that can render non-operative management less successful. The treatment of high-grade injuries with embolization remains controversial. Grade IV injuries can be embolized successfully, often when there is no large-volume haemoperitoneum or other intra-abdominal injuries that require abdominal exploration. Grade V injuries are generally unsuitable for embolization due to the degree of vascular disruption.

A haemodynamically unstable patient with suspected or radiologically proven splenic injury requires urgent abdominal exploration and either splenectomy or splenic salvage. Splenectomy is the safest option as the vast majority of patients requiring an urgent splenectomy for trauma are often physiologically unstable, hypothermic, coagulopathic, often with other injuries, and, therefore, would not tolerate recurrent haemorrhage.

Case continued

24 hours following admission to the high dependency unit, the patient began to complain of increasing abdominal pain. He remained haemo-dynamically stable, haemoglobin was 89 g/l, and lactate was normal. The pain was thought to be secondary to the chest and abdominal wall bruising from the seat-belt. He was reviewed again 4 hours later. He was now pyrexial and requiring additional IV fluid to maintain a normal urine output. Increased abdominal distension and tenderness, without peritonism, was noted. The patient continued to complain of severe pain despite large doses of morphine. An urgent repeat CT abdomen and pelvis was, therefore, performed. This revealed an increased amount of free fluid with locules of free gas within the small bowel mesentery (see Figure 7.6.1). The splenic injury remained unchanged. An urgent lapar-otomy was performed. At operation there was haemoperitoneum with active bleeding from a 2-cm laceration in the anterior spleen. There were four tears to the small bowel mesentery resulting in ischaemia to a 40-cm segment of jejunum 80 cm from the duodeno-jejunal flex-ure. The affected small bowel segment was necrotic with a contained perforation. Damage-control surgery was performed. The spleen was removed and the ischaemic jejunal segment was resected with a linear stapler. Intra-operatively the patient remained acidotic whilst requir-ing inotropic support to maintain blood pressure. Therefore a decision was made to not anastomose the two small bowel ends and instead the stapled ends were left in situ. The abdomen was washed out before the abdominal wall was closed with temporary fascial closure. The patient was stabilized on the critical care unit and a planned re-look lapar-otomy was performed 24 hours later once inotropes were no longer required and acidaemia had resolved. At the re-look laparotomy, the small bowel was well perfused and healthy. Intestinal continuity was, therefore, restored by performing a stapled functional end-to-end small bowel anastomosis with the remaining mesenteric tears also repaired. The patient made an uneventful post-operative recovery.

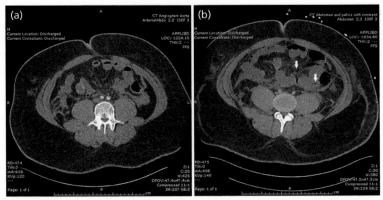

Figure 7.6.1 Images from the patient's serial contrast CT scans of the abdomen. Image A is taken from the CT scan performed on admission, which did not reveal any free air or abnormalities. Image B is taken from the repeat CT performed 24 hours later, which demonstrates free fluid with locules of extraluminal free gas (see arrows) within the small bowel mesentery in keeping with perforation of a hollow viscus.

Reproduced Courtesy of Mathew Kaduthodil.

Questions

5. What is the mechanism and pathophysiology of gastrointestinal injury following blunt abdominal trauma?

6. What are the key steps when performing a damage-control laparotomy?

Answers

5. What is the mechanism and pathophysiology of gastrointestinal injury following blunt abdominal trauma?

The mechanism of blunt gastrointestinal injury is typically due to a direct blow, such as the lower rim of a steering wheel, which can cause compression and crushing injuries to abdominal viscera. Patients involved in high-speed motor vehicle crashes may also sustain deceleration injuries, where there is a differential movement of fixed and non-fixed parts of the body.

Rupture of the stomach is uncommon due to its protected anatomical location. However, where present, it is associated with multiple injuries and trauma with higher injury severity scores. The anterior gastric wall is involved in 95% of stomach injuries with the risk of perforation more likely when there is pre-existing gastric distension, e.g. following a meal.

Common small bowel injuries are contusions limited to the serosa. However, one-third of mesenteric tears result in devascularization of bowel segments. Seatbelt trauma is a common mechanism of mesenteric injury, where both compression and deceleration forces cause bowel contusion, tearing of the bowel wall, shearing of the mesentery, and loss of blood supply. Mesenteric injuries can remain undetected for days until bowel necrosis occurs, leading to peritonitis.

Colonic and rectal injuries from blunt trauma are relatively uncommon. Colonic mesenteric injuries tend to occur at points where the mobile sections of the colon become fixed, such as at the ileo-caecal and recto-sigmoid junctions.

6. What are the key steps when performing a damage-control laparotomy?

A damage-control laparotomy has three stages:

1. Initial abbreviated operation to control haemorrhage and prevent contamination, with temporary abdominal closure.

2. Continued resuscitation with aggressive correction of coagulopathy, acidosis, and hypothermia.

3. Return to theatre once normal physiology has been restored for definitive repair of injuries with abdominal wall closure, if possible.

Operative control and cessation of haemorrhage is required, therefore patients should be transferred rapidly to the operating theatre without repeated attempts to restore circulating volume. Red blood cells, fresh frozen plasma, cryoprecipitate, and platelet transfusions need to be available, although clotting factors should only be administered once control of vascular haemorrhage has been achieved. Intravenous fluids should be warmed and the patients covered and warmed to minimize hypothermia and coagulopathy.

Skin should be prepped from neck to knees. A midline incision from xiphisternum to pubis should be made. Dramatic haemorrhage and hypotension may result once the abdomen is opened, as the intraperitoneal pressure is relieved by muscle paralysis and opening the abdominal cavity. Therefore, the surgeon must be ready with multiple, large abdominal packs to perform four-quadrant packing the moment the abdomen is opened. Once the abdomen is packed, this gives the anaesthetist time to stabilize the patient, if necessary.

The next step is to identify and control the main source of bleeding by carefully removing the packs one quadrant at a time. Direct pressure with surgeon's hands, swabs on sticks, and abdominal packs may be required to first control before addressing any bleeding identified. All intra-abdominal haematomas should be explored. All retroperitoneal haematomas in zone I (central region) should also be explored. Haematomas in zone II of the retroperitoneum (flank/perinephric region) should be explored only if the haematoma is expanding or pulsatile. Zone III (pelvic) retroperitoneal haematomas should be explored only in the presence of penetrating injuries. Non-expanding perinephric, retrohepatic, or blunt pelvic haematoma should be packed and subsequent angiographic embolization may be required.

The remaining viscera needs to be inspected systematically. Contamination should be controlled by the rapid closure of any hollow viscus injury. If there are a few small enterotomies, then these may be suture-repaired definitively. However, where bowel resection is required, then primary anastomosis should be avoided and instead bowel ends stapled or tied off. The bowel ends should be inspected and proceed on to re-anastomosis or stoma formation at a planned second procedure.

Rapid temporary abdominal closure (TAC) should then be performed and the patient transferred to the ICU for stabilization.

Further reading

American College of Surgeons (2012) *Advanced Trauma Life Support for Doctors (Student Course Manual)*, ninth edition. Chicago, IL: American College of Surgeons.

Hildebrand DR, Ben-Sassi A, Ross NP, Macvicar R, Frizelle FA, Watson AJ (2014) Modern management of splenic trauma. *British Medical Journal* **348**: g1864.

Hirshberg A, Mattox KL (2005) *Top Knife: Art and Craft in Trauma Surgery*. TFM Publishing: Harley UK.

Royal College of Radiologists (2011) *Standards of Practice and Guidance for Trauma Radiology in Severely Injured Patients*. London: Royal College of Radiologists, 2011. See: https://www.rcr.ac.uk/sites/default/files/publication/BFCR%2811%293_trauma.pdf Last accessed 18/09/2015.

Case history 7.7: Emergency: necrotizing soft-tissue infection

A 68-year-old male presented to the emergency department with acute confusion. A collateral history from the patient's partner was obtained. She reported that he had been unwell for 3 days, complaining of feeling feverish accompanied with increasing perianal pain and swelling that involved his scrotum. She had noted increasing redness over his abdominal wall over the last few hours. Past medical history included chronic pancreatitis secondary to alcoholism and pancreatogenic diabetes mellitus. He admitted to drinking approximately 22 units of alcohol per day and smoked 15 cigarettes a day. Drug history included metformin, thiamine, vitamin B, and Creon®.

On physical examination there was marked perianal swelling with fluctuance in the left ischiorectal fossa. There was marked cellulitis extending to the perineum, scrotum, and lower left anterior abdominal wall. Necrotic patches of skin were evident at the base of the scrotum and perianal region, with crepitus evident on palpation. Systemically there was evidence of severe sepsis: blood pressure was 105/70, pulse 120, temperature 38.7°C, oxygen saturations of 94% on air, and respiratory rate of 22 breaths per minute. The patient's blood results are show in Table 7.7.1.

A diagnosis of necrotizing fasciitis of the perineum (otherwise known as Fournier's gangrene) was made.

Table 7.7.1 Blood results

Blood results	
Hb	11.5
WCC	23.6
Platelets	260
Sodium	138
Potassium	5.2
Urea	5.2
Creatinine	130
INR	2.0
Lactate	4.5
CRP	351

Questions

1. What is necrotizing fasciitis?
2. How does necrotizing fasciitis present?
3. What is the pathophysiology of necrotizing fasciitis?
4. How is necrotizing fasciitis managed?
5. Is there a role for imaging in necrotizing fasciitis?
6. What operative strategy and techniques should be considered?

Answers

1. What is necrotizing fasciitis?

Although some deep soft-tissue infections remain localized, some can result in fulminant necrotizing spread with severe sepsis. When this rapid extensive infection involves the fascia deep to the adipose tissue, it is known as necrotizing fasciitis. When it involves muscles, it is known as necrotizing myositis. Common sites of necrotizing fasciitis are the perineum and external genitalia, where it is also known as Fournier's gangrene, and the abdominal wall. Approximately 500 cases of necrotizing fasciitis occur each year in the UK. Even with surgery it is associated with a mortality rate of 20–40% and long-term disability from extensive tissue loss, often requiring extensive surgery, amputation, and reconstruction. Mortality and significant disability from necrotizing fasciitis is prevented with prompt diagnosis and treatment.

2. How does necrotizing fasciitis present?

Necrotizing fasciitis can often be difficult to diagnose. Initial symptoms can be non-specific with the patient appearing relatively well until there is rapid deterioration with severe sepsis and confusion. The overall clinical picture is often more insidious. Fever and pain are an early feature, with the pain often disproportionate to the clinical findings. Cellulitis develops next, although again the severity of the infection is not always apparent early on in the clinical course, with skin necrosis and crepitus late signs. A high suspicion of necrotizing fasciitis is required for early diagnosis. Although 25% of cases occur in patients without any pre-existing illness or trauma, certain clues can be identified from the clinical history that may point towards a diagnosis of necrotizing fasciitis. Such risk factors are listed in Table 7.7.2.

Table 7.7.2 Risk factors for the development of necrotizing fasciitis

Skin injury to introduce infection	◆ Recent surgical procedure
	◆ IM injection
	◆ Acupuncture
	◆ Insect bite
	◆ Trauma
Underlying medical conditions	◆ Diabetes mellitus
	◆ Chronic liver disease
	◆ Iatrogenic immunosuppression
	◆ Obesity
	◆ Malignancy (particularly leukaemia)
	◆ Malnutrition
	◆ Peripheral vascular disease
	◆ Alcohol abuse
	◆ IV drug abuse
	◆ Smoking
	◆ NSAID use
Other	◆ Varicella infection (recognized risk factor in children)

Reproduced Courtesy of Jonathan Wild.

3. What is the pathophysiology of necrotizing fasciitis?

Necrotizing fasciitis is associated with a wide spectrum of causative organisms, which are classified into two groups:

◆ Type I (synergistic) necrotizing fasciitis:

◆ Mixed infection caused by anaerobic, aerobic, and anaerobic Gram-positive and Gram-negative bacteria.

◆ Most bacteria originate from gut flora, e.g. *E. coli*, *Pseudomonas* spp, *Bacteroides* spp, *Vibri* spp.

◆ Risk factors include recent gastrointestinal surgery, underlying abdominal and pelvic pathology, such as malignancy, perianal sepsis, or an immunocompromised state.

- ◆ Type II:

- ◆ Usually monomicrobial.

- ◆ Gram-positive bacteria.

- ◆ Most common pathogen is group-A β-haemolytic streptococcus, either alone or in combination with *Stapholococcus aureus.*

- ◆ Risk factors include lacerations, burns, or any trauma, including surgery, childbirth, IV drug abuse, or varicella infection that can cause a breach in the dermis.

In necrotizing fasciitis, the infection of the deeper tissues spreads to progressively destroy muscle, fascia, and subcutaneous fat. The muscle is often spared due to its good blood supply. Pain is caused by tissue necrosis but the cutaneous nerves can also become infarcted as perforating vessels thrombose, resulting in severe pain yet with paraesthesia in the overlying skin. Gas-producing organisms, such as *Clostridium*, produce crepitus with anaerobes producing a putrid odour.

Type I necrotizing fasciitis is normally slower in onset, as opposed to Type II, which progresses rapidly due in part to an endotoxin-driven toxic-shock syndrome. If left to progress, necrotizing fasciitis ultimately results in a systemic inflammatory response syndrome and multi-organ failure.

4. How is necrotizing fasciitis managed?

Key to successful management of necrotizing fasciitis is prompt recognition, broad-spectrum antibiotics, urgent aggressive surgical debridement, and haemodynamic support. Initial resection is followed by planned re-examination in the operating theatre and further debridement, as required.

In this case, the patient was immediately treated with high-flow oxygen, intravenous fluids, parenteral analgesia, and intravenous antibiotics (clindamycin, meropenem, and vancomycin) following discussion with a microbiologist. The patient was counselled pre-operatively for the potential need for repeated debridements, orchidectomy, and defunctioning colostomy, and was transferred directly from the emergency department to the operating theatre for urgent surgical debridement.

Hyperbaric oxygen is thought to be useful in treating synergistic infections by increasing the bactericidal effects of neutrophils and also by switching off the ability of *Clostridium perfringens* to produce α-toxins. Despite showing a reduction in mortality from necrotizing fasciitis, with the limited number of hyperbaric oxygen units with critical care facilities, in addition to the high costs involved, hyperbaric oxygen therapy is unlikely to become routine.

5. Is there a role for imaging in necrotizing fasciitis?

CT signs of necrotizing fasciitis include fascial swelling, inflammation, and soft-tissue gas. CT can also help identify an underlying source of infection, such as intra-abdominal sepsis, and may help plan surgery. Ultrasonography and MRI also have some diagnostic ability to detect necrotizing fasciitis. However, any radiological investigations should never delay surgery when the patient has advancing soft-tissue infection and systemic sepsis. A follow-up CT scan after the initial debridement, once the patient has been stabilized, is an option to rule out any suspected intraperitoneal collections. The mainstay of investigation and treatment is urgent surgical exploration and debridement.

6. What operative strategy and techniques should be considered?

In this case of perineal necrotizing fasciitis, the patient is placed in the lithotomy position and a urethral catheter inserted under anaesthetic. For suspected necrotizing fasciitis, an incision should be made over the site of maximal skin change in order to assess the viability of the underlying tissues. If healthy fascia and subcutaneous tissue is present, then further resection is not required. However, if necrotic fascia and fat is evident, often with the characteristic 'dishwater' appearance of liquefied necrotic tissue, debridement of non-viable tissue should be performed until healthy tissue is reached. Tissue samples and pus should be sent for culture and sensitivities.

In this case, a large left-sided ischiorectal abscess was found to be the underlying cause. This was drained and extensive areas of necrotic fascia, fat, and skin were debrided from the perineum, scrotum, and lower left anterior abdominal wall, and the resulting wounds were packed with ribbon gauze. The testes were viable and an orchidectomy was not required. The patient was then transferred to the intensive care unit for haemodynamic support with a planned return to theatre 24 hours later. At this point a small amount of debridement was required and a decision was made to perform a diagnostic laparoscopy and defunctioning loop colostomy in order to divert the faecal stream from the perineal wound to prevent repeated contamination. Following a second re-look, no further debridement was required and a negative pressure wound therapy (VAC®) was applied. After a prolonged period of hospitalization and intensive wound care, the patient was discharged to a rehabilitation unit. The wounds healed completely by secondary intention and did not require skin grafting. The patient has decided not to undergo colostomy reversal.

Further reading

Rhodes A, Evans LE, Alhazzani W, Levy MM, Antonelli M, Ferrer R et al. (2017) Surviving sepsis campaign: international guidelines for management of sepsis and septic shock: 2016. *Intensive Care Medicine* Mar;43(3):304–77.

Stevens DL et al. (2014) Practice guidelines for the diagnosis and management of skin and soft tissue infections: 2014 update by the infectious diseases society of America. *Clinical Infectious Diseases* Jul 15; 59(2): 147–59.

Sultan H, Boyle A, Sheppard N (2012) Practice pointer: necrotizing fasciitis. *British Medical Journal* 345: e4274.

Case history 7.8: Emergency: kidney transplant

A 30-year-old lady on haemodialysis for end-stage renal failure, secondary to IgA nephropathy, was called in for pre-transplant assessment. She had been on haemodialysis via a left brachio-cephalic fistula for over 6 months and peritoneal dialysis for 2 years prior to that. Apart from hypertension and anaemia, she had no other significant comorbidities and had been well recently. Physical examination revealed scars from previous operations where peritoneal dialysis catheters were inserted and subsequently removed. Her chest was clear to auscultation and her abdomen was soft and non-tender with no palpable masses. Kidneys were not palpable. She had good femoral and distal pulses. She underwent haemodialysis prior to theatre and her post-dialysis potassium was 4.8 mmol/l.

A deceased donor kidney was offered through the national organ allocation system from a 54-year old DBD (donation after brainstem death or heart-beating) donor. The cause of death was pneumococcal meningitis. The donor had no significant comorbidities. There was no history of cancer in the donor and virology was negative. On bench dissection of the right kidney, the anatomy was confirmed to be one artery on an aortic patch, one vein with a cuff of inferior vena cava, and one ureter with no lesions or iatrogenic damage.

Following induction of anaesthesia, administration of induction immunosuppression, and prophylactic antibiotics, implantation proceeded via a right Gibson incision with arterial anastomosis to the right common iliac artery and venous anastomosis to the right external iliac vein. Re-perfusion was initially patchy but quick to improve. The ureteric anastomosis to the bladder was performed over a J–J stent.

Post-operative recovery was uneventful and she was commenced on Tacrolimus monotherapy for immunosuppression. An ultra-sound Doppler scan performed on day 2 revealed a well-perfused kidney with patent artery and vein. Once discharge training was complete the recipient was discharged, to be followed up three times weekly in clinic in the first month.

Questions

1. What are the common causes of end-stage renal failure?

2. What options are available for renal replacement therapy (RRT), when would you consider this for a patient, and what are the benefits of renal transplantation over RRT?

3. What are the types of donors and how does this affect the function of the organ post-transplant?

4. What are the criteria for brain stem death certification?

5. How is organ retrieval co-ordinated in the United Kingdom?

6. How are organs preserved following retrieval until they are transplanted into the intended recipient?

7. What are the commonly used immunosuppressive agents in renal transplantation and what are their modes of action?

Answers

1. What are the common causes of end-stage renal failure?

Diabetic nephropathy is the commonest cause of end-stage renal failure, accounting for up to 25% of all cases. Up to a fifth of patients have an unknown aetiology. Glomerulonephritis, autosomal-dominant polycystic kidney disease, chronic pyelonephritis, hypertension, and renal vascular disease are also causes of chronic kidney disease that can lead to end-stage renal failure.

2. What options are available for renal replacement therapy (RRT), when would you consider this for a patient, and what are the benefits of renal transplantation over RRT?

Patients with advanced chronic kidney disease are followed up in low-clearance clinics with the focus being on delaying progression of disease and managing complications. Plans for RRT are made in anticipation of progression of renal failure and early referral for renal transplantation is considered. Choice of modality of dialysis depends on the patient's preference and their suitability for it. The RRT is usually commenced when glomerular filtration rate falls below 6–8 ml/min/1.73 m^2 or when clinically indicated (i.e. onset of uraemic symptoms, fluid overload, refractory hyperkalaemia or acidosis).

Elective

- *Haemodialysis (HD).* Surgical creation of a permanent arterio-venous fistula occurs in the months prior to commencement of haemodialysis, which allows time for the fistula to mature prior to use. The fistula can be accessed with two cannulae: one that removes blood slowly and transfers it to the dialysis machine, and the other that infuses 'clean' blood back to the patient. Synthetic arteriovenous (AV) grafts can also be used, if required, and accessed similar to fistulas for dialysis.

- *Peritoneal dialysis (PD).* Insertion of a peritoneal dialysis catheter (called a Tenckhoff catheter) into the peritoneal cavity can be performed via a laparoscopic approach or a mini-laparotomy.

Patients can opt to perform continuous ambulatory peritoneal dialysis (CAPD), which involves several short dialysis sessions throughout the day or automated peritoneal dialysis (APD), which involves overnight dialysis. Patient training is required for both methods as it is vital that the catheter is kept clean to prevent episodes of PD catheter-associated peritonitis.

Emergency

Emergency renal replacement therapy may be required for patients with severe hyperkalaemia resistant to medical treatment, refractory pulmonary oedema, or severe metabolic acidosis. Other indications are uraemic pericarditis or encephalopathy. This can be administered intermittently or continuously:

- *Intermittent haemodialysis.* Urgent haemodialysis can be achieved via a tunnelled central line (e.g. Vascath), which can be used for short-term haemodialysis.

- *Continuous veno-venous haemofiltration (CVVH) or haemodialysis (CVVHD).* This is used in patients with acute kidney injury requiring emergency RRT in a critical care setting. Vascular access is central venous, either through internal jugular or femoral line. CVVHD has the advantage of offering continuous volume control and responding to dynamic changes in physiology, as is the case with acutely ill patients, and is preferred over intermittent haemodialysis or peritoneal dialysis in critical care patients.

3. What are the types of donors and how does this affect the function of the organ post-transplant?

Organ donors can be either living or deceased but the gold standard is a living donor kidney from a healthy donor.

Living donors

- *Live-related donor.* Usually between close relatives like siblings, spouses, etc.

- *Live-unrelated donor.* When a close emotional relationship is confirmed between donor and recipient, despite being unrelated.

- *Altruistic donor.* Donor has no relationship to recipient and usually does not know the recipient nor has a say in who the recipient should be. Organs are usually allocated nationally to the best-matched recipient.

Deceased donors

- *Donation after brainstem death (DBD).* Any patient who has had two brainstem death tests independently by two clinicians with more than 5 years post-qualification experience and have been confirmed to be brain-dead, is a potential organ donor. Provided that consent to donation has been confirmed, and there are no objections from the coroner due to circumstances surrounding the death, organ donation can proceed. Once the donor's blood and tissue type are known, organs are offered to recipient centres by the national organ offering system. It is generally accepted that the 'quality' of DBD kidneys are better than DCD kidneys.

- *Donation after circulatory death (DCD).* These are donors who are not brain-dead but have an agreed terminal condition for which further medical intervention is futile. If consent is obtained for donation, with agreement from relatives, a plan is made for withdrawal of treatment. Once asystole is confirmed in the donor, death is confirmed and the retrieval operation begins swiftly in order to cannulate the aorta and infuse cold preservation fluid. Time to asystole from withdrawal impacts on graft function post-transplant and generally 3 hours is the accepted maximum.

- *Standard criteria versus extended/expanded criteria donors.* Extended criteria donors are generally defined as donors over 60 years of age with no comorbidities or those between 50 and 60 years of age with a history of hypertension, with terminal creatinine greater than 133 μmol/l, whose cause of death was a cerebrovascular accident. All other donors are considered standard criteria donors. Due to the shortfall of organs for transplantation and the ever-growing waiting list, extended-criteria kidneys are increasingly being utilized to expand the donor pool. Extended-criteria kidneys that are unlikely to render a recipient dialysis-free as a single graft can be consider for dual-renal transplantation in selected recipients.

4. What are the criteria for brainstem death certification?

Prior to attempting to confirm BSD, several criteria needs to be fulfilled. The irreversibility of brain damage and its aetiology should be known and any reversible causes (such as deep coma, metabolic/endocrine disturbances, depressant drugs, and hypothermia) are excluded. Tests have to be carried out by at least two medical practitioners who have been registered for more than 5 years and are competent to perform, as well as interpret, brainstem tests. Tests are performed to confirm the absence of the following brainstem reflexes:

- *Pupillary reflex.* Pupils fixed and dilated.
- *Corneal reflex.* No response to simulation of the cornea.
- *Absent oculo-vestibular reflex.* No eye movements in response to cold water in external auditory meatus.
- *Motor responses within cranial nerve distribution.* No motor response to application of supraorbital pressure.
- *Cough reflex.* No cough response to bronchial stimulation by suction catheter or gag response to stimulation of posterior pharynx.
- *No response to hypercarbia (apnoea test).* The final test to be performed involves cessation of ventilation and allowing the $PaCO_2$ to rise above 6.0 in an attempt to trigger respiratory response to hypercarbia.

5. How is organ retrieval co-ordinated in the United Kingdom?

The UK is divided geographically into seven abdominal organ retrieval zones and six cardiothoracic retrieval zones with an organ retrieval team comprising retrieval surgeons, scrub nurses, ambulance drivers, and a retrieval team co-ordinator. Each region has specialist nurses for organ donation (SNODs) who are called out to donor hospitals to assess potential donors and advise on donor management. The teams rely on the donor hospitals for theatre space and anaesthetic support. They have to face the challenge of working in unfamiliar hospitals and team-working within new teams.

The duty office of NHS Blood and Transplant co-ordinates the logistics of organ donation, retrieval, and allocation nationally. An electronic organ-offering system exists to ensure that there is consistency in the minimum required donor information for transplant centres accepting organs for their waiting-list patients.

6. How are organs preserved following retrieval until transplanted into the intended recipient?

Static, cold preservation remains the most commonly used method of organ preservation. Organs are maintained in solutions especially designed for organ preservation. University of Wisconsin (UW) solution is the oldest and most commonly used 'gold standard' preservation solution worldwide. The composition includes metabolically inert substances to maintain osmotic concentration, substances to scavenge free radicals to reduce free radical damage, as well as insulin and adenosine. The temperature is maintained just above freezing for optimal preservation while avoiding freezing. Freezing and subsequent thawing destroys the integrity of the cells and renders the organ non-transplantable.

Machine-perfusion is increasingly being used instead of cold-storage and has been shown to improve graft function post-transplant. Both hypothermic and normothermic perfusion methods have been developed.

7. What are the commonly used immunosuppressive agents in renal transplantation and what are their modes of action?

- *Basiliximab*. Anti-interleukin-2 (IL-2) receptor monoclonal antibody targeting the IL-2 receptor on activated lymphocytes. This is used as an induction immunosuppressive agent.

- *Methylprednisolone and prednisolone*. The immunosuppressive properties of steroids are still utilized in the induction of immunosuppression. Steroids are rarely used in recent times for maintenance immunosuppression due to long term side-effects. However, they still has a role in management of episodes of rejection.

- *Tacrolimus.* Calcineurin inhibitor that has similar anti-T-lymphocyte effects to the older drug ciclosporin. Calcineurin induces the transcription of IL-2. Tacrolimus is used as maintenance monotherapy as a steroid-sparing agent.

- *Mycophenolate mofetil.* Inhibitor of purine synthesis that has more potent effect on activated lymphocytes compared to other cell types. Generally added in to tacrolimus therapy for those patients with a higher HLA mismatch or following episodes of rejection.

- *Sirolimus.* Inhibitor of IL-2 leading to reduced activation of T- and B-lymphocytes.

- *Azathioprine.* This is an older drug. It is a purine analogue and the pro-drug of 6-mercaptopurine and exerts its immunosuppressive action via its effect on lymphocytes.

- *Ciclosporin.* Also an older drug and has a similar mechanism of action to tacrolimus.

Further reading

NHS Blood and Transplant (NHSBT) Organ Donation. https://www.organdonation.nhs.uk/ Last accessed 23/06/2017.

Immunosuppressive therapy for renal transplantation in adults. NICE guidance, TA85. https://www.nice.org.uk/guidance/TA85 Last accessed 23/06/2017.

Renal replacement therapy and transplantation. http://www.patient.co.uk/doctor/renal-replacement-therapy-and-transplantation Last accessed 23/06/2017.

Case history 7.9: Emergency: cutaneous abscesses

A 29-year-old man presents with a large painful swelling on his chest wall. This has developed over the course of 3 days, becoming progressively bigger and more painful. It has become hot and red over the last 24 hours. He denies any discharge. He has had no systemic features of sepsis. He has had a small lump at the area for a number of years that hasn't caused him any bother. He has no other past medical history. On examination he has a 4 × 4 cm raised erythematous tender swelling. There is a visible punctum with no discharge. There is no surrounding cellulitis. He was diagnosed with a chest wall abscess and underwent an incision and drainage.

This case covers the management of simple and uncomplicated skin abscesses. As part of clinical assessment of cutaneous sepsis, it is important to exclude necrotizing fasciitis as part of the differential diagnosis. This is covered in Case 7.7 in this chapter.

Questions

1. What is the aetiology of a cutaneous abscess?
2. What is the pathophysiology of a cutaneous abscess?
3. How should cutaneous abscesses be managed?

Answers

1. What is the aetiology of a cutaneous abscess?

Cutaneous abscess is a common emergency presentation to the general surgical acute take. Abscesses can arise from:

- A simple hair follicle that becomes obstructed and subsequently becomes inflamed and infected (termed folliculitis).

- On a background of hidradenitis suppurativa, a condition characterized by chronic inflammation within the apocrine glands in the follicular epithelium. Clinical history and examination of these patients can rapidly identify this, as the patient may have a history of developing multiple, small, erythematous papules or nodules, with or without discharge, and signs of sinus tracts and scarring in chronic and advanced disease at the sites where apocrine glands are found in the axillary and groin creases.

- Epidermal inclusion cysts, often referred to as sebaceous cysts. These arise from epidermal cell proliferation within the dermis, typically arising from the infundibulum of the hair follicle. The presence of an underlying epidermal inclusion cyst is suggested in the history, where patients may report the presence of a small, round, painless, and otherwise asymptomatic lump at the site of the abscess for some months or years before the formation of the abscess. It may have increased in size over recent months. The causative organism is usually a skin-derived organism such as *Staphylococcus aureus* and *Streptococcus pyogenes*, although the rate of community-acquired MRSA abscesses is increasing.

- Instrumentation. Pathogenic organisms may be introduced into soft tissue through instrumentation, e.g. port site insertion at laparoscopic surgery (resulting in port site infection and abscess) or injections, e.g. intravenous drug users.

2. What is the pathophysiology of a cutaneous abscess?

An abscess is the accumulation of both infective and inflammatory infiltrate within a tissue. Infective organisms penetrate a tissue and initiate an immune response. Mast cells produce histamine, which generates increased blood flow (hyperaemia) and redness to the area, as well as local vascular permeability. Neutrophils are drawn into the tissue through permeabilized blood vessels to attack the invading organisms, as well as bodily fluid that generates swelling. Over a couple of days, monocytes will also enter the area, converting into phagocytic macrophages in the process. Phagocytic response to the infection can cause cavitation of the tissue. An ongoing inflammatory process can produce fibrous or granulation tissue in an attempt to wall off the infection. Neutrophils have a short life-span, and the inflammatory process generally results in a collection of dead neutrophils and macrophages, cellular debris, and microorganisms, collectively termed pus, resulting in an abscess. Infection can penetrate the adjacent soft tissues resulting in cellulitis, which can be identified by the presence of erythema, heat, and tenderness.

It is important to differentiate the term abscess from the term empyema, which refers to an infective process and collection of pus in a hollow viscus rather than within a tissue, such as the gallbladder, appendix, or pleural space. Similar to an abscess, an empyema is the sequelae of suppurative inflammation involving the organ. An empyema also requires drainage for definitive treatment, but the approach is different than that for an abscess and is beyond the scope of this chapter.

3. How should cutaneous abscesses be managed?

Definitive management of all abscesses is incision and drainage. Infective collection at the site of instrumentation, such as port sites, may be managed simply by opening the wound cavity to allow pus and infection to drain. The immune response results in cavitation of subcutaneous tissue in which both infective organisms and pus become walled off by fibrous tissue into which antibiotics will not be able to penetrate. Adjuvant treatment with antibiotics is only warranted where there is evidence of cellulitis in the adjacent soft tissues or in immunocompromised patients. Common organisms are *Staphylococcus aureus* and streptococci, but may vary depending on location, route of entry, and whether the patient is immunocompromised.

Intravenous drug users can develop infection at injection sites, which commonly overlies arteries adjacent to the injected veins. It is, therefore, important to consider two things before proceeding to incision and drainage in these patients:

1. Whether the patient has developed a pseudoaneurysm (or false aneurysm) secondary to vascular injury during injection. These may or may not be pulsatile and may not be clinically distinguishable from a cutaneous abscess. They can present with concomitant infection, which can also advance into damaged arterial wall propagating a mycotic aneurysm. Proceeding to incision and drainage without identifying this can be disastrous. Therefore it is common practice to obtain imaging of the region, usually with ultrasound and vascular Doppler imaging, as part of surgical workup.

2. Whether the site may contain any remnant broken needles, which is an important consideration for the surgeon who would be at risk of a needlestick injury. A simple X-ray can help here.

Incision and drainage can be carried out under either local or general anaesthetic in small abscesses. However, this decision should be largely directed by the patient, as many will not be able to withstand incision under local anaesthetic. Local anaesthetic is not always as effective in the presence of acute inflammation. In addition, drainage under local anaesthesia may not be tolerated sufficiently to allow the surgeon to curette or incise the cavity sufficiently, which may result in a higher risk of recurrent infection. Very tender abscesses or those with associated cellulitis or sepsis should be drained under general anaesthesia.

The patient should be consented for the procedure regardless of whether they are drained under local or general anaesthesia. Patient consent should cover the immediate surgical risks of bleeding, pain, and anaesthetic risks, as well as delayed surgical risks of delayed wound healing, abscess recurrence, and scarring. Incision and drainage is a simple procedure comprising the following steps:

- *Incision.* The incision into the abscess should maintain an open wound and prevent apposition of the skin edges, as this can result in re-accumulation of the abscess. This can either use an elliptical incision or a cruciate incision with trimming of the four edges.

- *Microbiological culture.* A pus swab is routinely taken from the cavity at the time of drainage in most centres, which may be useful in localized or complicated infection. This is particularly important in abscess drainage in intravenous drug users, who may isolate multiple and atypical pathogenic organisms.

- *Curettage.* Loculations within the abscess cavity are broken down to prevent pockets of infection, which may result in persistence or recurrence of soft-tissue infection. Fibrous tissue should be removed by curettage.

- *Irrigation.* The wound is irrigated clean with copious amounts of saline with or without hydrogen peroxide.

- *Wound packing.* The resulting wound is left open to heal by primary intent. The resultant defect is packed gently with an absorbent dressing, such as sorbsan, to aid tissue drainage and promote healing. However, the surgeon should avoid splinting the wound with these dressings to keep it open as these increase patient discomfort. The incision should be adequate enough to keep the wound open.

An infected sebaceous cyst is apparent at the time of drainage as infected material is seen to be mixed with thick cheesy sebum that accumulates in obstructed epidermal inclusion cysts. It is very difficult to remove the entire cyst wall in the presence of acute infection, therefore, where this is not possible, as much cyst wall remnant is removed by excision and curettage as possible in order to prevent the cyst from persisting with the risk of recurrent infection.

Further reading

Bravo RD (2016) Abscess management, *in* Collins-Bride GM, Saxe JM, Duderstadt KG, Kaplan R. *Clinical Guidelines for Advanced Practice Nursing: An Interprofessional Approach*, third edition. Burlington, MA: Jones and Bartlett Publishers.

Index

abdominal pain
  acute 363–79
  chronic pancreatitis 147
  small bowel obstruction 408–9
abdominal radiographs
  acute abdominal pain 374
  acute appendicitis 387
  acute mesenteric ischaemia 261
  acute pancreatitis 161
  gallstones 93
  ileus 270
  inflammatory bowel disease 226
  large bowel obstruction 272
  pseudo-obstruction 270
  sigmoid volvulus 398–9
  small bowel obstruction 410
abdominal trauma
  blunt 423–36
  penetrating 426–7
ablation
  hepatocellular carcinoma 76
  peptic ulcer bleed 35
  thyroid cancer 333–4, 358
abscess
  anorectal 236, 237, 240
  breast 317–21
  cutaneous 455–9
  intersphincteric 237, 238, 240
  ischiorectal 237, 238, 239–40
  non-lactational breast 319–20
  pancreatic duct 175
  perianal 237, 238, 239–40
  pericolic 249, 251
  peridiverticular 271
  pilonidal 229–33
  supralevator 237, 238, 240
acalculous cholecystitis 92
ACE inhibitors 369
ACE procedure 184, 206
achalasia 3, 22
acute abdominal pain 363–79
acute appendicitis 381–92
acute ascending cholangitis 94–5,
  99–108, 135, 139
acute cholecystitis 91–2, 158

acute diverticulitis 243–52, 271
acute mesenteric ischaemia 253–63
acute pancreatitis
  compared to chronic disease 146, 148
  emergency presentation 155–65
  gallstones 94, 96
  serum amylase/lipase 92–3, 160–1
acute respiratory distress 360–1
acute severe pancreatitis 165
adenocarcinoma
  gastric 23
  oesophagus 22, 23
  pancreas 120, 135
adenomas, colorectal 195, 196
adjustable gastric band 3, 12, 13, 52, 53
adjuvant chemoradiotherapy, gastro-
    oesophageal cancer 27
adjuvant chemotherapy
  breast cancer 315–16
  cholangiocarcinoma 85–6
Adjuvant! Online 315
adrenaline
  peptic ulcer bleed 35
  variceal bleed 35
adrenal lesion 347–52
alanine aminotransferase (ALT) 66
alcohol intake
  bariatric surgery 12
  colorectal cancer 195
  gastro-oesophageal reflux disease 6
  Mallory–Weiss tear 31
  pancreatitis 147, 150, 165
  peptic ulcer disease 38
alpha fetoprotein (AFP) 72
Altemeier approach 287
Altemeier procedure 289
Alvarado score 388
American Association for the Surgery of
    Trauma (AAST) grading
  pancreatic injury 174
  splenic injury 429–30
American Society of Anesthesiologists
    (ASA) score 377
amylase, serum 92–3, 160–1, 171
anal advancement flap 210

anal fissure 180, 207–10, 236
anal fistula 185–90
analgesia, *see* pain control
anal pain 26
anal sphincter
  iatrogenic injuries 203
  mechanism 202
  repair 206
  replacement 206
anaplastic thyroid cancer 332–3
anastomotic bleed 53–4
anastomotic leak
  bariatric surgery 53–4
  oesophagogastric resections 47, 48–9
angiectasia
  radiation-induced 278
  upper gastrointestinal bleeding 31
angiodysplasia 278–9
angiography
  mesenteric 261
  pancreatic trauma 173
  see also CT angiography
angle of His 2
ankylosing spondylitis 224–5
annular pancreatitis 159
anococcygeal body (raphe) 285
anoplasty 210
anorectal abscess 236, 237, 240
anorectal fistula 236, 240
anorectal manometry 181, 204
anorectal sepsis 235–42
antegrade continence enema
    (appendicostomy) 184, 206
anterior overlapping
    sphincteroplasty 206
anticoagulation 369
anti-diarrhoeals 205
anti-platelets 369
anti-reflux surgery 7–8
anti-thyroid drugs 357
aortoenteric fistula 31
aphthous ulcers 224
apnoea test 451
appendicectomy 389, 390–1
appendicitis, acute 381–92
argon plasma coagulation 27
arterial ischaemia/spasm 257
arthropathies 11, 224
artificial sphincter 206
ASA score 377
ascending cholangitis 94–5, 99–108,
    135, 139

ascites 73, 147
autoimmune pancreatitis 159
autologous reconstruction 313
automated peritoneal dialysis 449
axillary surgery 304, 312
azathioprine 453

bacteria
  anorectal sepsis 237
  ascending cholangitis 103
  breast abscess 318
  gallstones 90, 92
  gangrenous and perforated
    appendicitis 385
  Helicobacter pylori 4, 23–4, 30, 31, 39
  necrotizing fasciitis 441, 442
  skin abscess 456
balloon tamponade 36
  bariatric surgery 9–18
  complications 3, 51–5
barium enema 250
barium fluoroscopy 226
barium swallow 4–5, 25, 54
Barrett's oesophagus 4, 6, 8, 23
Bascom's procedure 232
basiliximab 452
beta-blockers 357
bile
  constituents 90
  leak 112
  replacement 104
bile duct injury 112, 113, 114, 115–16
biliary colic 91, 96
biliary drainage 85, 104
biliary obstruction 85
biliary peritonitis 114
biliary reconstruction 115
biliary sludge 91
biliary stenosis 75, 153
biliary stent 85, 104, 140
biliary stricture 82, 132
biliary tract cancer 82, 85–6
biliopancreatic diversion 53, 54, 55
biofeedback therapy
  constipation 182
  faecal incontinence 205
biological therapy 190
biopsy, breast lump 293
Bismuth classification 113
bleeding
  anastomotic 53–4
  colonic ischaemia 277–8

diverticular 277
jaundice 135
lower gastrointestinal 276–9,
   280–2
oesophagogastric resections 47
rectal 208, 241–2, 275–82
upper gastrointestinal 29–36, 276
variceal 30, 31–2, 34, 35, 36, 73
blunt abdominal trauma 423–36
BOADICEA 295
body mass index (BMI) 10
bone mineral density 342–3
botulinum toxin 209
Bowel Cancer Screening
   Programme 196, 197
bowel injury, iatrogenic 112
bowel ischaemia 253–63
bowel obstruction
   diverticulitis 248–9
   hernia 219–20, 268
   large bowel 180, 219, 265–74
   pseudo-obstruction 268, 269–70,
      273–4, 396
   small bowel 219, 403–14
bowel resection 227
brainstem death 451
BRCA 1/2136, 297, 298
breast abscess 317–21
breast cancer 307–16
   aetiology 310
   chemoprevention 295–6, 297
   classification 310–11
   ductal carcinoma *in situ* 303–4
   familial 297–8
   genetic factors 296, 297–8
   HER-2 positive 311
   high risk patients 296–7
   luminal A 311
   luminal B 311
   prognostic indicators 314–15
   risk assessment 294–5
   Triple Negative 311
breast cyst 294
breast-feeding with breast
      abscess 319
breast fibroadenoma 292, 293–4
breast implants 313
breast lump 291–8
breast mouse 294
breast reconstruction 312–14
breast screening 296–7, 302–3, 304
bulk-forming agents 182

caecal volvulus 268–9
calculous cholecystitis 92
Calot's triangle 106, 112
campylobacter-like organism (CLO)
      biopsy 39
capsule endoscopy 226
carbimazole 357
carbohydrate antigen 19.9 (CA19.9) 138
carbon-13 urea breath test 39
carcinoembryonic antigen (CEA) 67,
      124, 138
catecholamines 349
cauda equina syndrome 286
caustic oesophageal injury 22
Chagas disease 397
Charcot's triad 102, 139
chemoprevention, breast
      cancer 295–6, 297
chemoradiotherapy
   colorectal cancer 199
   gastro-oesophageal cancer 27
chemotherapy
   biliary tract cancer 86
   breast cancer 315–16
   cholangiocarcinoma 85–6
chest radiographs
   acute abdominal pain 374
   acute appendicitis 387
   anastomotic leak 48
   gallstones 93
   large bowel obstruction 272
   perforated duodenal ulcer 41
   small bowel obstruction 410
Child–Pugh classification 73–4
cholangiocarcinoma 79–86
cholangitis 85
   ascending 94–5, 99–108, 135, 139
   primary sclerosing 225
cholecystectomy 96
   complication following 109–16
   laparoscopic 105–8, 109–16
   post-cholecystectomy syndrome 113
cholecystitis
   acalculous 92
   acute 91–2, 158
   calculous 92
   emphysematous 92
cholecystoenteric fistula 95
cholecystokinin 158
cholecystostomy, percutaneous 96–7
choledocholithiasis 132
cholestasis 135

cholestyramine 357–8
chronic mesenteric ischaemia 256
chronic pancreatitis 143–54
chylothorax 48
ciclosporin 453
cirrhosis 73–4
clotting disorders, jaundice 135
¹³C-mixed triglyceride breath test 152
coagulopathy 66
coeliac disease 195
'coffee bean' sign 398
colectomy
   sigmoid 288
   subtotal and end ileostomy 227
   subtotal with ilio-rectal
      anastomosis 184
colitis
   diverticular (segmental) 247
   ischaemic 278
colocutaneous fistula 249
colon cancer, large bowel
     obstruction 270–1
colonic blunt injuries 434
colonic fistula 249
colonic ischaemia 277–8
colonic pseudo-obstruction 396
colonic stents 272–3
colonic transit studies 180–1
colonic volvulus 271
colonoscopy
   anal fistula 188
   colorectal cancer 194
   constipation 180
   inflammatory bowel disease 225
   lower gastrointestinal bleeding 281
colorectal adenomas 195, 196
colorectal cancer 191–200
   liver metastases 57–68
colostomy
   diversion 206
   loop 189
   percutaneous endoscopic 402
colovaginal fistula 249
colovesical fistula 249
common bile duct stones 93–4, 103, 104,
   107–8, 112
complex reflux disease 7
compound volvulus 396
computed tomography (CT)
   acute abdominal pain 374–5
   acute appendicitis 387
   acute mesenteric ischaemia 261

acute pancreatitis 161
anastomotic leak 48–9
angiography 261, 281
blunt abdominal trauma 428
chronic pancreatitis 151
colonography 194
colorectal cancer 194
colorectal liver metastases 60
gallstones 94
gastro-oesophageal cancer 25
groin swelling 418
hepatocellular carcinoma 72
inflammatory bowel disease 225
large bowel obstruction 272
necrotizing fasciitis 443
pancreatic cancer 138
pancreatic mass 123, 124
pancreatic trauma 172
perforated duodenal ulcer 41
sigmoid volvulus 399
small bowel obstruction 410
constipation 177–84, 286
continuous ambulatory peritoneal
   dialysis 449
continuous positive airway pressure
   (CPAP) 11
contrast swallow 48, 49
corrosive oesophageal injury 22
cough, nocturnal 3
Courvoisier's sign 137
Cowden's syndrome 298
Creon 141, 153
Crigler–Najjar syndrome 133
Crohn's disease 197, 224, 227–8, 240
cryptoglandular sepsis 236
CT angiography
   acute mesenteric ischaemia 261
   lower gastrointestinal
     bleeding 281
CT colonography 194
Curling's ulcer 38
cutaneous abscess 455–9
cutting seton 188–9
cyst
   breast 294
   epidermal inclusion
     (sebaceous) 456, 459
   pancreatic 117–27

damage-control laparotomy 434–6
defaecating proctogram 182, 287–8
defunctioning stoma 189

delayed gastric emptying 3
  prokinetics 6
Delorme mucosal sleeve resection 289
depression
  obesity 11
  oesophagogastric resections 50
DEXA scan 342–3
diabetes
  chronic pancreatitis 148, 154
  delayed gastric emptying 3
  emphysematous cholecystitis 92
  obesity 11
  surgical emergencies 369
diagnostic laparoscopy
  acute abdominal pain 375
  acute appendicitis 387–8
  blunt abdominal trauma 428
  gastro-oesophageal cancer 25
  liver resection for
    cholangiocarcinoma 85
diet
  bariatric surgery 16
  colorectal cancer 195
  faecal incontinence 205
  gastric cancer 23
  gastro-oesophageal reflux disease 6, 8
  oesophageal cancer 22
Dieulafoy lesion 31
differentiated thyroid cancer 332
diltiazem 209
diversion colostomy 206
diverticulae 246
diverticular bleeding 277
diverticular colitis 247
diverticular disease 246–7
diverticulitis 243–52, 271
diverticulosis 246, 277
docusate sodium 182
donation after brainstem/circulatory
    death 450
drainage seton 188–9
drug-induced pancreatitis 159
dual X-ray absorptiometry
    (DEXA) 342–3
ductal carcinoma in situ 303–4
duct of Luschka injury 113, 114, 115
Duke's staging 197–8
dumping syndrome 17, 54
Dunphy sign 385
duodenal stenosis 153
duodenal ulcer 38, 39
  perforation 37–42, 158

dyslipidaemia 11
dyspepsia 3

embolus, mesenteric ischaemia 257, 258
emphysematous cholecystitis 92
empyema
  compared to abscess 457
  gallbladder 95, 108
endoanal ultrasound 204
endocrine neoplasm 120–1, 126
  functional 120–1
  non-functional 121
  somatostatinoma 121
endoscopic retrograde
    cholangiopancreatography (ERCP)
  acute ascending cholangitis 103, 104
  bile duct injury 114
  biliary drainage 85
  induced pancreatitis 160
  pancreatic cystic mass 124, 125
  pancreatic trauma 172–3
endoscopic ultrasound
  anorectal fistula 240
  chronic pancreatitis 152
  gallstones 94
  gastro-oesophageal cancer 25
  pancreatic cancer 138
  pancreatic mass 124
endoscopy
  capsule 226
  inflammatory bowel disease 226
  mucosal resection 25, 27
  pancreatic cancer 138
  perforated duodenal ulcer 41
  upper gastrointestinal bleed 34–5
  upper gastrointestinal
    malignancy 24–5
end-stage renal failure 448
environmental factors
  gastric cancer 23
  pancreatic cancer 136
epidermal inclusion (sebaceous)
    cyst 456, 459
epigastric pain 39
erosive gastritis/oesophagitis 31
erythema nodosum 225
erythromycin 6
exocrine neoplasm 120
extended criteria donors 450–1
external anal sphincter 202
external beam radiotherapy 334
external laryngeal nerve injury 330

extra-adrenal
    phaeochromocytoma 348–52
extra-hepatic cholangiocarcinoma 82, 83
eye inflammation 225

faecal fat 152
faecal incontinence 179, 201–6
faecal occult blood tests 196
faecal peritonitis 248, 249, 375
false aneurysm (pseudoaneurysm)
    intravenous drug users 458
    peripancreatic arteries 148
false diverticulae 246
familial adenomatous polyposis 195
familial breast cancer 297–8
familial hyperparathyroidism 344
familial hypocalciuric (benign)
    hypercalcaemia 341
familial pancreatitis 136
fat malabsorption 135
femoral canal 218
femoral hernia 218–19
    obstructed 415–22
^{18}F-FDG 61, 83
fibrin glue 189
fibroadenoma, breast 292, 293–4
fine needle aspiration cytology 327–8
fissurectomy 209
fissure in ano 180, 207–10, 236
fistula
    anal 185–90
    anorectal 236, 240
    aortoenteric 31
    cholecystoenteric 95
    colocutaneous 249
    colonic 249
    colovaginal 249
    colovesical 249
    pancreatic duct 175
    plug 189
fistulotomy 188
flaps
    anal advancement 210
    breast reconstruction 313
    pilonidal abscess 232–3
    rectal advancement 189
flexible sigmoidoscopy
    decompression of sigmoid
        volvulus 401
    faecal incontinence 204
[18]flurodeoxyglucose 61, 83
focused assessment with sonography for
    trauma (FAST) 428

folliculitis 456
Fournier's gangrene 440
Frey's procedure 153
Frimann Dahl's sign 398
Frykman–Goldberg procedure 288
functional endocrine neoplasm 120–1

gallbladder
    carcinoma 82
    empyema 95, 108
    perforation 95
gallstone ileus 95
gallstones 82, 87–97, 103, 108, 165
gastrectomy
    sleeve 12, 14, 16, 17, 53
    subtotal (partial) 26
    total 26
gastric band 3, 12, 13, 52, 53
gastric bypass, Roux-en-Y 12, 14, 16, 17,
    53, 54, 55
gastric cancer 23–4
    hereditary diffuse 298
gastric conduit necrosis 47
gastric resection 26
gastric ulcers 38, 39
gastric wall injuries 434
gastrinoma 121
gastritis
    erosive 31
    NSAID-associated 38, 39
Gastrografin® 411, 412
gastrointestinal bleeding
    lower 276–9, 280–2
    upper 29–36, 276
gastrointestinal blunt injury 434
gastrointestinal stromal tumour
    (GIST) 278
gastro-oesophageal cancer 19–28
gastro-oesophageal reflux disease 1–8
genetic factors
    acute pancreatitis 160
    breast cancer 296, 297–8
    colorectal cancer 195
    oesophageal cancer 22
    pancreatic cancer 136
Gilbert's syndrome 133
glucagonoma 121
goitre 323–35
Goodsall's rule 186
gracilis muscle transposition 206
graft dysfunction, liver
    transplantation 75
Graves' disease 356, 359

groin lump 216, 418
growth hormone 321

H2 receptor antagonists 6
haematoma
　inguinal hernia repair 221
　intra-abdominal 435
　neck 329, 360, 361
haemodialysis 448
　continuous veno-venous 449
　intermittent 449
haemorrhoidal artery ligation operation
　(HALO) 214
haemorrhoids
　constipation 179
　differentiating from rectal
　　prolapse 284
　elective surgery 211–14
　lower gastrointestinal bleeding 277
　non-surgical treatment 213
　prolapse 236
　thrombosed 236
hair follicle obstruction 456
HALO 214
Hannover classification 113
Hartmann's pouch 91
Hartmann's procedure 252, 375
Hasson technique 413
Helicobacter pylori 4, 23–4, 30, 31, 39
hemi-thyroidectomy 333
hepatic artery stenosis/thrombosis 75
hepatic jaundice 133
hepatitis B 73, 77
hepatitis C 73, 78
hepatitis D 73
hepatocellular carcinoma 69–78
HER2-positive breast cancer 311
hereditary non-polyposis colorectal
　cancer 195
hernias 215–22
　bowel obstruction 219–20, 268
　direct inguinal 218–19
　femoral 218–19, 415–22
　hiatus 2, 4
　incarcerated 219
　incisional 55
　indirect inguinal 218–19
　inguinal 216, 218–19, 220–2
　internal 54
　obstructed femoral 415–22
　strangulation 220, 419
Hesselbach's triangle 219
hidradenitis suppurativa 456

Hinchey classification 250
Hirschsprung's disease 204, 397
HIV 78
Huber needle 53
human placental lactogen 321
hungry bone syndrome 330, 343–4
hyperbaric oxygen 443
hypercalcaemia
　familial hypocalciuric (benign) 341
　post-operative 343–4
hyperemesis gravidarum 31
hyperparathyroidism 340–1, 342,
　343, 344
hyperparathyroidism–jaw tumour
　syndrome 344
hypertensive crisis 351
hyperthyroidism 357
hypertriglyceridaemia 160
hypocalcaemia 330
hypoparathyroidism 330, 343

iatrogenic injury
　anal sphincter 203
　bile duct 112, 113, 114, 115–16
　bowel 112
IBIS II 295, 304
ileal pouch-anal anastomosis 227
ileosigmoid knot 396
ileus 270, 273, 274
　gallstone 95
　paralytic 407
iliococcygeus 285
immunosuppression/immunodeficiency
　jaundice 135
　long-term risks 75
　renal transplantation 452–3
　surgical emergencies 369
indirect inguinal hernia 218–19
infarction
　mucosal 258–9
　mural 259
　tissue 258–9
　transmural 259
infertility 12
inflammatory bowel disease 195,
　197, 223–8
infliximab 190
inguinal canal 216–18
inguinal hernia 216, 218–19, 220–2
insulinoma 121
intermittent haemodialysis 449
internal anal sphincter 202, 204
interventional radiography 281

intra-abdominal sepsis 375
intraductal papillary mucinous neoplasm (IPMN) 122, 123, 126
intra-hepatic cholangiocarcinoma 82, 83
intra-operative ultrasound 61
intravenous drug users 458
iodine
  deficiency 326
  radioactive ablation 333–4, 358
  thyrotoxicosis treatment 357
iodine-131-labelled meta-iodobenzylguanidine (MIBG) scan 349
ischaemic bowel 253–63
ischaemic colitis 278
ischaemic colon 277–8
ischiorectal abscess 237, 238, 239–40
islet cell neoplasm 120–1
ispaghula husks 182
Ivor–Lewis oesophagogastrectomy 26, 46, 48

jaundice
  classification 132–3
  hepatic 133
  obstructive 85, 95, 135
  post-hepatic 134
  pre-hepatic 133
Johnson classification 40
junctional oesophageal adenocarcinoma 23

Karydakis procedure 233
Kausch–Whipple's procedure 140, 154
kidney transplantation 445–53
Klatskin tumour 82

lactation 320–1
lactulose 183
laparoscopy/laparoscopic surgery
  adjustable gastric band 3, 12, 13, 52, 53
  appendicectomy 390–1
  cholecystectomy 105–8, 109–16
  common bile duct exploration 105
  diverticulitis 252
  inguinal hernia repair 220–1
  pregnancy 392
  small bowel obstruction 413
  ventral mesh rectopexy 288
  see also diagnostic laparoscopy

laparotomy
  damage-control 434–6
  emergency, mortality 376, 377
lateral internal sphincterectomy 209
laxatives 182–3, 213
lifestyle
  bariatric surgery 12
  constipation 182
  gastro-oesophageal reflux disease 6
  pancreatic cancer 136
Li-Fraumeni syndrome 298
ligation of the intersphincteric fistula tract (LIFT) 189
linaclotide 183
lipase, serum 92–3, 160–1
liver cirrhosis 73–4
live-related donors 449
liver flukes 103
liver metastases 57–68
liver resection
  cholangiocarcinoma 83–5
  follow-up 67–8
  hepatocellular carcinoma 74–5
  patient assessment 61–2
  post-operative management 65–7
  risks and benefits 65
  types of 64
liver-shrinking diet 16
liver transplantation
  bile duct injuries 116
  cholangiocarcinoma 86
  eligibility (Milan) criteria 77
  graft dysfunction 75
  hepatocellular carcinoma 75–6
  variceal bleed 36
live-unrelated donors 449
Lockwood's infra-inguinal approach 420–1
Long–Myer's procedure 140
loop colostomy 189
loperamide 205
LORIS 304
Lotheissen's trans-inguinal approach 421
lower gastrointestinal bleeding 276–9, 280–2
lower oesophageal sphincter 2
lubiprostone 183
Lugol's iodine 357
luminal A breast cancer 311
luminal B breast cancer 311
lung metastases 67–8
lymphadenectomy 26
lymphoma, thyroid 333
Lynch syndrome 136

McBurney's point 385
McEvedy's high approach 421
magnetic resonance
   cholangiopancreatography
   (MRCP) 94, 103, 152, 161, 173
magnetic resonance
   enterography 410–11
magnetic resonance imaging (MRI)
   anal fistula 188
   anorectal fistula 240
   breast cancer screening 296–7
   chronic pancreatitis 151–2
   colorectal cancer 194
   colorectal liver metastases 60
   gallstones 94, 103
   hepatocellular carcinoma 72
   inflammatory bowel disease 225
   necrotizing fasciitis 443
   pancreatic cancer 138
   pancreatic mass 123, 124
malaena 276
Mallory–Weiss tear 31
mammography
   screening 296–7, 302
   triple assessment 293
M-ANNHEIM classification 150
Marlex rectopexy 288
marsupialization 232
mastectomy 303, 312
   reconstruction after 312–314
   risk-reducing 297
Meckel's diverticulum 277
medication management
   bariatric surgery 16–17
   surgical emergencies 368–9
medullary thyroid cancer 332
megacolon 397
mega-rectum 396
MELD score 74
MEN syndromes (MEN 1/2)120, 344
mesenchymal neoplasm 121, 126
mesenteric adenitis 384
mesenteric angina 256
mesenteric angiography 261
mesenteric ischaemia
   acute 253–63
   chronic 256
   non-occlusive 258, 259, 260
   occlusive 256–8, 259, 260, 262
mesenteric venousthrombosis 257
mesh infection 222
metabolic surgery 9–18
   complications 3, 51–5

metaclopramide 6
metanephrines 349
metastases
   liver 57–68
   lung 67–8
   pancreas 120
   thyroid 333
methimazole 357
methylprednisolone 452–3
MIBG scan 349
microdochectomy 301
migratory thrombophlebitis 137
Milan criteria 77
Milligan–Morgan procedure 213
Minnesota tube 36
mixed gallstones 90
mixed triglyceride breath test 152
Modified End-stage Liver Disease
   (MELD) score 74
MR enterography 410–11
mucin 122, 124
mucinous cystic neoplasm
   (MCN) 122, 126
mucocele 91
mucosal infarction 258–9
multiple endocrine neoplasia (MEN 1/
   2)120, 344
mural infarction 259
Murphy's sign 91–2
mycophenolate mofetil 453
myocutaneous flaps 313

near-total thyroidectomy 333, 358–9
necrosis
   gastric conduit 47
   pancreatic 163
   tissue 258–9
necrotizing fasciitis 437–44
neoadjuvant chemoradiotherapy
   colorectal cancer 199
   gastro-oesophageal cancer 27
neoadjuvant short-course
   radiotherapy 199
neosphincter 206
neuroendocrine tumours 120
NHS Bowel Cancer Screening
   Programme 196, 197
NHS Breast Cancer Screening
   Programme 302–3, 304
NICE
   obesity classification 10
   weight-loss drug therapy 10–11
   weight-loss surgery 11

nipple discharge 299–305
nipple reconstruction 313–14
Nissen fundoplication 7
nocturnal cough 3
non-alcoholic fatty liver disease 73
non-lactational breast abscess 319–20
non-steroidal anti-inflammatory drugs
  (NSAIDs)
  gastritis 38, 39
  peptic ulcer disease 30, 38
non-variceal bleed 34, 35, 36
Nottingham prognostic index 314
nutrition
  acute pancreatitis 162
  bariatric surgery 17, 54
  chronic pancreatitis 152–3
  liver resection 67
  oesophagogastric resections 50

obesity
  comorbidities 10–12
  NICE classification 10
obstetric trauma 203
obstructive jaundice 85, 95, 135
obstructive sleep apnoea 11
obturator sign 386
occlusive mesenteric ischaemia 256–8,
  259, 260, 262
ocular inflammation 225
oesophageal cancer 22–3, 24, 30–1
oesophageal dysmotility 5, 8
oesophageal manometry 5, 8
oesophageal pH 5
oesophageal resection 25–6
oesophagectomy, trans-hiatal/
  trans-thoracic 26
oesophagitis 4, 6, 22
oesophagogastrectomy 26, 46, 48
oesophagogastric resections,
  complications 46–7, 50
oesophagogastroduodenoscopy 4
oesophagostomy 50
oestrogen 321
online prognostic calculators 315
online risk calculators 295
open haemorrhoidectomy 213
ophthalmological disease 225
oral aphthous ulcers 224
oral pancreatic enzyme
  supplement 141, 152–3
organ donors 449–51
organ preservation 452
organ retrieval 451–2

Osler–Weber–Rendu syndrome 31
osmotic agents 183
osteopenia 224
osteoporosis 224
ovarian cancer risk 297
oxytocin 321

pain control
  chronic pancreatitis 152
  liver resection 67
  pancreatic cancer 141
palliative care 26, 27–8
pANCA 226
pancreatectomy, total 141
pancreatic adenocarcinoma 120, 135
pancreatic ascites 147
pancreatic cancer 129–42, 148, 154
pancreatic cystic mass 117–27
pancreatic diversum 159
pancreatic duct
  abscess 175
  decompression 153
  fibrosis 147
  fistula 175
  injuries 174, 175
pancreatic enzyme
  supplement 141, 152–3
pancreatic metastases 120
pancreatic necrosis 163
pancreatic neoplasm 120–1
pancreaticoduodenectomy 140
pancreaticojejunostomy 153, 173
pancreatic pleural effusion 147
pancreatic pseudocyst 123, 126–7, 153,
  164, 175
pancreatic stellate cells 149
pancreatitis
  acute 92–3, 94, 96, 146, 148, 155–65
  acute severe 165
  annular 159
  autoimmune 159
  chronic 143–54
  drug-induced 159
  ERCP-induced 160
  familial 136
  gallstones 94, 96, 165
  post-trauma 175
  serum amylase/lipase 92–3
panproctocolectomy and end
  ileostomy 227
papaverine 263
paralytic ileus 407
parathyroid disease 337–45

parathyroid surgery 342, 343
parietal pain 371
Parks classification 186–7
partial gastrectomy 26
PEG 183
pelvic floor
    anatomy 285
    dysfunction 179
    surgery 286
    trauma 286
penetrating abdominal
    trauma 426–7
peptic ulcer disease 30, 35, 36, 38–40,
    42, 121
percutaneous cholecystostomy 96–7
percutaneous endoscopic
    colostomy 402
percutaneous trans-hepatic
    cholangiography (PTC) 85,
    103, 104–5
perforation
    appendicitis 385
    duodenal ulcer 37–42, 158
    gallbladder 95
    stercoral 180
    viscus 256
perianal pain 236
pericolic abscess 249, 251
peridiverticular abscess 271
perineal proctosigmoidectomy 289
perinuclear ANCA 226
peri-operative mortality risk
    estimation 376–9
peripancreatic collections 163
peristalsis 3
peritoneal dialysis 448–9
peritonism 373
peritonitis
    biliary 114
    faecal 248, 249, 375
    stercoral 180
PET-CT
    colorectal liver metastases 61
    liver resection for
        cholangiocarcinoma 83
Peutz–Jeghers syndrome 136, 298
pH, oesophageal 5
phaeochromocytoma 348–52
phenol injections 213
phlegmon 248, 249
physical fitness for surgery 25
pilonidal disease 230–1
pilonidal sinus 231–2

plain radiographs, trauma
    assessment 172; see also abdominal
    radiographs; chest radiographs
Plummer–Vinson syndrome 22
polyethylene glycol 183
portal hypertension 30, 31–2, 73
portal vein
    stenosis 75
    thrombosis 75, 116
positron emission tomography (PET)
    gastro-oesophageal cancer 25
    pancreatic cancer 138
post-cholecystectomy
    syndrome 113
post-hepatic jaundice 134
post-trauma pancreatitis 175
P-POSSUM 377–9
Predict 315
prednisolone
    renal transplantation 452–3
    surgical emergencies 369
pregnancy, acute appendicitis 391–2
primary sclerosing cholangitis 225
procedure for prolapsing
    haemorrhoids 213–14
progesterone 321
prognostication, breast cancer 314–15
prokinetics 6
prolactin 321
prolapse
    haemorrhoids 236
    rectal 283–9
    visceral 180
propylthiouracil 357
proton pump inhibitors 6
PRSS 1136, 160
prucalopride 183
pseudoaneurysm
    intravenous drug users 458
    peripancreatic arteries 148
pseudocyst, pancreas 123, 126–7, 153,
    164, 175
pseudo-obstruction 268, 269–70,
    273–4, 396
psoas sign 386
psychological issues, bariatric
    surgery 13, 55
PTEN 298
pubococcygeus 285
puborectalis 202, 285
pubovisceralis 285
pulmonary metastases 67–8
pyoderma gangrenosum 225

radiation-induced conditions
  angiectasia 278
  colorectal cancer 196
radioactive iodine ablation 333–4, 358
radiofrequency ablation 76
radionuclide transit studies 181
ranitidine 6
rectal advancement flap 189
rectal bleeding 208, 241–2, 275–82
rectal blunt injuries 434
rectal irrigation 205
rectal procidentia 284, 286, 287
rectal prolapse 283–9
  concealed 284, 286
  full-thickness 284, 286, 287
  incomplete 284, 286
  internal 284, 286
  mucosal 284, 286
recto-anal angle 202
rectopexy 288
recurrent laryngeal nerve injury 48,
    329–30, 360, 361
red flag symptoms 24
referred pain 371
renal replacement therapy 448–9
resection rectopexy 288
respiratory disease, post-
    oesophagogastric resections 46
respiratory distress, thyroid
    surgery 360–1
resuscitation
  anastomotic leak 49
  perforated duodenal ulcer 41
  upper gastrointestinal bleed 33–4
Reynold's pentad 102
right iliac fossa pain 384
rigid sigmoidoscopy
  anorectal sepsis 239
  decompression of sigmoid
    volvulus 399, 401
  use in general surgery 240–2
Rigler's sign 172, 410
Ripstein procedure 288
risk stratification
  breast cancer 294–5
  peri-operative mortality 376–9
  upper gastrointestinal bleed 32
Rockall score 32
Roux-en-Y gastric bypass 12, 14, 16, 17,
    53, 54, 55
Roux-en-Y hepaticojejunostomy 115
Roux-en-Y
    pancreaticojejunostomy 153, 173

Roux-en-Y reconstruction 26
Rovsing sign 385
rubber band ligation 213

sacral nerve stimulator 184, 205
Schatzki ring 4
sclerosant
  haemorrhoids 213
  variceal bleed 35
scorpion bite 160
screening
  breast cancer 296–7, 302–3, 304
  colorectal cancer 196–7
  WHO criteria 301–2
sebaceous cyst 456, 459
secretin MRCP 152
segmental colitis 247
Sengstaken tube 36
senna 183
sentinel lymph node biopsy 304, 312
sentinel pile 208
sepsis
  anorectal 235–42
  intra-abdominal 375
seroma, inguinal hernia repair 221
serous cystadenoma 123
serum amylase 92–3, 160–1, 171
serum lipase 92–3, 160–1
seton insertion 188–9
shoulder tip pain 171
Siewert and Stein classification 23
sigmoid colectomy 288
sigmoidoscopy
  anal fistula 188
  anorectal sepsis 239
  decompression of sigmoid
    volvulus 399, 401
  faecal incontinence 204
  use in general surgery 240–2
Sipple syndrome 344
sirolimus 453
Sister Mary Joseph's nodule 137
skin abscess 455–9
skin-removal surgery 18
skip lesions 224
sleeve gastrectomy 12, 14, 16, 17, 53
sliding hiatus hernia 2
slow transit constipation 179
small bowel
  blunt injuries 434
  obstruction 219, 403–14
smoking
  bariatric surgery 12

breast abscess 319–20
colorectal cancer 195
gastro-oesophageal reflux disease 6
oesophageal cancer 22
pancreatitis 147
peptic ulcer disease 38
social history 370
SOCRATES 370–2
solid pseudopapillary neoplasm 122
somatic pain 371
somatostatin 175
somatostatinoma 121
sorafenib 77
sphincter repair/replacement 206
spicy food 6
spina bifida 204
spinal cord injury 286
SPINK 1 136, 160
splenectomy 430
splenic injuries 429–30
splenic vein thrombosis 148
squamous cell carcinoma
    gastric 23
    oesophagus 22
standard criteria donors 450
stapled haemorrhoidopexy 213–14
steatorrhoea 135
stenosis
    biliary 75, 153
    duodenal 153
    hepatic artery 75
    portal vein 75
stents
    anastomotic leak 49
    biliary 85, 104, 140
    gastro-oesophageal cancer 26, 28
    large bowel obstruction 272–3
stercobilinogen 132
stercoral perforation 180
steroids
    renal transplantation 452–3
    surgical emergencies 369
    thyrotoxicosis 357
Stewart–Way classification 113
stimulant laxatives 183
STK 11 136, 298
stoma, defunctioning 189
stool antigen test 39
stool softeners 182
strangulation
    hernia 220, 419
    rectal prolapse 287
Strasberg classification 113

strictuloplasty 227–8
strictures
    anastomotic line 54
    biliary 82, 132
subtotal colectomy
    and end ileostomy 227
    with ilio-rectal anastomosis 184
subtotal gastrectomy 26
supralevator abscess 237, 238, 240
suture rectopexy 288
systemic inflammatory response
        syndrome (SIRS) 159, 162–3

TACE 76
tacrolimus 453
Tenckhoff catheter 448
tenesmus 271
testicular complications, hernia
        repair 222
thionamides 357
thromboembolism
    bariatric surgery 16
    oesophagogastric resections 46
thromboprophylaxis
    bariatric surgery 16
    liver resection 66–7
    oesophagogastric resections 46, 50
thrombosis
    hepatic artery 75
    mesenteric ischaemia 257, 258
    portal vein 75, 116
    splenic vein 148
Thy category 328–9
thyroid cancer 323–35
    anaplastic 332–3
    differentiated 332
    medullary 332
    metastases 333
thyroidectomy
    acute respiratory distress
        following 360–1
    hemi-thyroidectomy 333
    near-total 333, 358–9
    patient preparation 359
    total 333, 358–9
thyroid lymphoma 333
thyroid stimulating hormone 321, 333
thyroid storm 331, 359
thyroid surgery
    peri-operative management 353–61
    respiratory distress following 360–1
    risks 329–31, 360
thyrotoxic crisis 331, 359

thyrotoxicosis 330, 356–8
thyroxine 333
tissue infarction 258–9
tissue necrosis 258–9
TNF monoclonal antibodies 190
TNM classification 197–8
tobacco, *see* smoking
total gastrectomy 26
total pancreatectomy 141
tracheomalacia 330, 360, 361
trans-arterial chemoembolization
    (TACE) 76
transcatheter embolization 281
trans-hiatal oesophagectomy 26
transjugular intra-hepatic portosystemic
    shunt (TIPS) 36
transmural infarction 259
trans-rectal ultrasound 194
trans-thoracic oesophagectomy 26
trauma
    blunt abdominal 423–36
    FAST scan 428
    obstetric 203
    pancreatic 167–76
    pelvic floor 286
    penetrating abdominal 426–7
triple assessment 292–3
Trousseau sign 137
trypsin 158, 159
trypsinogen 158, 159
T-tube 49
tylosis 22

UK model for End-stage Liver Disease
    (UKELD) score 74
ulcer
    Curling's 38
    duodenal 38, 39
    gastric 38, 39
    oral aphthous 224
    peptic ulcer disease 30, 35, 36, 38–40,
        42, 121
    perforated duodenal 37–42, 158
ulcerative colitis 197, 224, 226–7
ultrasound
    acute abdominal pain 374
    acute appendicitis 387
    acute pancreatitis 161
    aspiration of breast abscess 318
    breast lump 293
    chronic pancreatitis 151
    colorectal cancer 194

faecal incontinence 204
FAST scan 428
gallstones 93–4
groin swelling 418
hernias 219
    intra-operative 61
    necrotizing fasciitis 443
    pancreatic cancer 137–8
    pancreatic mass 124
    parathyroid disease 342, 343
    see also endoscopic ultrasound
unconjugated hyperbilirubinaemia 133
University of Wisconsin solution 452
upper gastrointestinal
    haemorrhage 29–36, 276
    non-variceal 34, 35, 36
    variceal 30, 31–2, 34, 35, 36, 73
upper gastrointestinal resectional
    surgery, complications 43–50
upper oesophageal sphincter 2
urea breath test 39
urobilinogen 132–3
UW solution 452

variceal banding 35
variceal bleed 30, 31–2, 34, 35, 36, 73
vasoactive intestinal peptide (VIP) 158
vasopressin, intra-arterial infusions 281
VIPoma 121
viral hepatitis 73, 77–8
viral pancreatitis 160
Virchow's node 137
visceral pain 371
viscus perforation 256
vitamin deficiency, jaundice 135
vitamin K 135, 139
vitamin supplements, bariatric
    surgery 17
volvulus 268–9
    caecal 268–9
    colonic 271
    compound 396
    sigmoid 242, 393–402

water-soluble contrast
    anastomotic leak 48–9
    sigmoid volvulus 399
    small bowel obstruction 411
weight loss
    drug therapy 10–11
    gastro-oesophageal reflux disease 6
    see also bariatric surgery

Werner syndrome 344
Whipple's procedure 140, 173
Whipple's triad 121
whirl sign 399
wide local excision 303, 311–12
Wolff–Chaikoff effect 357

X-rays, *see* abdominal radiographs; chest
    radiographs

Zollinger–Ellison
    syndrome 39, 121
zymogen granules 158